RESPIRATORY DISEASES

Edited by **Mostafa Ghanei**

Respiratory Diseases
Edited by Mostafa Ghanei

Published by InTech
Janeza Trdine 9, 51000 Rijeka, Croatia

Publishing Process Manager Ivana Zec

Technical Editor Teodora Smiljanic

Cover Designer InTech Design Team

Additional hard copies can be obtained from orders@intechopen.com

Respiratory Diseases, Edited by Mostafa Ghanei
p. cm.
ISBN 978-953-307-964-6

For EU product safety concerns:
IN TECH d.o.o., Prolaz Marije Krucifikse Kozulić 3, 51000 Rijeka, Croatia,
info@intechopen.com or visit our website at intechopen.com.

Meet the editor

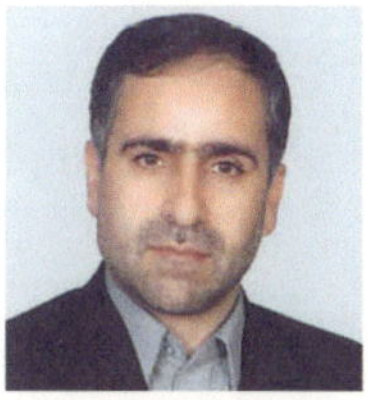

Professor Mostafa Ghanei, MD, was born in 1962 in Esfahan, Iran. He obtained his PhD in medicine in 1988, and obtained his specialty certification in internal medicine in 1993 from Esfahan University of Medical Sciences, Esfahan, Iran. He has been practicing as a pulmonologist since 1997. He is now Vice Chancellor in Research of Ministry of Health of Iran and Head of Research Center of Chemical Injuries, Baqiyatallah Medical Sciences University, Tehran, Iran. Additionally, he is a member of the European Respiratory Society, Iranian Lung Society, Iranian Executive Board of Lung Society, National Board Exam in Respiratory Medicine, American College of Chest Physicians, and American Thoracic Society. He has many articles in the field of basic and clinical aspects of respiratory diseases, and is one of the most distinguished researchers in the field of chemical inhalation toxicology.

Contents

Preface

Medicine is an ever-changing science. In this regard, Respiratory medicine is not an exception and has been evolving during recent years. As new research broadens our knowledge, advanced methods for diagnoses are better understood, providing genetic and underlying pathophysiology of diseases and new clinical experiences. Consequently, publications of new resources along with revisions of previous ones are required. Although respiratory textbooks might clearly describe several aspects of respiratory disease, most of them contain significant information regarding both common and uncommon diseases and disorders. Additionally, some of them are not available or easily accessible in all countries.

In *Respiratory Diseases,* we introduce and describe common respiratory disorders in a more simplistic manner. Before being published, we reviewed different proposals of different chapters from several authors. Accepted proposals were then developed into chapters for this book which opens with a clinical scenario that presents the results of these authors' findings.

There are many disorders we have not yet reviewed and many more to come. After years of producing systematic reviews, which will include the article that launched the evidence-based medicine movement, it is time for us to update and combine our work in one resource for learners and clinicians to enjoy in upcoming editions. However, the edition of this book provides more room to move and opportunity for young researchers and scientists through the world to gather, classify, and present their knowledge in this field.

I would like to thank my colleagues around the world who have encouraged this work and contributed to it. I give my thanks to Dr Ali Amini Harandi for his loyal assistance.

I am grateful to my family, who supported my work on many nights and weekends in order to complete my portion of the book.

I would like to especially thank Ivana Zec, Publishing Process Manager and InTech for their support and organization.

Dr Mostafa Ghanei
Baqiyatollah University, Teheran,
Iran

Part 1

Respiratory Defense Mechanisms and Immunology

1

Cordyceps Extracts and the Major Ingredient, Cordycepin: Possible Cellular Mechanisms of Their Therapeutic Effects on Respiratory Disease

Chun-kit Fung and Wing-hung Ko
School of Biomedical Sciences, The Chinese University of Hong Kong, Shatin, N.T. Hong Kong

1. Introduction

Cordyceps militaris (CM), also known as the caterpillar fungus, is a well-known, traditional Chinese medicine that can be artificially cultivated on a large scale (Fig. 1). In recent decades, CM extract has been reported to have different biological activities, such as anti-tumor activity (Park et al., 2009) and immunomodulation (Shin et al., 2010). Similar to *Cordyceps sinensis* (CS), an expensive, wild-fruiting species of *Cordyceps*, CM can be used to treat certain respiratory diseases, such as asthma, bronchitis, and chronic obstructive pulmonary disease (COPD) (Paterson, 2008). In contrast to CS, CM can be artificially cultivated on a large scale and hence is much cheaper to produce. While CM has medicinal properties similar to CS, it is widely used as a substitute for CS in health supplements. A recent clinical trial demonstrated that naturally grown and cultivated mycelia of *Cordyceps* are effective for the treatment of asthma (Wang et al., 2007). In addition to the treatment of respiratory diseases, CM has beneficial therapeutic effects for patients with influenza A viral infections (Ohta et al., 2007).

Recently, we demonstrated that the water extracts of both CS and CM can stimulate anion secretion across Calu-3 airway epithelia with similar prosecretory activities (Yue et al., 2008). Calu-3 monolayers have characteristics of both serous and mucus cells and more closely resemble submucosal glands (Shan et al., 2011). Therefore, our recent paper has challenged the traditional belief that natural *Cordyceps* has better therapeutic medicinal value than cultivated *Cordyceps*. We show that the two have similar pharmacological properties in stimulating transepithelial anion secretion in airway epithelia. While both CS and CM have established efficacies for the treatment of pulmonary disorders, the cellular mechanisms that are responsible for the medicinal properties of *Cordyceps* are not entirely clear. The aim of this chapter is to discuss the potential cellular mechanisms and signal transduction pathways underlying the prosecretory action of CS and CM extracts and their major ingredient, cordycepin. We propose that the activation of ion transport processes by *Cordyceps* extracts and cordycepin in airway epithelia may have clinical relevance and partly explain their traditional use in the treatment of respiratory diseases, such as asthma and COPD. In addition, the purported therapeutic effects of CS, CM, and cordycepin may be due to their anti-inflammatory effects on airway epithelial cells. Asthma is now defined as a chronic inflammatory disorder of the airways, in which many immune cells (e.g. mast cells, eosinophils) are involved. There are many similarities and differences between asthma and COPD, but a full description of their pathophysiology and management is beyond the scope of this chapter.

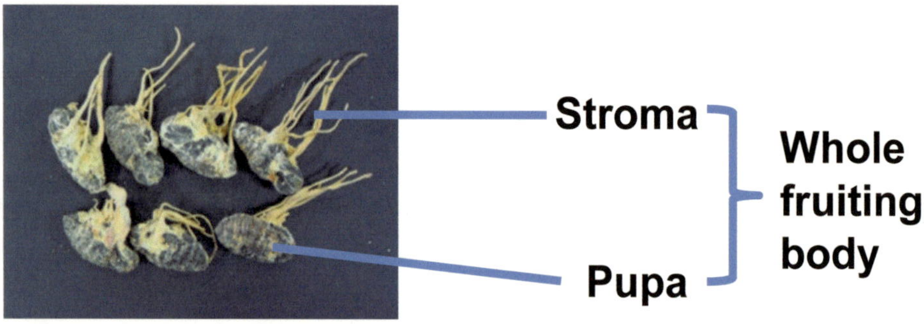

Fig. 1. Photograph of *Cordyceps militaris*, showing the different parts of the fruiting bodies.

2. Ion transport in airway epithelia

2.1 Role of airway epithelia in transepithelial electrolyte and fluid transport

Epithelial cells characteristically grow as distinct sheets that form the anatomical boundaries between the relatively stable internal environment of the body and the constantly changing environment of the outside world. Many epithelia have become specialized to permit the controlled secretion and/or absorption of salt and water. These transport processes can be controlled by hormones and neurotransmitters that bind to specific cell surface receptors. Receptor occupation causes the production of characteristic 'second messenger' signals within the cytoplasm, which then modifies cellular metabolism and evokes ion transport. This regulated transport of salt and water is essential to the integrated function of many organ systems, including the respiratory tract.

The hydration of the normal airway surface is dependent on the active ion transport processes of the airway epithelia, which are highly water-permeable (Chambers et al., 2007). Airway fluid secretion is a passive process that is driven by osmotic forces generated by ion transport. The main determinant of a luminally directed osmotic gradient is the mucosal transport of chloride ions (Cl^-) into the lumen. Airway Cl^- secretion is an energy-dependent process that generates an electrical potential across the mucosal epithelium (i.e., electrogenic). Cations are drawn into the lumen by the established electrochemical gradient, and water loss is an obligatory consequence of the efflux of salt. The coordinated regulation and balance of Cl^- secretion and Na^+ reabsorption, therefore, controls the mass of salt (NaCl) on airway surfaces. This is important in maintaining the thickness and composition of airway surface liquid (ASL), which in turn affects airway mucus clearance (Tarran et al., 2006). Mucus clearance is an important component of the innate defense of the lungs against disease. Abnormal ASL volume, salt content, or mucus clearance can compromise airway immunity and predispose the airway to various respiratory diseases and infection (Danahay and Jackson, 2005).

2.2 Stimulation of Cl^- secretion by cAMP and Ca^{2+}

The mechanism of airway Cl^- secretion is well understood. Increases in cAMP levels activate Cl^- secretion via luminal cystic fibrosis transmembrane conductance regulator (CFTR) Cl^- channels (Boucher, 2002). In addition, cAMP also increases basolateral K^+ conductance, probably via K_vLQT_1-type K^+ channels, which hyperpolarize the membrane and increase the driving force for apical Cl^- exit (Bardou et al., 2009). Calcium-activated Cl^- channels (CaCCs) are also involved in Cl^- secretion, and their molecular identity has recently been determined (Caputo et al., 2008). Increases in intracellular Ca^{2+} concentrations ($[Ca^{2+}]_i$) lead to the opening of CaCCs and basolateral SK4-type K^+ channels (Bardou et al., 2009), which provide an additional driving force for Cl^- exit through apical Cl^- channels (i.e., CFTR and CaCCs). Therefore, $[Ca^{2+}]_i$ and cAMP are the two major signal transduction cascades involved in the regulation of airway ion transport.

3. Stimulation of ion transport by CM extract and its active ingredient, cordycepin, in Calu-3 and 16HBE14o- cells

3.1 Calu-3 cells

To study the effects of extracts of CS and CM, and its active ingredient, cordycepin, on ion transport activities in Calu-3 epithelia, the cells were grown on permeable supports (Transwell-COL membranes) until confluent (Wong et al., 2009a). Calu-3 cells have many properties of serous cells of the submucosal glands and express the highest levels of natural CFTR of any known immortalized cell line (Haws et al., 1994; Shen et al., 1994). The monolayers were mounted in Ussing chambers and bathed in normal Krebs-Henseleit solution with a basolateral-to-apical Cl^- gradient. An increase in short-circuit currents (I_{SC}), which is an index of electrogenic ion transport, was measured by an electrophysiological technique. Our data demonstrate that extracts of CS and CM, as well as its isolated compound, cordycepin, all stimulate ion transport in a dose-dependent manner in Calu-3 monolayers. Apical application of 300 µg/ml CM extract or 300 µM cordycepin stimulates the highest peak increase in I_{SC}. The transport mechanisms involve both basolateral Na^+-K^+-$2Cl^-$ cotransporters and apical CFTR Cl^- channels for the uptake and exit of Cl^-, respectively (Yue et al., 2008). These data indicate for the first time that extracts of CS and CM, and cordycepin could stimulate transepithelial Cl^- secretion and may therefore promote fluid secretion by human airway epithelial cells. Insufficient fluid secretion leads to airway dehydration, which hampers clearance of secreted mucus and promotes airway inflammatory conditions, such as asthma and bronchitis. In addition, the fluid lining the airway serves as an anatomical barrier between inspired pathogens/particulates and the epithelial surface. Decreased ion transport activity of the surface epithelium may therefore compromise its innate lung defense function and exacerbate airway inflammation (Clunes et al., 2008). Since *Cordyceps* has proven clinically efficacy for treating patients with chronic bronchitis and COPD, the effects observed in promoting Cl^- secretion may partially explain the mechanism that underlies this efficacy.

3.2 16HBE14o- cells

Apart from the recent data on Calu-3 cells, our laboratory has further investigated the cellular signal transduction mechanisms underlying the prosecretory effects of CM extract and cordycepin in 16HBE14o- cells, an immortalized cell line that was derived from human bronchial surface epithelium (Cozens et al., 1994). It is a good model to study transepithelial Cl^- secretion (Bernard et al., 2003; Bernard et al., 2005), airway inflammation, and airway remodeling (Holgate et al., 1999; Kidney and Proud, 2000; Puddicombe et al., 2000). An electrophysiological technique, similar to that described above, was employed to examine the prosecretory effects of CM extract and cordycepin on 16HBE14o- cells. The involvement of various ion channels located at the apical and basolateral membranes was investigated by pharmacological approaches. Different ion channels inhibitors, such as $CFTR_{inh-172}$ (CFTR inhibitor), DIDS (Ca^{2+} activated Cl^- channel inhibitor), 293B (cAMP-dependent K^+ channel blocker), etc., were used to delineate the transport mechanism. The involvement of different second messengers, such as Ca^{2+} or cAMP, was examined by fluorescence imaging techniques using specific pathway inhibitors. Our data suggest that CM extract stimulated transepithelial Cl^- secretion in 16HBE14o- cells through apical CFTR Cl^- channels and/or CaCCs. Basolateral cAMP- or Ca^{2+}-activated K^+ channels were activated by CM extract to provide a driving force for apical Cl^- secretion. The underlying signal transduction mechanisms involve both cAMP- and Ca^{2+}-dependent pathways (Fung et al., 2011).

The pharmacological properties of CM have been studied for more than 50 years since cordycepin (3'-deoxyadenosine) was isolated from CM (Cunningham et al., 1950). Cordycepin is a major bioactive component of CM and has been detected in different parts of the CM fruiting body, ranging from 0.16 to 0.25% (w/w) (Yue et al., 2008). In 16HBE14o- cells, apical or basolateral application of cordycepin resulted in a stimulation of I_{SC}, which has been shown to be due to Cl^- secretion (Fung et al., 2011). Both apical and basolateral addition of cordycepin stimulates a concentration-dependent increase in I_{SC} (Fig. 2).

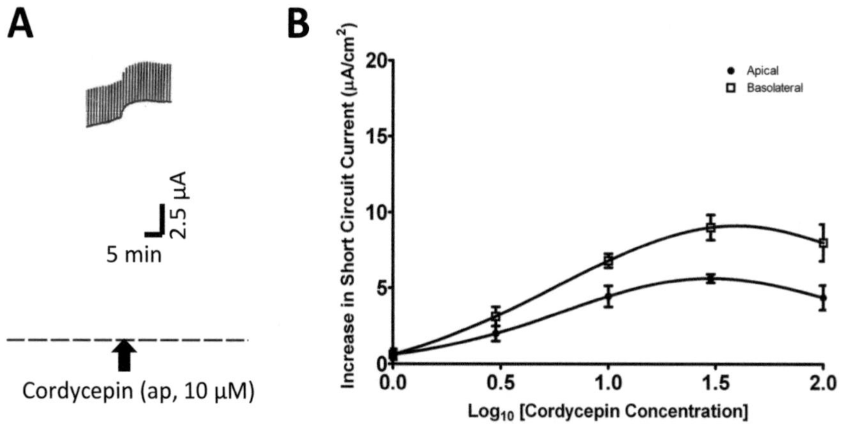

Fig. 2. Stimulation of Cl^- secretion by cordycepin in 16HBE14o- cells. (A) A representative I_{SC} trace in response to cordycepin applied apically to 16HBE14o- epithelia (ap, 10 µM). The horizontal dotted line represents zero I_{SC}. The transient current pulses are the result of intermittently clamping of the potential at 1 mV for the calculation of transepithelial resistance using Ohm's law. The record is representative of six experiments.
(B) Concentration-response curves for changes in I_{SC} in response to cordycepin added either apically or basolaterally. Each point represents the mean ± S.E. for at least six experiments.

In order to ascertain which types of Cl^- and/or K^+ channels mediated the stimulation of Cl^- secretion caused by cordycepin, the CFTR Cl^- channel ($CFTR_{inh172}$) and CaCC (DIDS) blockers as well as the intermediate conductance Ca^{2+}-dependent (TRAM-34) and cAMP-dependent K^+ channel (293B) blockers were used. As shown in Figure 3, the current evoked by cordycepin could be significantly inhibited in the presence of Ca^{2+}- and cAMP-dependent Cl^- and K^+ channel blockers.

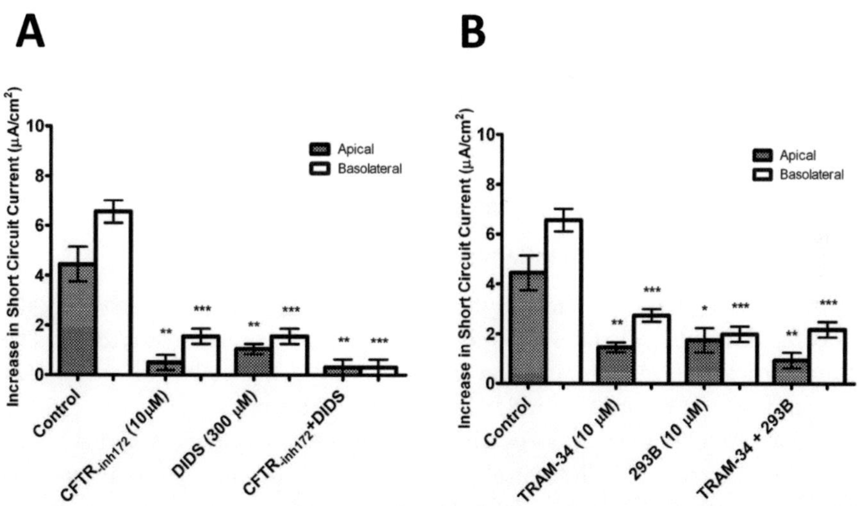

Fig. 3. Effects of Cl^- (A) and K^+ (B) channel blockers on I_{SC} responses to cordycepin. The control was the apical or basolateral application of cordycepin (10 µM) alone. Each column represents the mean ± S.E. (**$p < 0.01$, ***$p < 0.001$, Student's t test compared with control, $n = 4–5$).

The cordycepin-evoked I_{SC} was sensitive to both cAMP- and Ca^{2+}-dependent channel blockers, suggesting that Cl^- secretion was mediated by these two signaling molecules. Indeed, the cordycepin-evoked I_{SC} could be inhibited by the adenylate cyclase inhibitor, MDL-12330A, and the protein kinase A inhibitor, H-89. Adenylate cyclase is responsible for the generation of intracellular cAMP, while protein kinase A is the downstream signaling target of cAMP. Therefore, both CFTR Cl^- channels and cAMP-dependent K^+ channels expressed in 16HBE14o- cells could by stimulated by cordycepin through the activation of the cAMP/protein kinase A signaling pathway (Bleich and Warth, 2000; Li and Naren, 2010). In addition to the activation of the cAMP-dependent pathway, cordycepin evoked a concentration-dependent increase in intracellular [Ca^{2+}] as measured by Fura-2 imaging (Lau et al., 2011) (Fig. 4). Our experimental data, therefore, indicate that cordycepin exerts a similar prosecretory action and activates the same signal transduction pathways, namely Ca^{2+} and cAMP, in human airway epithelia compared with CM extract, suggesting that cordycepin is responsible, at least in part, for the medicinal effects of CM.

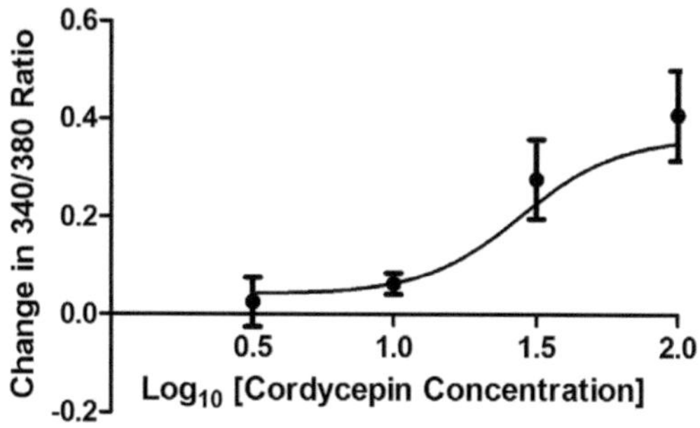

Fig. 4. Concentration-response curve for changes in $[Ca^{2+}]_i$ (represented by 340/380 nm Fura-2 ratio) elicited by cordycepin (in μM). Changes in $[Ca^{2+}]_i$ were plotted against the logarithm of cordycepin concentration (n = 4–9). Each data point represents the mean ± S.E.

4. Anti-inflammatory effects of CM extract

4.1 Role of airway epithelium in inflammation

In addition to the regulation of electrolyte and fluid transport, airway epithelia also play a key role as regulators of inflammation and immunity (Bals and Hiemstra, 2004). The airway epithelium participates in inflammation in many ways. The cells can act as targets that respond to exposure to a variety of inflammatory mediators and cytokines by altering one or several of their functions, such as mucin secretion or ion transport (Adler et al., 1994). Moreover, the surface epithelium itself is responsible for the synthesis and release of cytokines that cause the selective recruitment, retention, and accumulation of various inflammatory cells (Jeffery, 2000). Certain inflammatory cytokines alter the fluid and electrolyte transport of the airway epithelium. Therefore, airway diseases, such as asthma, can be considered diseases of the bronchial epithelium, which could contribute to the pathophysiology of airway inflammation (Holgate et al., 1999).

4.2 Cytokines as bronchial epithelial ion transport regulators

Recent studies suggest that certain inflammatory cytokines affect transepithelial ion transport. The T-helper 1 cytokine, interferon-γ (IFN-γ), inhibits both Na^+ reabsorption and cAMP-mediated Cl^- secretion in human bronchial epithelial cells (Galietta et al., 2000). This is due to the downregulation of epithelial Na^+ channel and CFTR activities. In contrast, IFN-γ upregulates the Ca^{2+}-dependent Cl^- secretion that is stimulated by UTP (Galietta et al., 2000), which binds to $P2Y_2$ receptors (Mason et al., 1991). The net effect is a reduction in fluid absorption, which favors the hydration of mucus secretion. In 16HBE14o- cells, both IL-9 and IL-13 augment UTP-induced Cl^- secretion via the increased expression of hCLCA1, a Ca^{2+}-activated Cl^- channel (Endo et al., 2007). Inhibition of CaCCs by niflumic acid has been shown to control IL-13-induced asthma phenotypes by suppressing JAK/STAT6 activation (Nakano et al., 2006). Therefore, certain cytokines change the balance between fluid absorption and secretion to favor hydration of the airway surface and, consequently, mucus clearance (Galietta et al., 2004).

4.3 Anti-inflammatory effects of CM extract

Both CM and cordycepin have been shown to possess anti-inflammatory activities against *in vitro* and *in vivo* models of inflammation (Cheng et al., 2011; Han et al., 2011; Jeong et al., 2010). CPS-1, a polysaccharide purified from CM extract, was shown to have anti-inflammatory effects in mice, possibly via the suppression of humoral immunity (Yu et al., 2004). Similar anti-inflammatory effects of CM extract and cordycepin were also observed in a study by Won and Park (Won and Park, 2005). CM extract also suppressed intestinal inflammation in an acute colitic mouse model by inhibiting the level of pro-inflammatory cytokine mediators, such as TNFα (Han et al., 2011). In microglia, cordycepin is capable of inhibiting the expression of pro-inflammatory cytokines, such as TNFα and IL-1β (Jeong et al., 2010). However, there have been very few studies addressing the anti-inflammatory effects of *Cordyceps* extracts or cordycepin in the respiratory system. Hsu et al. reported that CM extract can modulate airway inflammation in a mouse model of asthma, but the therapeutic effects are less than those of two commonly used western medicines, namely prednisolone and montelukast (Hsu et al., 2008). On the contrary, a recent randomized, double-blind, placebo-controlled trial in asthmatic children (Wong et al., 2009b) challenged the use of CS extract as an asthma therapy. In this study, children with asthma were treated with a herbal formula of dried aqueous extracts of five herbs containing CS. However, no significant differences were found between the treated group and the placebo group (Wong et al., 2009b). Therefore, there is still controversy over the treatment of asthma using *Cordyceps* extracts.

5. Conclusion

In summary, CM extract stimulates anion secretion from both surface epithelia of the airways (16HBE14o- cells) and submucosal glands (Calu-3 cells). Figure 5 shows the cellular signaling mechanisms underlying the effects of CM extract and cordycepin. Enhancing fluid and electrolyte transport may improve both airway surface hydration and mucus clearance, which becomes hypersecreted in various respiratory diseases, such as asthma and COPD. Therefore, this stimulatory effect of CM extract and cordycepin on major secretory cell types of the upper airways may account for its traditional use in treating different respiratory diseases. Our previous study suggests that 16HBE14o- cells can secrete interleukin- (IL-) 6 and IL-8, two important pro-inflammatory cytokines, towards the mucosal side in a polarized fashion (Chow et al., 2010). This phenomenon may contribute to the pathophysiology of asthmatic inflammation and the development of other inflammatory lung diseases (Chow et al., 2010). Therefore, the therapeutic effects of CM and cordycepin on airway diseases may be attributed to their influences on immune response regulation (Das et al., 2010), although the detailed molecular mechanisms await to be elucidated.

Further study is required to delineate the immunomodulatory effects of CM extract and cordycepin in both normal and diseased airway epithelia. In particular, it would be interesting to determine whether the stimulatory effects on ion transport could be attributed to cytokine secretion. Further experiments are needed to purify and characterize the other active component(s) present in the CM extract and determine the mechanisms of action for their therapeutic effects since the prosecretory action of CM extract is not solely explained by the presence of cordycepin. Calu-3 and 16HBE14o- cells are models for submucosal glands and airway surface epithelium, respectively. The airway consists of different cell types, such as goblet (mucous) cells, which secrete mucins. Goblet cell hyperplasia or metaplasia is commonly seen in airway diseases, such as asthma, COPD, and chronic bronchitis (Rogers, 2007). It is important to examine whether CM extract or cordycepin has any effect on mucus secretion by goblet cells. Finally, more carefully conducted clinical trials should be performed to evaluate the therapeutic potential of CM extract and its major ingredients in the treatment of respiratory diseases.

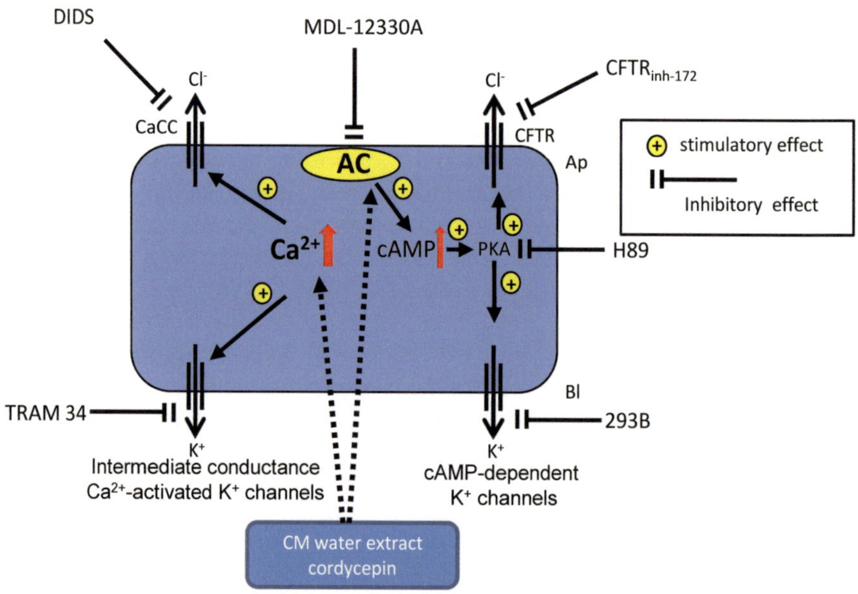

Fig. 5. Cellular mechanisms underlying the prosecretory effects of CM extract and cordycepin.

6. Acknowledgement

The work was supported by a Direct Grant for Research, CUHK (#2041539), RGC General Research Fund (#2140595), and Research Fund for the Control of Infectious Diseases (#10090872). The CS and CM extracts were kindly provided by Dr. Grace Gar-Lee Yue and Prof. Kwok-Pui Fung from Institute of Chinese Medicine, The Chinese University of Hong Kong.

7. References

Adler, K.B., Fischer, B.M., Wright, D.T., Cohn, L.A., & Becker, S. (1994). Interactions between respiratory epithelial cells and cytokines: relationships to lung inflammation. *Annals of the New York Academy of Sciences*, Vol.725, pp.128-145.

Bals, R., & Hiemstra, P.S. (2004). Innate immunity in the lung: how epithelial cells fight against respiratory pathogens. *European Respiratory Journal*, Vol.23, pp.327-333.

Bardou, O., Trinh, N.T., & Brochiero, E. (2009). Molecular diversity and function of K^+ channels in airway and alveolar epithelial cells. *American Journal of Respiratory Cell and Molecular Biology*, Vol.296, pp.L145-L155.

Bernard, K., Bogliolo, S., & Ehrenfeld, J. (2005). Vasotocin and vasopressin stimulation of the chloride secretion in the human bronchial epithelial cell line, 16HBE14o-. *British Journal of Pharmacology,* Vol.144, pp.1037-1050.

Bernard, K., Bogliolo, S., Soriani, O., & Ehrenfeld, J. (2003). Modulation of calcium-dependent chloride secretion by basolateral SK4-like channels in a human bronchial cell line. *Journal of Membrane Biology,* Vol.196, pp.15-31.

Bleich, M., & Warth, R. (2000). The very small-conductance K^+ channel KvLQT1 and epithelial function. *Pflügers Archiv European Journal of Physiology,* Vol.440, pp.202-206.

Boucher, R.C. (2002). An overview of the pathogenesis of cystic fibrosis lung disease. *Advanced Drug Delivery Reviews,* Vol.54, pp.1359-1371.

Caputo, A., Caci, E., Ferrera, L., Pedemonte, N., Barsanti, C., Sondo, E., Pfeffer, U., Ravazzolo, R., Zegarra-Moran, O., & Galietta, L.J. (2008). TMEM16A, a membrane protein associated with calcium-dependent chloride channel activity. *Science,* Vol.322, pp.590-594.

Chambers, L.A., Rollins, B.M., & Tarran, R. (2007). Liquid movement across the surface epithelium of large airways. *Respiratory Physiology & Neurobiology,* Vol.159, pp.256-270.

Cheng, Z., He, W., Zhou, X., Lv, Q., Xu, X., Yang, S., Zhao, C., & Guo, L. (2011). Cordycepin protects against cerebral ischemia/reperfusion injury *in vivo* and *in vitro*. *European Journal of Pharmacology,* Vol.664, pp.20-28.

Chow, A.W., Liang, J.F., Wong, J.S., Fu, Y., Tang, N.L., & Ko, W.H. (2010). Polarized Secretion of Interleukin (IL)-6 and IL-8 by Human Airway Epithelia 16HBE14o- Cells in Response to Cationic Polypeptide Challenge. *PLoS ONE,* Vol.5, e12091.

Clunes, M.T., Bove, P.F., & Boucher, R.C. (2008). Integration of Epithelial Ion Transport Activities into Airway Surface Liquid Volume and Ion Composition Regulation, In: *The Pulmonary Epithelium in Health and Disease,* D. Proud, (Ed.), 89-110, ISBN 978-0-470-05951-7, West Sussex, John Wiley & Son.

Cozens, A.L., Yezzi, M.J., Kunzelmann, K., Ohrui, T., Chin, L., Eng, K., Finkbeiner, W.E., Widdicombe, J.H., & Gruenert, D.C. (1994). CFTR expression and chloride secretion in polarized immortal human bronchial epithelial cells. *American Journal of Respiratory Cell and Molecular Biology,* Vol.10, pp.38-47.

Cunningham, K.G., Manson, W., Spring, F.S., & Hutchinson, S.A. (1950). Cordycepin, a metabolic product isolated from cultures of *Cordyceps militaris* (Linn.) Link. *Nature,* Vol.166, pp.949.

Danahay, H., & Jackson, A.D. (2005). Epithelial mucus-hypersecretion and respiratory disease. *Current Drug Targets – Inflammation & Allergy,* Vol.4, pp.651-664.

Das, S.K., Masuda, M., Sakurai, A., & Sakakibara, M. (2010). Medicinal uses of the mushroom *Cordyceps militaris*: current state and prospects. *Fitoterapia,* Vol.81, pp.961-968.

Endo, Y., Isono, K., Kondo, M., Tamaoki, J., & Nagai, A. (2007). Interleukin-9 and Interleukin-13 augment UTP-induced Cl ion transport via hCLCA1 expression in a human bronchial epithelial cell line. *Clinical & Experimental Allergy,* Vol.37, pp.219-224.

Fung, J.C., Yue, G.G., Fung, K.P., Ma, X., Yao, X., & Ko, W. (2011). *Cordyceps militaris* extract stimulates Cl^- secretion across human bronchial epithelia by both Ca^{2+}- and cAMP-dependent pathways. *Journal of Ethnopharmacology*, In Press.

Galietta, L.J., Folli, C., Caci, E., Pedemonte, N., Taddei, A., Ravazzolo, R., & Zegarra-Moran, O. (2004). Effect of inflammatory stimuli on airway ion transport. *Proceedings of the American Thoracic Society,* Vol.1, pp.62-65.

Galietta, L.J., Folli, C., Marchetti, C., Romano, L., Carpani, D., Conese, M., & Zegarra-Moran, O. (2000). Modification of transepithelial ion transport in human cultured bronchial epithelial cells by interferon-gamma. *American Journal of Physiology – Lung Cellular and Molecular Physiology,* Vol.278, pp.L1186-L1194.

Han, E.S., Oh, J.Y., & Park, H.J. (2011). *Cordyceps militaris* extract suppresses dextran sodium sulfate-induced acute colitis in mice and production of inflammatory mediators from macrophages and mast cells. *Journal of Ethnopharmacology,* Vol.134, pp.703-710.

Haws, C., Finkbeiner, W.E., Widdicombe, J.H., & Wine, J.J. (1994). CFTR in Calu–3 human airway cells: channel properties and role in cAMP–activated Cl^- conductance. *American Journal of Physiology – Lung Cellular and Molecular Physiology,* Vol.266, pp.L502–L512.

Holgate, S.T., Lackie, P.M., Davies, D.E., Roche, W.R., & Walls, A.F. (1999). The bronchial epithelium as a key regulator of airway inflammation and remodelling in asthma. *Clinical & Experimental Allergy,* Vol.29, Suppl 2, pp.90-95.

Hsu, C.H., Sun, H.L., Sheu, J.N., Ku, M.S., Hu, C.M., Chan, Y., & Lue, K.H. (2008). Effects of the immunomodulatory agent *Cordyceps militaris* on airway inflammation in a mouse asthma model. *Pediatrics & Neonatology,* Vol.49, pp.171-178.

Jeffery, P.K. (2000). Pathological spectrum of airway inflammation. In: *Cellular Mechanisms in Airways Inflammation,* C.F. Page, K.H. Banner, & D. Spina, (Eds.) 1-52, ISBN 3-7643-5852-1 Basel - Boston – Berlin, Birkhauser Verlag.

Jeong, J.W., Jin, C.Y., Kim, G.Y., Lee, J.D., Park, C., Kim, G.D., Kim, W.J., Jung, W.K., Seo, S.K., Choi, I.W., & Choi, Y.H. (2010). Anti-inflammatory effects of cordycepin via suppression of inflammatory mediators in BV2 microglial cells. *International Immunopharmacology,* Vol.10, pp.1580-1586.

Kidney, J.C., & Proud, D. (2000). Neutrophil transmigration across human airway epithelial monolayers: mechanisms and dependence on electrical resistance. *American Journal of Respiratory Cell and Molecular Biology,* Vol.23, pp.389-395.

Lau, W.K., Chow, A.W., Au, S.C., & Ko, W.H. (2011). Differential Inhibitory Effects of $CysLT_1$ Receptor Antagonists on $P2Y_6$ Receptor-Mediated Signaling and Ion Transport in Human Bronchial Epithelia. *PLoS ONE*, Vol.6, e22363.

Li, C., & Naren, A.P. (2010). CFTR chloride channel in the apical compartments: spatiotemporal coupling to its interacting partners. *Integrative Biology (Camb.),* Vol.2, pp.161-177.

Mason, S.J., Paradiso, A.M., & Boucher, R.C. (1991). Regulation of ion transport and intracellular calcium by extracellular ATP in normal human and cystic fibrosis airway epithelium. *British Journal of Pharmacology,* Vol.103, pp.1649–1656.

Nakano, T., Inoue, H., Fukuyama, S., Matsumoto, K., Matsumura, M., Tsuda, M., Matsumoto, T., Aizawa, H., & Nakanishi, Y. (2006). Niflumic acid suppresses interleukin-13-induced asthma phenotypes. *American Journal of Respiraotry and Crictical Care Medicine,* Vol.173, pp.1216-1221.

Ohta, Y., Lee, J.B., Hayashi, K., Fujita, A., Park, D.K., & Hayashi, T. (2007). *In vivo* anti-influenza virus activity of an immunomodulatory acidic polysaccharide isolated from *Cordyceps militaris* grown on germinated soybeans. *Journal of Agricultural and Food Chemistry,* Vol.55, pp.10194-10199.

Park, S.E., Kim, J., Lee, Y.W., Yoo, H.S., & Cho, C.K. (2009). Antitumor activity of water extracts from *Cordyceps militaris* in NCI-H460 cell xenografted nude mice. *Journal of Acupuncuture and Meridian Studies,* Vol.2, pp.294-300.

Paterson, R.R. (2008). *Cordyceps*: a traditional Chinese medicine and another fungal therapeutic biofactory? *Phytochemistry,* Vol.69, pp.1469-1495.

Puddicombe, S.M., Polosa, R., Richter, A., Krishna, M.T., Howarth, P.H., Holgate, S.T., & Davies, D.E. (2000). Involvement of the epidermal growth factor receptor in epithelial repair in asthma. *FASEB J,* Vol.14, pp.1362-1374.

Rogers, D.F. (2007). Physiology of airway mucus secretion and pathophysiology of hypersecretion. *Respiratory Care,* Vol.52, pp.1134-1146.

Shan, J., Huang, J., Liao, J., Robert, R., & Hanrahan, J.W. (2011). Anion secretion by a model epithelium: More lessons from Calu-3. *Acta Physiologica (Oxf.),* Vol.201, pp.523-531.

Shen, B.Q., Finkberger, W.E., Wine, J.J., Mrsny, R.J., & Widdicombe, J.H. (1994). Calu-3: a human airway epithelial cell line that shows cAMP–dependent Cl^- secretion. *American Journal of Physiology – Lung Cellular and Molecular Biology,* Vol.266, pp.L493–L501.

Shin, S., Kwon, J., Lee, S., Kong, H., Lee, S., Lee, C.K., Cho, K., Ha, N.J., & Kim, K. (2010). Immunostimulatory Effects of *Cordyceps militaris* on Macrophages through the Enhanced Production of Cytokines via the Activation of NF-kappaB. *Immune Network,* Vol.10, pp.55-63.

Tarran, R., Button, B., & Boucher, R.C. (2006). Regulation of normal and cystic fibrosis airway surface liquid volume by phasic shear stress. *Annual Review of Physiology,* Vol.68, pp.543-561.

Wang, N.Q., Jiang, L.D., Zhang, X.M., & Li, Z.X. (2007). Effect of dongchong xiacao capsule on airway inflammation of asthmatic patients. *Zhongguo Zhong Yao Za Zhi,* Vol.32, pp.1566-1568.

Won, S.Y., and Park, E.H. (2005). Anti-inflammatory and related pharmacological activities of cultured mycelia and fruiting bodies of Cordyceps militaris. *Journal of Ethnopharmacology,* Vol.96, pp.555-561.

Wong, A.M., Chow, A.W., Au, S.C., Wong, C.C., & Ko, W.H. (2009a). Apical versus basolateral $P2Y_6$ receptor-mediated Cl^- secretion in immortalized bronchial epithelia. *American Journal of Respiratory Cell and Molecular Biology,* Vol.40, pp.733-745.

Wong, E.L., Sung, R.Y., Leung, T.F., Wong, Y.O., Li, A.M., Cheung, K.L., Wong, C.K., Fok, T.F., & Leung, P.C. (2009b). Randomized, double-blind, placebo-controlled trial of herbal therapy for children with asthma. *Journal of Alternative and Complementary Medicine,* Vol.15, pp.1091-1097.

Yu, R., Song, L., Zhao, Y., Bin, W., Wang, L., Zhang, H., Wu, Y., Ye, W., & Yao, X. (2004). Isolation and biological properties of polysaccharide CPS-1 from cultured *Cordyceps militaris. Fitoterapia,* Vol.75, pp.465-472.

Yue, G.G., Lau, C.B., Fung, K.P., Leung, P.C., & Ko, W.H. (2008). Effects of *Cordyceps sinensis*, *Cordyceps militaris* and their isolated compounds on ion transport in Calu-3 human airway epithelial cells. *Journal of Ethnopharmacology*, Vol.117, pp.92-101.

2

Cellular Defences of the Lung: Comparative Perspectives

J.N. Maina
Department of Zoology,
University of Johannesburg,
Johannesburg,
South Africa

'Our lungs are highly complex organs that are exquisitely specialized for gas exchange and host defense.'
Rawlins (2010)

1. Introduction

1.1 General considerations

The most important function of the lung is to acquire molecular oxygen and eliminate carbon dioxide. Except probably for the gastrointestinal system, no other organ in the body interacts with the external environment as constantly and as intimately as the respiratory system. For example, during a 24 hour period, at rest, the human lung is ventilated ~25,000 times with ~20,000 L of air (e.g. Burri, 1985; Brain, 1996), it has a respiratory surface area (RSA) of ~140 m^2 (about the size of a tennis court) which is located in the acini that lie no more than 40 to 50 cm from the external environment (air) (e.g. Weibel, 1984), and the thickness of the blood-gas (tissue) barrier (BGB) (harmonic mean thickness, τht) is 0.62 µm, a value about one-fiftieth of the thickness of a foolscap paper or that of a human head hair (Gehr et al., 1978, 1990a). By weight, each day, more than 20 kg of air enters and leaves the human body, a load that far exceeds that of food and water ingested during the same time period (Brain, 1996). Depending on the level of air pollution, different types and quantities of foreign particulates and microbial pathogens are inhaled. While large RSA and thin BGB increase gas exchange, the concomitant downside to these structural properties is that they make the lung a leading portal of entry and therefore attack by pathogenic micro-organisms, damage by allergens and particulates, and injury by noxious gases (e.g. Brain, 1984, 1992; Lambrecht et al. 2001; Garn et al., 2006). The inhaled particulates are deposited on the epithelial lining of the conducting airways and that of the peripheral air spaces where they are retained for various durations before they are removed or destroyed (e.g. Geiser et al., 1988; Gehr et al., 1990 a, b). Brain (1996) observed that *'the lung is unique in that the marriage between environment and lung disease is profound.* The respiratory system threfore forms a huge challenge to the body's immune integrity (e.g. von Garnier and Nicod, 2009).

According to the United Nations Environmental Program (UNEP) and the WHO Report of 1994 (UNEP-WHO, 1994), annual averages of 600 mg/cm^3 and peak concentrations that may exceed 1,000 mg/cm^3 of solid particles occur in the air that covers many of the world's large metropolis. The frequency and severity of respiratory diseases that arise from inhalation of airborne particles are on the increase (e.g. EPS, 1996; Peters et al., 1997; Wichman and Peters, 2000; Warheit et al., 2009). Epidemiological studies have shown that even moderate inhalation of particulates, especially those of a diameter <10µm (PM_{10}), cause high morbidity and mortality not only from respiratory but also from cardiovascular diseases, especially in individuals with pre-existing medical conditions (e.g. Dockery et al., 1993; Schwartz, 1994; Brunekreef et al., 1995; Ware, 2000; Pope, 2000; Nemmar et al., 2002; Pope et al., 2002; Suwa et al., 2002; Schulz et al., 2005; Kaufman, 2010; Brook et al., 2010; van den Hooven et al., 2011; Kampfrath et al., 2011). $PM_{2.5}$ cause airway inflammation that presents in form of influx of committed monocytes, even in healthy individuals (Schaumann et al., 2004). Pulmonary afflictions and diseases have considerable socioeconomic impact. For example, in the United Kingdom, in 2006 more people died from respiratory diseases than from coronary disease or cancer and the cost to the National Health Service (NHS) was over £6.6 billion (BTS, 2006). According to the National Institutes of Health (NIH), in the United States, people suffer an average 1 billion colds per year and in 2006 the country spent more than 3 billion dollars to investigate respiratory-related diseases (http://www3.niaid.nih.gov/topics/commonCold/). Over 10% of hospitalizations and in excess of 16% of deaths in Canada are attributed to respiratory diseases (http://www.phac-aspc.gc.ca/ccdpc-cpcmc/crd-mrc/facts_gen_e.html). According to the Canadian Lung Association (CLA), the economic burden of respiratory disease in the Country is ~3 billion ($US) dollars (http://www.bukisa.com/articles/455926_lung-health-occupational-health-incidence#ixzz1I4jwMvBX). Based on net changes in gross domestic product (GDP) growth forecasts, the estimated annual cost of SARS (Sudden Avian Respiratory Syndrome) in Asia exceeds 10 billion dollars ($US) (Lee and McKibbin, 2003; Fan, 2003; McKibbin and Sidorenko, 2006) and according to the World Bank's estimates, an influenza pandemic may result in a loss (expenditure) of 800 billion dollars ($US) (Brahmbhatt, 2005): each year, seasonal influenza affects 5%-15% of the population in the northern hemisphere, with some some 3-5 million infections worldwide requiring hospitalization or leading to death (Sanders et al., 2011; http://www.euro.who.int/en/what-we-do/health-topics/diseases-and-conditions/influenza/seasonal-influenza 2010). For poultry, an important relatively more affordable source of animal protein, worldwide losses from respiratory diseases are estimated to cost the broiler industry over 1 billion dollars ($US) annually (e.g. Dekich, 1997; Currie, 1999; Wideman, 2005). Because avian species form an important reservoir of human infections, it is vital to study and understand avian toll-like receptors and related recetors so as to both design vaccine adjuvants and substitutes to the widespread application of antibiotics and in selection of strains of birds with augmented pathogen resistance.

By exerting direct selective pressure and evolving novel strategies of evading and surviving host defences (e.g. Litman et al., 1993; DuPasquier, 1993; Bartl et al., 1994; Beck and Habicht, 1996; Spurgin and Richardson, 2010; Finlay and Buckner, 2011), microbial pathogens have directly and indirectly fundamentally shaped the genetic and the phenotypic diversity of life. One of the most complex and astounding biological designs - the immune system - by which 'non-self' is recognized, neutralized, and eliminated has developed to counter continuous assaults (e.g. Janeway, 1993; Beck et al. 1994; Litman, 1996; Beck and Habicht, 1996; Wang et al., 2011; Yewdell and Dolan, 2011; McClung, 2011). In vertebrates, the genes for the major histocompatibility complex show how natural selection maintains variation in wild-populations of animals (e.g. Klein, 1986; Hughes and Neil, 1989; Apanius et al., 1997; Hughes, 1999; Meyer and Thompson, 2001; Hess and Edwards, 2002; Meyer and Mack, 2003). A diverse and extensive immune defence system that comprises of cellular (innate = natural)- and immunological (adaptive = acquired = specific) immunities have formed for protection (Fig. 1). The innate immune system which predominates in plants, fungi, insects, and the primitive multicellular organisms is believed to have formed first (e.g. Litman et al., 1993; DuPasquier, 1993; Bartl et al., 1994; Beck and Habicht, 1996; Hazlett and Wu, 2011). Invertebrates lack lymphocytes and antibody (immunoglobulin) based humoral immune system while lectins which are found in plants, bacteria, invertebrates, and vertebrates should have developed earlier (e.g. DuPasquier 1993; Beck et al., 1994). In certain interesting ways, the immunities of the sharks and skates are similar to the human one (e.g. Litman 1996). Many aspects of the invertebrate host defense mechanisms and their control signals have been conserved and carried over from lower to higher orders of animals (e.g. Mulnix and Dunn, 1995; Brownlie and Allan, 2011).

While among vertebrates host defences have been well-studied, mainly in the laboratory mammals and in the humans (e.g. Green et al., 1977; Johnson and Philip, 1977; Geiser, 2002; Whitset, 2002; Alexis et al., 2006), birds have only been modestly investigated (e.g. Ochs et al., 1988; Maina and Cowley, 1998; Nganpiep and Maina, 2002; Reese et al., 2006), and only scanty details exist on amphibians and reptiles (e.g. Bargmann, 1936; Grant et al., 1981; Welsch, 1981, 1983; Maina, 1989; Conlon, 2011). The need to understand immunological- and cellular defences in different animal taxa is becoming more important because of the most recent flare-up of high morbidity and mortality zoonotic infectious diseases, e.g., bovine spongiform encephalopathy, hemorrhagic fever, swine influenza, avian influenza H5N1, hantavirus, West Nile virus disease, Nipah virus, Rabies, leptospirosis, Rift Valley fever, and lyme disease (e.g. Rehman, 1998; Field et al., 2001; Cleaveland et al., 2001; Burroughs et al., 2002; Krauss et al., 2003; Chen et al., 2004; Brown, 2004; Chomel et al., 2007; Greger, 2007). The term 'zoonosis' was coined by Rudolph Virchow (1821-1902) in his studies of the pig muscle parasite, *Trichnella*. Factors like increase of human population and consequently ecological pressures on land leading to relocation to totally new habitats (e.g. Tilman et al., 2001; Daszak et al., 2001; Patz and Wolfe, 2002; Patz et al., 2004) and globalization with its rapid mass movement of people, animals, animal products, and global warming (e.g. IPCC, 2007; Sachan and Singh, 2010; Mills et al., 2010) are some of the factors that have been implicated in the recent outbreaks of zoonotic diseases (e.g. Burroughs et al., 2002). Comparative immunology has shown some esoteric immune related systems and substances that have potential for use as medications for humans (Boman and Hultmark, 1987; Hoffman and Hetru, 1992; Litman, 1996; Beck and Habicht, 1996).

The term 'macrophage', which derives from Greek, means 'large eaters'; a phagocyte literally means 'eating cell'; and, to 'phagocytose' means 'to eat'. Large leukocytic cells which in tissues differentiate into organ- specific (dedicated) subpopulations, macrophages move between tissue compartments in pursuit of invading pathogens and harmful particulates. The phagocytic cells of the immune system include macrophages, neutrophils, and dendritic cells. On activation by an antigen, phagocytes release and/or react to a group of highly specialized molecular signals called cytokines, e.g., interferons, interleukins (e.g. IL-1 and IL-6), and tumour necrosis factor (TNF) (e.g. Beck and Habicht, 1991; Gerlach et al., 2011). They also recognize and usually eliminate 'altered self', i.e., cells or tissues that have died, commonly by programmed cell death (apoptosis) or have changed by injury or disease like cancer.

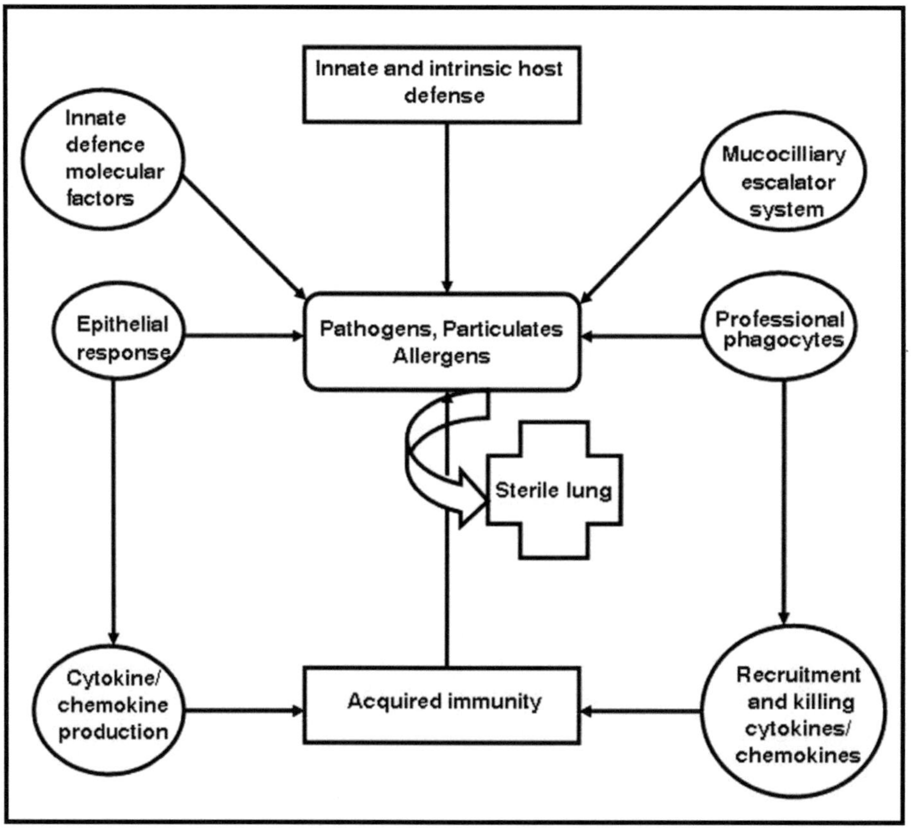

Fig. 1. The sterility of the lung is maintained by complex and efficient interplay of innate-(cellular) and acquired immune factors/systems. Pathogens and particulates that gain enty into it are neutralized, removed or sequestered.

Macrophages form an important part of the innate immune system that comprises of a group of cells that instantly defend the host from infection in a non-specific (generic) manner. In contrast to acquired immunity, macrophages don't confer long-lasting or protective immunity to the host. The common strategies by which bacteria become pathogens were comprehensively reviewed by Finlay and Falkow (1997). It is evident that pathogenic bacteria evolved from related non-pathogenic microorganisms by genetically gaining relatively large parts of genetic material that encode for virulence factors rather than by slow, adaptive evolution of pre-existing genes (e.g. Blum et al., 1994, 1995; Lee, 1996; Cheetham and Katz, 1995; Finlay and Falkow, 1997) and that the relentless nature of the challenge (selective pressure) posed by pathogens on animals (and even on plants) affected the evolution of host genes, conceivablyby selecting for changes (genetic) that promote survival (Finlay and Falkow, 1997). This may have lead to sudden radical changes in the way antibody genes are organized (Litman, 1996). Pathogenic microorganisms appear to evolve in quantum leaps, normally by their gaining genetic segments (factors acquired from unrelated organisms) that encode for multiple virulences (Finlay and Falkow, 1997).

Definition of abbreviations	
AM	Alveolar macrophage
BEC	Bronchial epithelial cell
BGB	Blood-gas (tissue) barrier
BM	Bronchial macrophage
BMM	Bone marrow monocyte
DC	Dendritic cell
PIM	Pulmonary interstitial macrophage
PM	Pulmonary macrophage
PIVM	Pulmonary intravascular macrophage
PlM	Pleural macrophage
PSM	Pulmonary surface macrophage
ROS	Reactive oxygen species

1.2 Pulmonary defences and macrophages

Having a lot to do with the fact that it is continuously exposed to insults from inhaled particulates, allergens, noxious gases, and pathogens over a large surface area and across thin BGB (e.g. Gehr et al., 1978; Meban, 1980; Maina and King, 1982; Rohmann et al., 2011), directly and indirectly, the respiratory system is exceptionally well-defended (e.g. Brain, 1980, 1992; Bedoret et al., 2009) (Figs. 1, 2). Directly, it is endowed with a formidable number of mechanical, physical, and cellular defences which are augmented by inflammatory and immune responses (e.g. Nicod, 2005). The inventory includes: a) a cough reflex that mechanically removes deposited irritants (Eckert et al., 2006; Canning, 2008; Poth and Matfin, 2010); b) a surface lining (surfactant) (Schürch et al., 1990; Gehr et al., 1990a, b; Geiser et al., 2003; Gehr et al., 2006), c) the BGB (e.g. Gil and Weibel, 1971; Maina and King, 1982; Gehr et al., 1990a, b; Maina and West, 2005); d) ciliated, mucus covered epithelium that traps, destroys, and clears deposited particulates through a mucociliary escalator system (e.g. Kilburn, 1968; Lippmann and Schlesinger, 1984; Geiser et al., 1990, 2003; Whitsett, 2002; Callaghan and Voynow, 2006) (Figs. 3-6); e) motile phagocytic cells (macrophages) that engulf, destroy, and sequester harmful particulates and pathogens (e.g. Geiser et al., 1990; Nicod, 2005) (Figs. 7-14); f) epithelium endowed with tightly packed cells that physically stop and destroy harmful agents (e.g. Breeze and Wheeldon, 1977; Harkema et al., 1991; Godfrey, 1997; Maina and Cowley, 1998; Nicod, 2005; Nganpiep and Maina, 2002) (Fig. 4), and; g) strategically placed mucosal and bronchial lymphatic tissue that is involved in the dissolution and antibody labelling of foreign particulates (Fagerland and Arp, 1990, 1993; Crapo et al., 2000; Reese et al., 2006).

Considering the intensity and the regularity of daily attacks to which it is exposed, its capacity of adapting to shifting environmental conditions, and the relative infrequency of diseases, the efficiency of the defences of the respiratory system is bewildering. In actual fact, the mechanisms and processes are so proficient that when pulmonary diseases and/or other pathologies are absent, the respiratory system is practically sterile below the larynx (e.g. Laurenzi et al., 1964; Green and Kass, 1964; Brain, 1980, 1984; Fawcett, 1986; Warheit et al., 1988; Brain, 1988; Steinmüller et al., 2000; Whitsett, 2002). This level of 'cleanliness' emanates from the diverse, well-coordinated pulmonary host defences that adeptly neutralize pathogenic microorganisms like bacteria, fungi, viruses, and harmful particulates that are inhaled or brought to the lung through blood (e.g. Zetterberg et al., 1998; Laskin et al., 2001; Whitsett, 2002; Pabst and Tschernig, 2002; Camner et al., 2002; Tschernig et al., 2006; Moniuszko et al., 2007; Tschernig and Pabst, 2009).

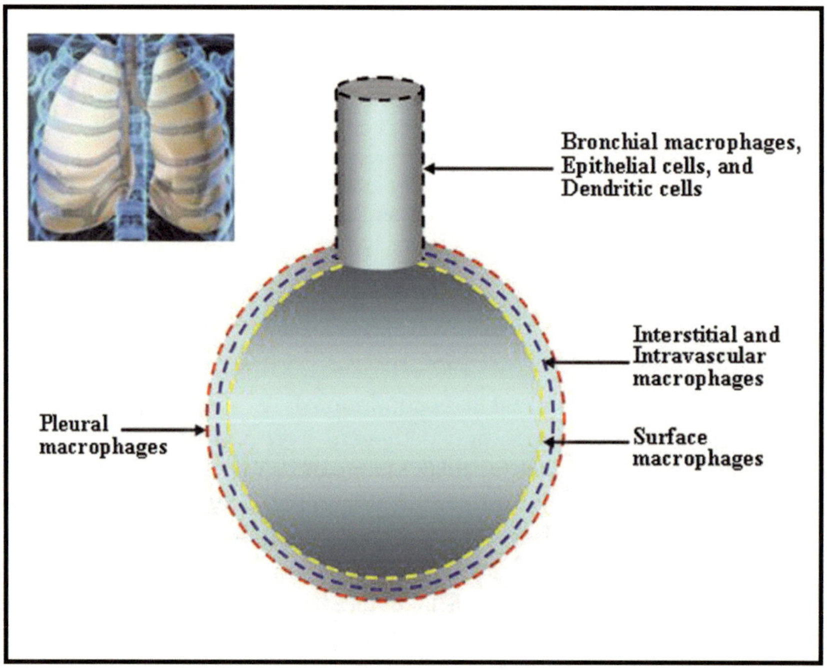

Fig. 2. Cellular defences of the respiratory system. Consistent with its high exposure to particulate matter and pathogenic microorganisms, the lung is very well-protected by various populations of phagocytic cells. Depending on need and circumstances, the cells can transfer from one compartment to another.

Among the cellular defences of the respiratory system, at the gas exchange level, pulmonary surface macrophages (PSMs) form the frontline defence of the lung. Highly specialized cells, macrophages clear dead host cells while defending against infection by broad range of pathogen-recognition receptor and their ability to produce inflammatory cytokines and chemokines that control the replication of the invaders (e.g. Gordon, 2002; Hazlett and Wu, 2011). Macrophages are highly specialized, robust motile cells that belong to a range of subpopulations: in different forms and locations, they display different behaviours and functions (e.g. Bowden, 1976; Dougherty and McBride, 1984; Lehnert, 1992; Brain, 1992; Gordon, 2002; Gordon and Taylor, 2005; Geissmann et al., 2010a, b; Schneberger et al., 2011). By detecting injurious agents, phagocytosing them, and acting as effector cells for both humoral and cell-mediated immune responses, macrophages serve as the frontline innate defence cells of the lung and as sentinels of the immune system of the body (e.g. Fels and Cohn, 1986; Peão et al., 1993; Warheit and Hartsky, 1993; Yamaya et al., 1995; Rubovitch et al., 2007). A relationship exists between the numbers of PSMs [like the alveolar macrophages (AMs)] with the level of environmental pollution (Brain, 1971, 1987; Nagdeve, 2004; Sichletidis et al., 2005; Mateen and Brook, 2011; Conklin, 2011). Even with an elegant defence inventory, respiratory diseases, especially those caused by air pollution, are on the increase (e.g. Peters et al., 1997; Mateen and Brook, 2011; Conklin, 2011). After the particles or pathogens have eluded or overwhelmed the epithelial barrier of the upper airways, they come into contact with the dedicated antigen presenting dendritic cells (DCs) (e.g. Steinman and Cohn, 1973; Nicod, 1997; Lipscomb and Masten, 2002; Holt, 2005) which are highly phagocytic (Dreher et al., 2001; Kiama et al., 2001, 2006; Walter et al., 2001). If they reach the alveolar surface, they are dealt with by the PSMs (e.g. Bowden, 1976; Goldstein and Bartlema, 1977; Geiser, 2002).

While macrophages are central to the defence of the lung from assaults by injurious materials and pathogenic agents (e.g. Holt et al., 1982; Brain, 1984; Weissler et al., 1986), their roles extend beyond engulfing (phagocytosing) and neutralizing harmful agents. They are secretory and regulatory and control activities of other cells like neutrophils, lymphocytes, and fibroblasts (e.g. Adamson and Bowden, 1981). Contrary to their well-serving protective activities, under certain conditions, macrophages function as a 'double-edged sword': they can initiate, exacerbate, and prolong inflammatory responses that cause immune suppression and progression of pathologies like cancer, leading to higher morbidity and mortality (e.g. Brain, 1976, 1980, 1984, 1986, 1992; Brain et al., 1984; Bowden, 1987; Warner, 1996; Yanagawa et al., 1996; Fireman et al., 1999; Ishii et al., 2005; Parbhakar et al., 2005; Rubovitch et al., 2007; Shimotakahara et al., 2007; Sica and Bronte, 2007; Kaczmarek et al., 2008; Gill et al., 2008; Biswas et al., 2008; Aharonson-Raz and Singh, 2010; De Palma and Lewis, 2011).

In spite of their widely accepted common origin from the bone marrow, their hematogenetic origin (e.g. Brain, 1976, 1984; van Furth, 1982; Geiser, 2010), macrophages display great phenotypic and functional heterogeneity (Krombach et al., 1977; Nguyen et al., 1982; Lehnert, 1992; Warheit and Hartsky, 1993; Kiama et al., 2008). Local environments largely determine the structural and functional differences (e.g. Morrissette et al., 1999). Within and between animal species, the immune reactions, phagocytic competences, and the cytoenzymological properties of different groups of macrophages have been shown to be spatially compartmentalized: observations made on one population of macrophages may therefore not correctly apply to another. For example, the AMs have slower rate of phagocytosis, higher motility, and faster particle clearance compared to the pulmonary intervascular macrophages (PIVMs) (Molina and Brain, 2007). Compared to the human ones, the dog's AMs have relatively less cytoplamic motility when acutely exposed to cigarette smoke (Yamaya et al., 1989) and during acute asthmatic attack (Yamaya et al., 1990). Among rodents, the AMs of the rat lung are the most efficient in clearing inhaled iron particles while the hamster ones are recruited to the site of particle deposition by noncomplement-mediated mechanism (Warheit and Hartsky, 1993) while the hamster and guinea pig's AMs best respond to bacteria (Warheit et al., 1988). Compared to those of the rat, the PSMs of the bird lung phagocytose polystylene particles more efficiently (Kiama et al., 2008).

The term 'pulmonary macrophage' (PM) loosely refers to cells that occupy two anatomical compartments of the lung: in the upper airways are the bronchial macrophages (BMs) and in the lower respiratory tract are the surface (free) macrophages (SMs) (e.g. Crowell et al., 1992). Other groups of phagocytes, however, exist in other parts of the lung. These are the dendritic cells (DCs), the pleural macrophages (PlMs), the pulmonary interstitial macrophages (PIMs), and in the lungs of certain species of animals the pulmonary intravascular macrophages (PIVMs). The structural attributes and the functional roles of these groups of cells are succinctly described below. To the best of my knowledge, this is the first comprehensive review of the biology of the PMs from a comparative perspective.

2. Pulmonary surface (free) macrophages (PSMs)

Acting as scavengers on the respiratory surface, the highly motile PSMs phagocytose, neutralize, and sequester harmful foreign materials (e.g. Sibille and Reynolds, 1990; Kelley, 1990; Lohmann-Matthes et al., 1994; Steinmüller et al., 2000). Also, by having receptor sites for immunoglobulins and complement on their cell membranes, PSMs contribute to the health of the lung by passing on specific information to immunologically competent cells like neutrophils, lymphocytes, and plasma cells, in so doing promoting antigen-antibody response (e.g. Said and Foda, 1989; Ooi et al., 1994). PSMs appear to stimulate and promote repair of epithelial cells after injury by releasing a growth factor (e.g. Takizawa et al., 1990). Interaction between PSMs and bronchial epithelial cells (BECs) during exposure to particulates with a diameter of less than 10 µm (PM_{10}) contributes to production of mediators (molecular factors) that induce a systematic inflammatory response (e.g. Hirano, 1996; Fujii et al., 2002; Ishii et al., 2005; Rubovitch et al., 2007).

Large, mononuclear cells, PSMs consist of several subtypes that can be categorized by criteria like size, morphology, numbers, motility, ingestion and handling of foreign materials, adherence onto surfaces, and expression of surface receptors (e.g. Brain, 1976, 1980, 1992; Zwilling et al., 1982; Nguyen et al., 1982; Holt et al., 1982; Warheit et al., 1984, 1986; Sebring and Lehnert, 1992; Spiteri et al., 1992; Lavnikova et al., 1993; Johansson et al., 1997). The existence of subpopulations of macrophages that have functionally distinct roles in airway immunity derives from the individual bone marrow precursor cells and the environment that they reside in (Gant and Hamblin 1985). Compared to the PIVMs, the rat PSMs exhibit marked microbial activity through high production of reactive oxygen species (ROS), nitric oxide (NO), and tumour necrotic factor-α (TNF-α) (Steinmüller et al., 2000). Exposure of rats to NO induces infiltration of AMs that are phenotypically and functionally different (regarding mediator mRNA expression and production as well as mRNA expression for several matrix metalloproteinases) from the resident AMs (Garn et al., 2006). Ensuing from infection or overwhelming by irritants, need for more macrophages is met by *in situ* replication of existing cells, release of pre-existing cells from various compartments (reservoirs) within the lung, increased production from macrophage precursors in the lung interstitium, and increased flux of monocytes from blood to the lung (e.g. Brain, 1980, 1992). The PSMs are renewed at a rate of ~1-2% of the total number of cells in the lung (e.g. Shellito et al., 1987) daily.

The temporal sequence of particle clearance by phagocytes entails particle identification, endocytosis, and transport from the alveolar surface (Green, 1973, 1984; Warheit et al., 1984). Resting freely on the respiratory surface, PSMs are directly exposed to particulates,

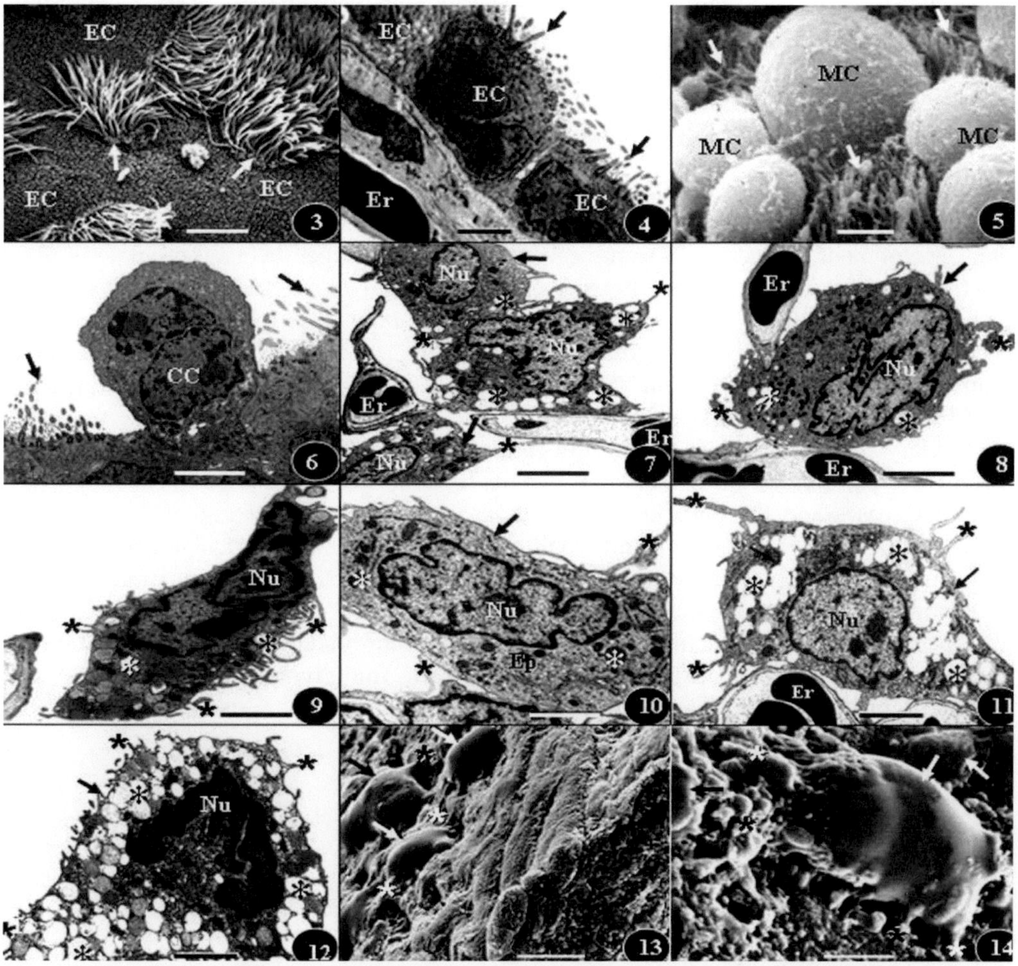

Fig. 3.-4. Bronchial epithelial cells (EC) that comprise of ciliated cells (arrows) and mucus secreting cells (MC). Er, erythrocyte. Fig. 5.-6. Respiratory epithelium at the bronchiole level showing Clara cells (CC) interspersed between ciliated cells (arrows). Figs. 7.-14. Surface macrophages (arrows) of the mammalian- (Figs. 7-12) and the frog lungs (Fig. 13. -14.). Stars, filopodia (feet); Er, erythrocyte; asterisks, lysosomes; Nu, nucleus; Ep, epithelial cell. Scale bars: Figs. 3, 30 µm; 4, 45 µm; 5, 30 µm; 6, 50 µm; 7, 10 µm; 8, 25 µm; 9, 10 µm; 10, 10 µm; 11, 10 µm; 12, 15, µm; 13, 20 µm; 14, 10 µm.

environmental toxicants, and pathogens. In contrast to fixed or interstitial macrophages that are attached to the collagenous fibers of the tissue matrix, they (PSMs) actively move over the respiratory surface by ameboid movement that entails formation of deformations of the cell membrane, leading to cytoplasmic extensions (advancing lamella = filopodia = pseudopodia) in the direction of the movement, pulling the main part of the cell with it (Figs. 10, 11, 13, 14). Actin-binding protein and myosin advance in the tips of the filopodia (Reaven and Axline, 1973; Stossel and Hartwig, 1976; Hartwig et al., 1977). In addition to effecting movement, formation of filopodial extensions by contractile proteins is involved in phagocytosis of foreign agents (Stossel, 1978; Zigmond and Hirsch, 1979). Cytoplasmic motility corresponds with phagocytic activity of PSMs: both cytoplasmic movement and phagocytosis may be regulated by similar mechanism in the cytoskeletal system (Yamaya et al., 1995). Once the phagocytosed particle is engulfed, i.e., is enclosed within the invaginated cell membrane and transferred to a cytoplasmic location, it is called a phagosome.

Macrophages are chemotactically driven to foreign materials/agents. The terms 'free', 'wandering', and 'fixed' macrophages refer to different functional states and/or stages of the development of cells of same cell phagocytic lineage. When stimulated, fixed macrophages detach from collagenous fibers and migrate as free macrophages to sites of pathogen invasion, injury, or irritation. PSMs remain motile up to a certain particle loading and beyond that the mobility is greatly inhibited (e.g. Yu et al., 1989; Lehnert et al., 1990; Kiama et al., 2008). For the avian PSMs (Kiama et al., 2008), the cells burst after ingesting high loads of polystylene particles (Figs. 15-17). Inability of dust-laden AMs to reach the mucociliary escalator system of the upper airways correlates with the particle loading (Morrow, 1988). In the Fischer 344 rat, when the loading exceeds ~600 μm^3 per cell, particle clearance ceases and the particle laden cells remain in the alveolar region. Interestingly, PSMs can be overwhelmed by even small amounts of ingested particulates, e.g., carbon particles (concentration 0.2 $\mu m.10^{-6}$) and also by long term (22-44 hr) incubation with low concentrations (12.5 $M.ml^{-1}$) of interferon-γ (IFN-γ) (Lundborg et al., 1999, 2001). PSMs may also be rendered non-functional by exposure to inordinately high concentration of particulates or pathogens, especially where there are underlying infections that invoke increase in production of IFN-γ (Baron et al., 1991; Cuffs et al., 1997; Camner et al., 2002).

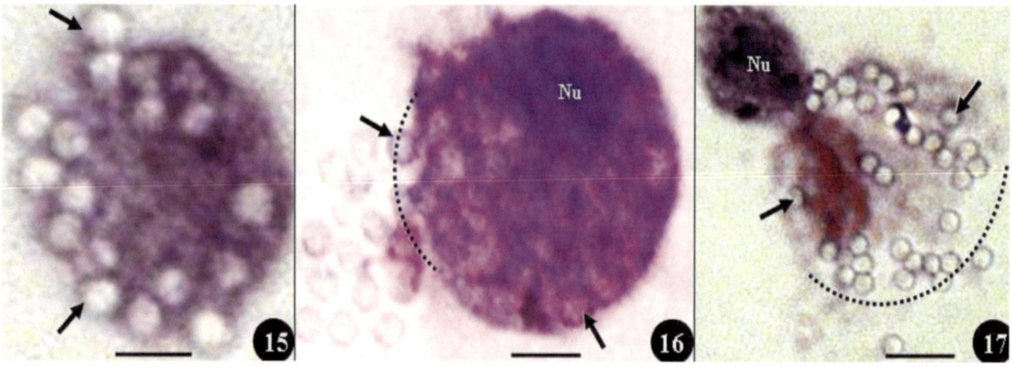

Fig. 15.-17. Pulmonary surface macrophages of the avian lung showing various stages of uptake of polystylene particles (arrows). At a certain critical point of particulate ingestion, the cells burst (dashed line). Nu, nucleus. Scale bars: 3μm.

The ultrastructural morphology of the AMs has been well-documented (e.g. Weibel, 1984, 1985). Remarkably heteromorphic, they vary in size from 10 to 40 μm in diameter, constitute 2 to 9% of the pneumocytes, and have an indented (bean = horse shoe-shaped) eccentrically located nucleus (e.g. Sebring and Lehnert, 1992; Weibel, 1984, 1985) (Fig. 12). The nuclear indentation contains numerous vacuoles, Golgi apparati, rough endoplasmic reticulum, and mitochondria. The most striking structural features of the PSMs are the large number of membrane bound cytoplasmic inclusions that include lysosomes, phagososmes, vacuoles, and lipid droplets (Figs. 7, 11, 12). Many of the vacuoles are about 0.5 μm or less in diameter and are oblong or spherical in shape. They contain high concentrations of various strong hydrolytic enzymes which are synthesized in the rough endoplasmic reticulum and packaged in the Golgi complex, forming the primary lysosomes. When the primary lysosomes combine with the phagosomes, they form the secondary lysosomes. The broken-down/detoxified foreign agents are either discharged from the cell or are stored in membrane bound granules called residual bodies. The foreign indigestible materials, e.g., carbon- and heavy metal particles, are sometimes permanently stored in the phagocytic cells of the lung. When macrophages are overwhelmed by large foreign materials that cannot be efficiently phagocytosed by individual cells, they form multinucleated giant cells that sequester such factors. Nodular inflammatory lesions that contain these cells are termed granulomas (e.g. Fawcett, 1986).

Although different views have been expressed by, e.g., Sorokin et al. (1984), it is now widely accepted that PSMs do not form *in situ*, i.e., in the lung: they belong to the general mononuclear phagocyte (formerly reticuloendothelial) system of the body and originate from stem cells in the bone marrow from where they are transported in blood as monocytes. On entering the interstitium of the lung they undergo a series of maturational stages before transferring to the surface (e.g. van Furth, 1970; Bowden and Adamson, 1980; Blussé van Oud Alblas et al., 1983; Bowden, 1987; Sebring and Lehnert, 1992; Brain et al., 1999; Geiser, 2010). The turnover time of the PSMs is ~6 days and amounts to 15.10^3 cells per hour (Blussé van Oud Alblas et al., 1983). The fate of PSMs is varied: a) many of the cells leave the peripheral air spaces via the bronchi where they are transported by the mucociliary escalator system to the oral pharynx (e.g. Spritzer et al., 1968) to be swallowed or expectorated; b) others move to the interstitium and either settle there or leave via the lymphatics (e.g. Sorokin and Brain, 1975). Compared to the PIMs, AMs have greater phagocytic activity and faster attachment and ingestion properties (Franke-Ullmann et al., 1996; Fathi et al., 2001).

While pulmonary cellular defence appears to exist in the amphibian- (e.g. Welsch, 1981, 1983; Maina and Maloiy, 1988; Maina, 1989) (Figs. 13, 14) and reptilian lungs (Grant et al., 1981), PSMs are rare in the lungs of the lower vertebrates (Bargmann, 1936). Welsch (1983) experimentally stimulated a macrophagic response in the lung of *Xenopus laevis* after exposure and aspiration of carbon particles. In the caecilian lung, macrophages contain acid phosphatase, β-glucosaminidae, and unspecific esterase (Welsch, 1981). In the lungs of the lower vertebrates (Welsch and Müller 1980), epithelial cells (pneumocytes) contain acid phosphatase and have a phagocytic capacity. No resident surface macrophages occur in a nonchallenged lung of the snake, *Boa constrictor* (Grant et al., 1981): unphagocytosed materials remained on the respiratoty surface for up to 4 days. Challenge of the snake lung with inspirable particles increases surfactant secretion, elicits surfacing of nonphagocytic eosinophilic granulocytes, but interestingly doesn't set off release of mononuclear phagocytic macrophages (Grant et al., 1981).

While the biology of the AMs has been well-studied (e.g. Bowden, 1987), relatively little is known about the SMs of the avian respiratory system. Paucity of SMs (e.g. Stearns et al., 1986; Toth et al., 1988; Klika et al., 1996; Maina and Cowley, 1998; Nganpiep and Maina, 2002; Kiama et al., 2008) and even lack of them was reported by, e.g., Lorz and López (1997). In mice, rats, and guinea pigs, respectively, yields of $0.55\text{-}1.55.10^6$, $2.86\text{-}4.43.10^6$, and $1.08\text{-}1.77.10^7$ AMs were determined by Holt (1979). Some of these values are 20 times greater than those determined in much larger birds (e.g. Toth and Siegel, 1986). The average number of SMs in the lung of the pigeon, *Columba livia* is 1.6.10^5 (Maina and Cowley, 1998), in the domestic fowl, *Gallus gallus* variant *domesticus* it is 2.5.10^5 (Toth and Siegel, 1986; Toth et al., 1987), and in the turkey, *Meleagris gallopavo* is 1.15.10^6 (Ficken et al., 1986). The number of SMs per unit body mass in the rat was significantly greater than that of the domestic fowl and the duck, *Cairina moschata* (Nganpiep and Maina 2002) (Fig. 18). In a 30 year-old smoker and a nonsmoker, respectively, 1.5.10^7 and 5.2.10^7 AMs were harvested by bronchopulmonary lavage by Hof et al. (1990). Regarding cellular defence strategies, mechanisms, and proficiencies, it has been contended by different investigators, e.g., Klika et al. (1996) and Spira (1996) that compared to mammals, birds are relatively more susceptible to pulmonary diseases and afflictions. In the poultry industry, huge economical losses have been ascribed to mortalities arising from respiratory diseases (e.g. Mensah and Brain, 1982; Toth et al., 1988). Scarcity of SMs in the avian lung (e.g. Stearns et al., 1986; Maina and Cowley, 1998; Nganpiep and Maina, 2002; Kiama et al., 2008) and enzymatic deficiencies in the oxidative metabolism of the SMs (e.g. Penniall and Spitznagel, 1975; Bellavite et al., 1977) have been reported.

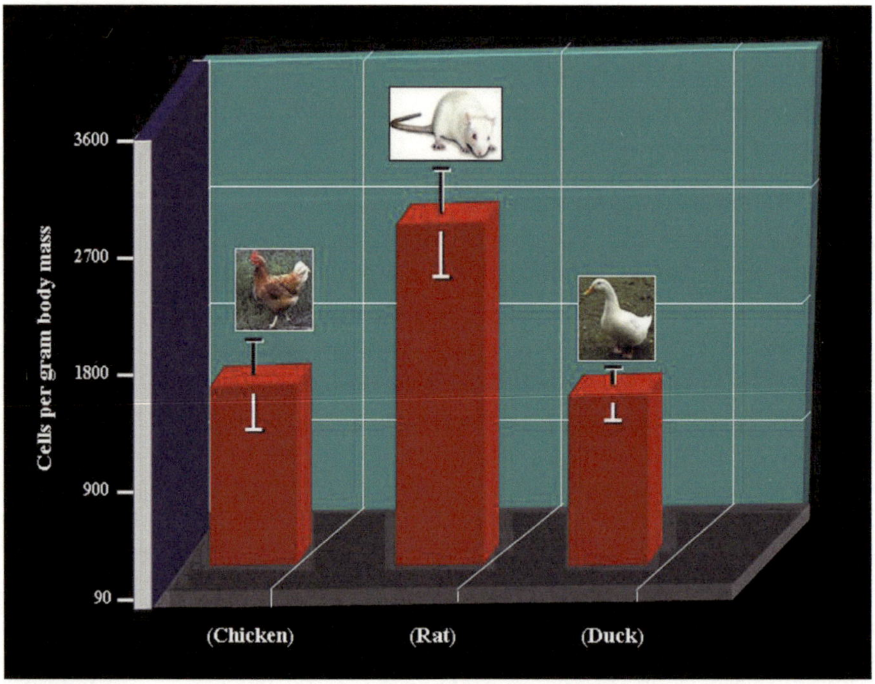

Fig. 18. Comparison between the numbers of pulmonary surface macrophages (PSMs) in the chicken (domestic fowl) (*Gallus domesticus*), the rat (*Rattus rattus*), and the duck (*Cairina moschata*). Birds have relatively fewer PMS compared to mammals. From Nganpiep and Maina (2002).

The foremost morphological and physiological factors that may predispose the avian respiratory system to injury by inspired foreign agents are: a) a relatively thin BGB and extensive RSA (e.g. Maina et al., 1989), b) large tidal volume and continuous and unidirectional ventilation of the lung (e.g. Fedde 1980, 1997; Brown et al., 1997), and c) in some species, e.g., the ostrich, *Struthio camelus* (Bezuidenhout et al., 2000), the air sacs extend out of the coelomic cavity to lie subcutaneously, where they are highly susceptible to trauma and infection: in such cases, air sacculitis (infection of the air sacs) can easily spread to the lung.Categorical proof that the avian lung is relatively more susceptible to infection by inhaled biological pathogens is lacking. It was argued by Maina (2005) that in the bird lung, PSMs, cells that are abundantly endowed with lysosomes (Nganpiep and Maina 2002) (Fig. 19-24) and have greater motility and phagocytic capacity (Kiama et al., 2008) may be so efficient that only few of them are required to reside on the respiratory surface and provide adequate protection. Pulmonary cellular defence is reinforced by capacity of rapidly mobilizing and transferring PIMs, PIVMs and probably blood monocytes to the respiratory surface (Nganpiep and Maina, 2002). Under similar conditions, birds may not be any more susceptible to pulmonary diseases than mammals. Factors like extreme genetic manipulation for faster growth and weight gain and the intensive and stressful regimes of battery production and management may explain the high incidence of aerosol transmitted pulmonary diseases, particularly in poultry.

3. Pulmonary interstitial (subepithelial) macrophages (PIMs)

Mainly because they are relatively less accessible, compared to the PSMs which are easily harvested by pulmonary lavage (e.g. Holt et al., 1985; Steinmüller et al., 2000), the PIMs have been relatively less well-studied. They are found in the peribronchial and perivascular spaces, in the interstitial spaces of the lung parenchyma (Fig. 25), in the lymphatic channels, and in the visceral pleural region (e.g. Bedoret et al., 2009; Nganpiep and Maina, 2002). Occurring in substantial numbers, PIMs provide bactericidal and immune mediated protection against particles and pathogens that escape the PSMs and penetrate the epithelium: there, they are sequestered or removed via the lymphatic channels. In the rat lung, PIMs form a substantial fraction of the PMs (e.g. Sebring and Lehnert, 1992): they comprise from 37% to 40% of the PMs (Lehnert et al., 1985; Crowell et al., 1992). However, using a different method, Blussé van Oud Alblas and van Furth (1979) determined that PIMs form only 7% of the PMs in the mouse-, rat-, and hamster lungs. In normal and injured lungs, PIMs exceed the number of PSMs (e.g. Thet et al., 1983).

Phenotypical and functional differences occur between the PIMs and the PSMs: PIMs are smaller in diameter (7.6 µm versus 16 µm for the PSMs), are more homogenous in size, have a smoother outline [i.e., they have fewer and blunter filopodia (pseudopodia)], have an indented (kidney-shaped) nucleus and greater nuclear to cytoplasm ratio, the primary lysosomes and phagososmes are fewer and larger, mitochondria and rough (granular) endoplasmic reticulum are scanty, Golgi bodies are rare, the cells are less phagocytic, they possess greater antigen presenting capability to T-cells, when they are activated they can release different cytokines [particularly TGF-β, TNF-α, and metalloproteinases-1 (MCP-1) and IGF-1], and the cells resemble the peripheral monocytes (e.g. Kobzik et al., 1988; Sebring and Lehnert, 1992; Lavnikova et al., 1993; Wizemann and Laskin, 1994; Prokhorova et al., 1994; Johansson et al., 1997; Fathi et al., 2001). Antigenic differences occur between the PIMs and the PSMs (e.g. Kobzik et al., 1986). In the rat lung, regarding the mechanisms that are mainly involved in the induction and the furtherance of specific immune reactions, e.g., the major histocompartibility complex (MHC) class-II expression and interleukin (IL-1) and IL-6 production, the PIMs are more efficient than the PSMs (Steinmüller et al., 2000). Since they

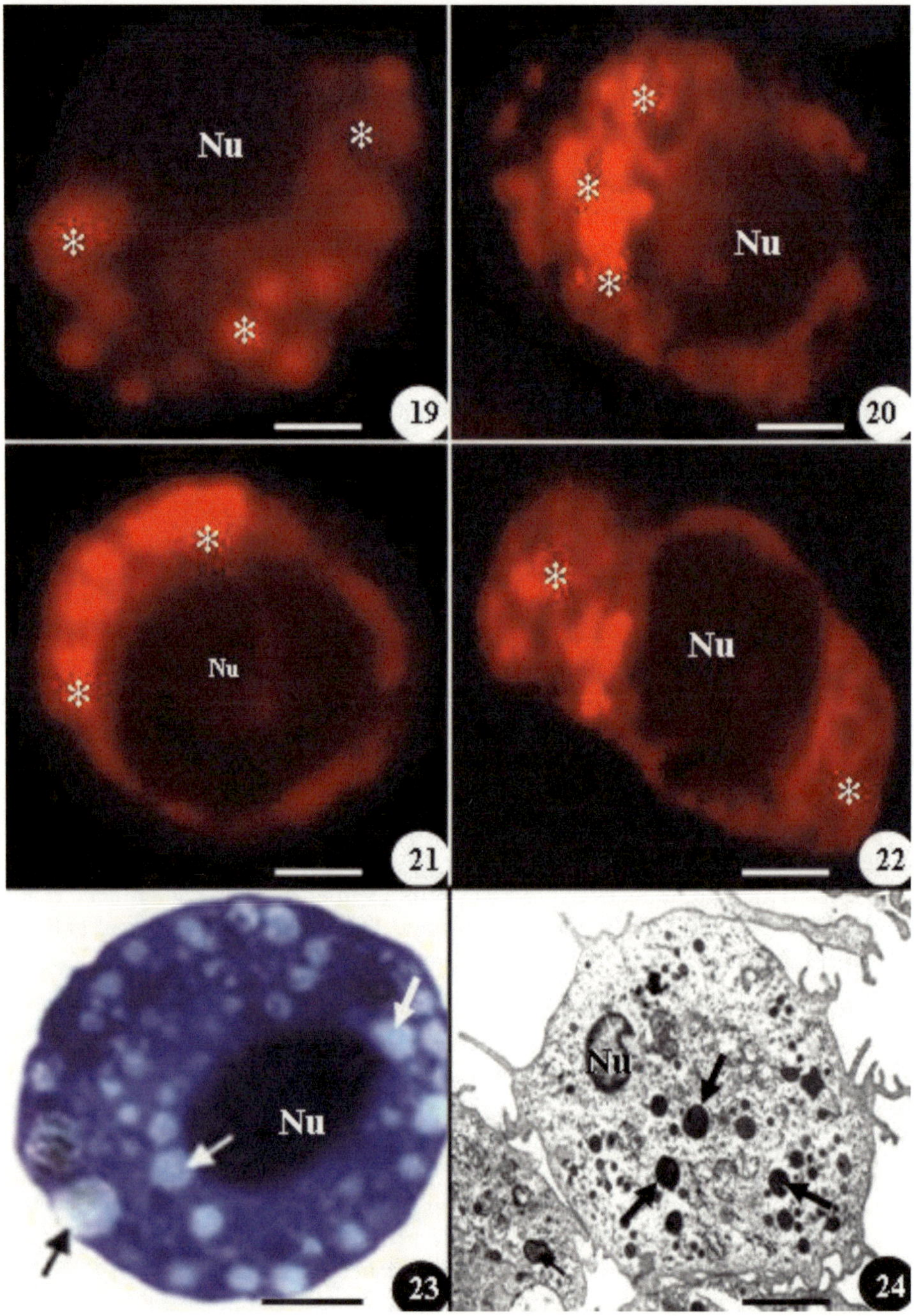

Fig. 19.-24. Pulmonary surface macrophages of the chicken (domestic fowl) (*Gallus domesticus*) showing the concentration of lyric vesicles in the cytoplasm in Figs. 19-22) (asterisks) and arrows (Figs. 23 and 24). Nu, nucleus. Scale bars: 4 μm. Figs. 19-22 from Nganpiep and Maina (2002) and Figs 23 and 24 from Kiama et al. (2008).

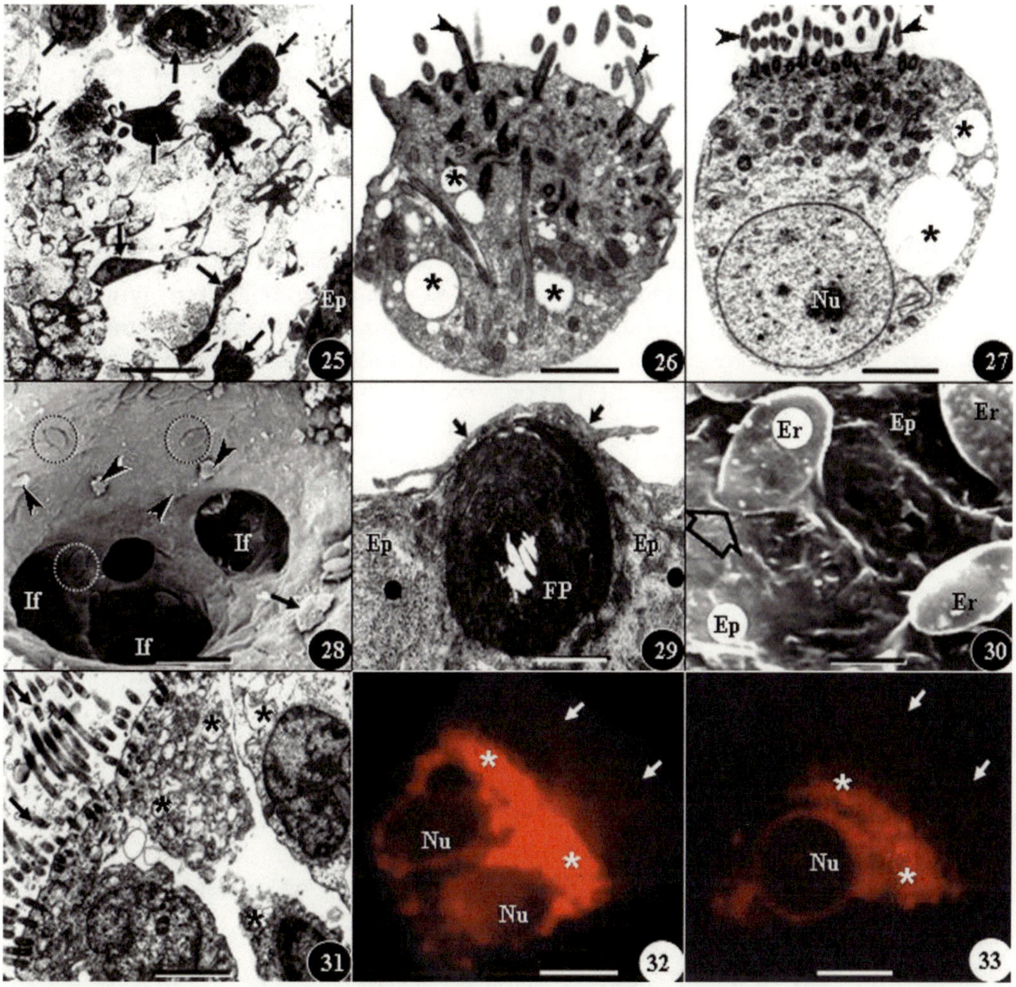

Fig. 25. Subepithelial macrophages in the lung of the chicken, *Gallus domesticus* (arrows). Ep, respiratory epithelium. Figs. 26 & 27: Bronchial epithelial cells of the chicken's lung which have phagocytosed polysylene particles (stars). Arrow heads, cilia. Fig. 28: Surface of an atrium of a parabronchus of the lung of the chicken showing a surface macrophage (arrow), particles (arrow heads), and extravasated red blood cell (dashed circles) that are about to be phagocytosed by the epithelial cells. If, infundibulum. Fig. 29: Close-up of a foreign particle (FP) being engulfed by an epithelial cell (Ep) in the chicken lung. Arrows, cytoplasmic extensions of the epithelial cell. Fig. 30: Close-up of extravasated erythrocytes (Er) on the epithelial surface (Ep) of the lung of the duck, *Cairina moschata*. One of the erythrocytes (arrow) is being engulfed by the epithelial cell. Figs. 31-33: The ciliated bronchial epithelial cells (arrows) of the lung of the domestic fowl, *Gallus gallus* are well-endowed with lysosomes (stars). Nu, nuclei of the epithelial cells. Scale bars: Figs. 25, 50 µm; 26 & 27, 10 µm; 28, 50 µm; 29, 10 µm; 30, 10 µm; 31-33, 10 µm. From Nganpiep and Maina (2002).

are set in the lung tissue, the cytotoxic or inflammatory mediators released by the PIMs have greater biological and/or pathological effects on the surrounding lung tissue than those released by the PSMs (Steinmüller et al., 2000; Laskin et al., 2001). In the murine lung, PIMs exhibit immunoregulatory and phagocytic functions (e.g. Bilyk et al., 1988; Franke-Ullman et al., 1996). Increased numbers of PIMs appear within active lesions of the injured lung (e.g. Brain, 1988). There is ample evidence that PIMs replicate *in situ* (e.g. Bowden and Adamson, 1980). Compared to the PSMs, the PIMs exhibit a significantly greater proliferative capacity (Johansson et al., 1997), a process that maintains the lung macrophage pool in the lung tissue compartment (Adamson and Bowden, 1981).

The PIMs can be discriminated from the PSMs by their unique capacity of inhibiting the maturation of the lung's DCs and their migration on stimulation with lipopolysaccharides (LPS) like those located in the outer membrane of gram positive bacteria which act as endotoxins that elicit strong immune responses that prevent sensitization to prevailing antigens (e.g. Buckner and Finlay, 2011). In presence of LPS, PIMs and not PSMs disrupt the link between the innate and the adaptive immunity, allowing inhaled antigens to escape from T-cell dependent responses (e.g. Bedoret et al., 2009). The PIMs are morphologically more like the BMs than they are to PSMs (Sebring and Lehnert, 1992). It has been suggested by some investigators, e.g., Holt et al. (1982), Bluseé van Oud Alblas and van Furth (1982), and Sebring and Lehnert (1992) that PIMs are an intermediate maturation stage (from the bone marrow monocytes) of the PSMs, i.e., they are precursors of the PSMs before the cells transfer to the respiratory surface. There is, however, contrary evidence that PIMs represent a distinct population of cells with dedicated pulmonary inflammatory and immunoregulatory roles of defending the lung (e.g. Chandler et al., 1988; Dethloff and Lehnert, 1988; Lehnert, 1992; Prokhorova et al., 1994; Johansson et al., 1997; Zetterberg et al., 1998; Steinmüller et al., 2000). Although concerning inflammation and antimicrobial defense AMs exhibit greater functional repertoire related to and including increased chemotaxis, phagocytosis, cytotoxicity, and release of ROSs, PIMs express higher quantities of C3-receptor and intercellular adhesion molecule-1 and are more active in producing interleukins-1 and -6 (IL-1 and -6) and exhibit greater I-a antigen expression (Chandler and Brannen, 1990; Franke-Ullmann et al., 1996; Steinmüller et al., 2000).

4. Bronchial epithelial cells (BECs) and bronchial macrophages (BMs)

The ciliated BECs and the nonciliated cells of the upper airways of the lung are the first cellular entities that interact and deal with the inhaled particulates and pathogenic microorganisms (Figs. 31-34). They secrete inflammatory cytokines that initiate and ultimately aggravate host innate inflammatory responses that may cause harmful immune-mediated pathologies (e.g. Yoshikawa et al., 2010) and afterwards initiate remodelling of the lung (Altraja et al., 2009). In the bronchial tree, macrophages are suspended in the mucus carpet while others lie under the layer, directly attached onto the epithelial substratum (e.g. Sorokin and Brain, 1975; Brain et al., 1984; von Garnier and Nicod, 2009) (Fig. 34). A highly active group of cells, ciliated BECs and non-ciliated BECs may ingest and degrade antigens that land on the surface of the airways and/or may release mediators that attract lymphocytes, neutrophils, or mast cells to the airways and regulate their activities there (Geiser et al., 1988). On their depositing on the airway epithelium, inhaled bacteria soon loose their replicative capacity (e.g. Laurenzi et al., 1964; Brain et al., 1984). Particulates with a diameter of less than 10 μm (PM_{10}) stimulate epithelial cells to produce ROS and inflammatory mediators/cytokines (Carter et al., 1997; Fujii et al., 2001; Schaumann et al.,

2004; Ishii et al., 2005). In the avian lung, ciliated epithelial cells particularly phagocytose inhaled atmospheric particles (Fedde, 1997; Maina and Cowley, 1998; Fujii et al., 2001; Nganpiep and Maina, 2002) (Figs. 26, 27). Ciliated BECs express an oxidative stress response that is different from that of the PSMs by rapidly shifting from cytoprotective to cytotoxic responses but are incapable of converting *N*-acetylcysteine to cytoprotective glutathione (Li et al., 2002). A mucus escalator system, which is maintained by the motility of cilia (Fig. 34), transports particulates and pathogens that settle on the airways towards the mouth. Normal motility of cilia is vital to the preservation of the integrity of the mucus conveyer-belt system. Infectious diseases and genetic conditions that reduce or abolish cilia motility, e.g., Kartagener's syndrome (e.g. Mahsud and Din, 2006; Kapur et al., 2009), and those that increase the consistency (viscosity) of the mucus, e.g., cystic fibrosis (Chmiel and Davis, 2003; McShane et al., 2004) lead to higher incidence of pulmonary infections, as they decrease the removal of particulates and pathogens by the mucus escalator system.

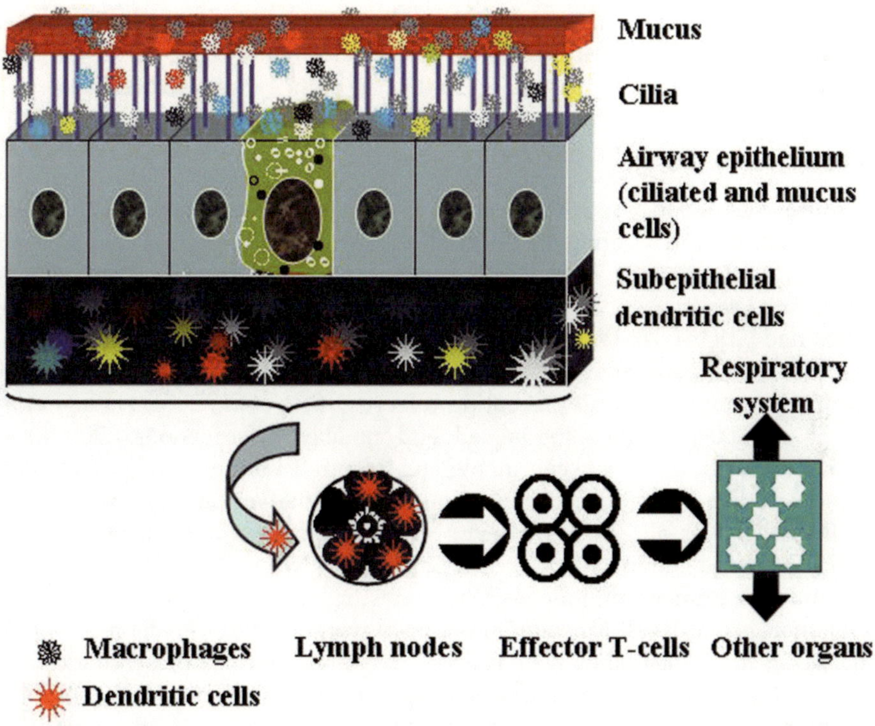

Fig. 34. Schematic diagram of the bronchial epithelium. Bronchial macrophages are located in the mucus carpet and on the epithelial cells themselves. Dendritic cells are located in the subepithelial space from where they send their long projections between the epithelial cells to sense foreign agents.

According to Fireman et al. (1999), 'asthma may be defined as failure to regulate T-cell mediated immunoreactivity within the bronchial wall of hyperreactive airways'. Inadequate regulation of the T-cell response by suppressive macrophages may set off allergic bronchial inflammation. The BMs of asthmatics are functionally modulated (e.g. Fireman et al., 1999:

they have lower suppressive activity. Probably caused by T-helper cell cytokines (Th-2), this explains the bronchial hyperactivity displayed by asthmatics (Fireman et al., 1999; Alexis et al., 2001). Different subsets of the BMs may to different extents regulate the inflammatory response in allergic asthma and respond to immunomodulatory signals, especially those mediated by interleukin 10 (IL-10) (Moniuszko et al., 2007). Power et al. (1994) observed that in normal human bronchial wall, a small number of T-cells, the majority of which were $CD8^+$ cells existed: $CD4^+$ cells predominated in the subepithelial tissue and a small number of macrophages were present. In individuals with sarcoidosis, compared to healthy subjects, Hawley et al. (1979) observed physical interaction between the BMs and the lymphocytes, the BMs presented a more highly irregular cell surface, and more membrane bound inclusions and fewer lysosomes and phagolysosomes were present: no significant differences were observed in the nuclear or cellular diameters of the BMs from normal- and sarcoidosis affected individuals. In patients with chronic obstructive pulmonary disease (COPD), the BMs were relatively small in size, contained little cytoplasm, and had a markedly high kario-cytoplasmic ratio (Fedosenko et al., 2010): these features improved after treatment with the drug tiotropium. In the bronchial mucosa of patients with chronic bronchitis, there was a significant number of BMs and T-lymphocytes in the lamina propria (Saetta et al., 1993): these cells may be involved in the pathogenesis of the disease.

5. Dendritic cells (DCs)

The DCs derive from bone marrow precursor cells and with their maturation, dependent on the extracellular microenvironments establish themselves as immature cells in tissues (e.g. Steinman, 1991; Reid, 1997; Hart, 1997; Banchereau and Steinman, 1998; Austyn 1998; Satthaporn and Eremin, 2001; Lipscomb and Masten, 2002; Geurtsvankessel and Lambrecht, 2008; Fries and Griebel, 2011). Under appropriate signals, monocytes can differentiate into DCs (e.g. Banchereau and Steinman, 1998; Satthaporn and Eremin, 2001) which are potent antigen uptake, processing, and presenting cells (e.g. Belz et al., 2004; Harada et al., 2009; Bedoret et al., 2009). Highly specialized and notably heterogenous, DCs function as messengers and regulators between innate and acquired immunity (e.g. Reid, 1997; Hart, 1997; Banchereau and Steinman, 1998; Austyn, 1998; Satthaporn and Eremin, 2001; Dzionek et al., 2000; Webb et al., 2005; McKenna et al., 2005; Lommatzsch et al., 2007, 2010; GeurtsvanKessel and Lambrecht, 2008; von Garnier and Nicod, 2009). Because DCs have the ability to induce a primary immune response in resting naïve T-lymphocytes and play a role in the maintenance of B-cell function and antigen memory (recall) responses (e.g. Webb et al., 2005; Bessa et al., 2009), they were called 'professional antigen presenting cells' by, e.g., Lipscomb and Masten (2002) and Liu (2005). To better assess incoming antigens for possible threat, mature DCs particularly occur in tissues that interface between the external- and the internal environments and are therefore greatly exposed to microbial pathogens, harmful particulates, and injurious gases. These include the skin, where the cells are called Langerhan's cells [named after Paul Langerhan (1847-1888), a German physician, who first described them in the late 19th Century], the inner lining of the nose, the lungs, the stomach, and the intestines (e.g. Satthaporn and Eremin, 2001; Sallusto and Lanzavecchia, 2002; von Garnier and Nicod, 2009). Notable exceptions are the complete absence of the DCs in the cornea and the central nervous system (e.g. Steinman, 1991). DCs are a major source of many cytokines, e.g., interferon-α (IFN-α) and the inflammatory protein MIP1g: both of these molecular factors are important in effecting primary immune response (e.g. Zhou and

Tedder, 1995; Devergne, 1996). In the different sites where they are located, DCs differentiate and become active in acquiring and processing antigens. The subsequent presentation on the host cell surface is associated with the major histocompatibility molecules (e.g. Meyer and Mack, 2003).

The DCs are found in immature form in blood (e.g. Dzionek et al., 2000) (Fig. 35) and once they are activated, they migrate to the lymph nodes where they interact with the T- and B-cells to initiate acquired immune response. In the lung, DCs exist in many subpopulations that are fine-tuned to different roles that maintain immune homeostasis. Infectious and inflammatory conditions can profoundly change functions, with steady-state DC subsets resulting in recruitment of inflammatory type DCs (e.g. Geurtsvankessel and Lambrecht, 2008) which exert specific functions that can be associated with distinct expression of endocytotic receptors and cell-surface molecules, and the topographical location in the lung. During DC trafficking into the lung, blood DCs are preferentially recruited over blood monocytes (Klinke, 2006): for short-lived antigens, lung epithelial DCs that are derived from blood DCs exhibit a 62.5% increase in antigen density compared to those derived from the blood monocytes. The cells (DCs) are located within the bronchial epithelium and the pulmonary interstitium where they impinge on the innate immune system. CD11c-positive DCs are widely distributed in the alveolar region of the lung, with most of them displaying an immature phenotype (Gonzalez-Juarrero and Orme, 2001): the cells are capable of phagocytosing live *Mycobacterium tuberculosis* bacteria, leading to secretion of interleukin-12 (IL-12) and stimulation of CD4-T cells to produce gamma interferon (IFN-γ). In steady-state (homeostatic) conditions, fine balance exists between the various functions of lung's DC populations, a feature necessary for the maintaintence of immune homeostasis in the lung (GeurtsvanKessel and Lambrecht, 2008). On identification and internalization of pathogens, DCs move to the draining lymph nodes of the lung to instigate specific cellular and humoral immune responses. Extensive network of bone marrow-derived DCs exist in the mucosa of the nose and the large conducting airways, the alveolar lumen, and the connective tissue surrounding the blood vessels and the pleura (Holt et al., 1988, 1994; Schon-Hegrad et al., 1991; van Haarst et al., 1994; Lambrecht et al., 1998; Gonzalez-Juarrero and Orme, 2001; von Garnier and Nicod, 2009). The migration of the airway DCs in response to an immunogenic stimulus is rapid (e.g. Havenith et al., 1993; Xia et al., 1995): within 12 hours, the lung derived DCs can be found in the T-cell area of draining mediastinal lymph nodes of the lung. Inflammatory diseases of the human lung are associated with the different phenotypes and the process of the recruitment of the airway DCs (Lommatzsch et al., 2007, 2010; Geurtsvankessel and Lambrecht, 2008; Vassallo et al., 2010). Regulation of galectin-3 in the lungs may represent one of the multiple potential mechanisms by which galectins contribute to modulation of the innate and acquired immune responses (Maldonado et al., 2011).

The classical morphology of the DCs, i.e., that of having numerous membranous processes (projections) that extend out of the main cell body (Fig. 35), makes them highly motile. Also, it endows them with very large surface-to-volume ratio that permits them to contact and therefore adeptly sample (sense) vast parts of the surrounding environment. DCs contain abundant antigen processing organelles that include endosomes, lysosomes, and special granules. From their distinctive projections, the designation 'dendritic cell' was coined by Steinman and Cohn (1973) since the cells (DCs) resemble the dendrites of the neurones, although DCs are not associated with the nervous system and by extension the neuronal dendrites.

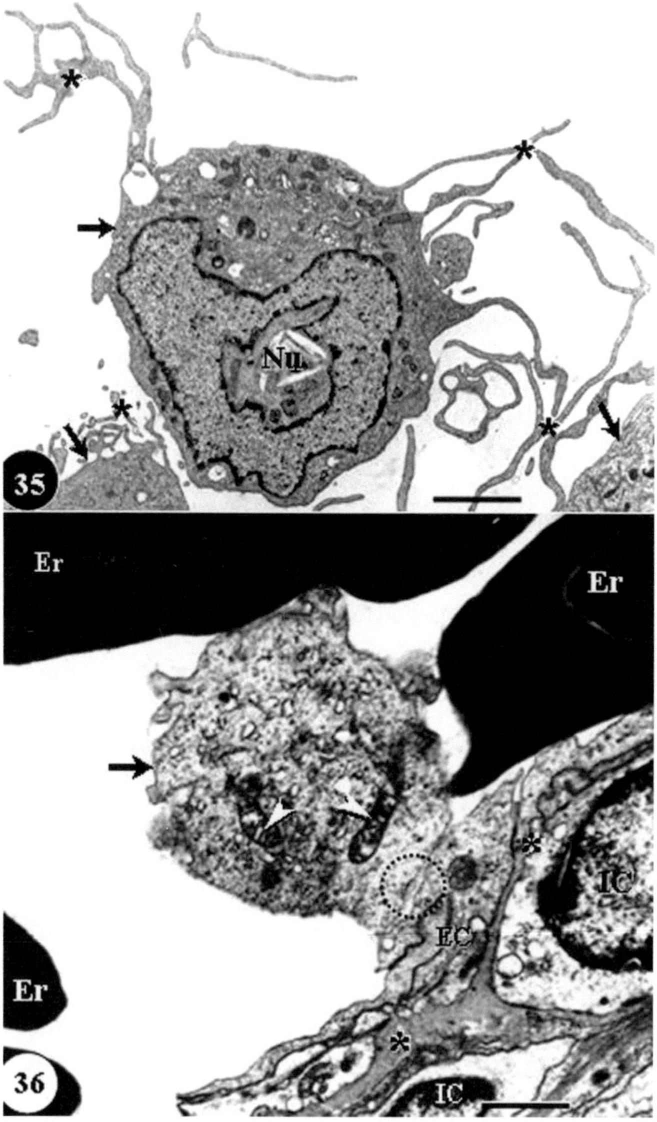

Fig. 35. Dendritic cells from the peripheral blood (arrows) showing cytoplasmic extensions (stars) that the cells use to move and sense the surrounding environment. Nu, nucleus. Courtesy of Dr. S.G. Kiama, University Nairobi, Kenya. Fig. 36: A pulmonary intravascular macrophage (arrow) in the lung of the rock dove, *Columba livia,* attached to the vascular endothelial cell (dashed circle). EC, endothelial cell; Er, erythrocyte; asterisk, basement membrane; arrow heads, mitochondria; IC, interstitial cells. Scale bars: Fig. 35, 15 µm; 36, 10 µm.

Depending on species, DCs are classified into myeloid DCs (mDCs) and plasmacytoid DCs (pDCs) (e.g. McKenna et al., 2005; Geurtsvankessel and Lambrecht, 2008; von Garnier and Nicod, 2009). The former are more common and are divided into an mDC-1 subpopulation which is the foremost stimulator of T-cells and the mDC-2 which are involved in wound healing. Both groups of cells secrete IL-12 (interleukin-12) and express TLR-2 and TLR-4 receptors (e.g. Sallusto and Lanzavecchia, 2002). The pDCs resemble plasma cells but have certain features similar to the mDCs (Vanbervliet et al., 2003; Liu, 2005): they can produce large amounts of interferon-α. The functional specialization and the degree of maturation of the DCs are determined by the tissue environment and the tissue cells that DCs directly interact with (Wu and Liu, 2007). In the airways, DCs sense incoming airborne antigens by extending their dendrites through the epithelial cells that line the airway lumen (e.g. Jahnsen et al., 2006; Holt et al., 2008). Under normal (healthy = steady-state) conditions, in the alveolar space, 80% of the cells are PSMs, with the remainder comprising of T-cells and DCs (von Garnier et al., 2005). In the respiratory tract, resident DCs are deemed to be immature (von Garnier and Nicod, 2009). This signifies that the cells have optimal capacity of detecting, capturing, and processing inhaled antigens but have a low capacity of stimulating T-cells. In contrast to the B and T-lymphocytes, DCs have retained many of the pattern recognition receptors and are thus uniquely capable of sensing stimuli such as tissue damage, necrosis, and bacterial and viral infection (Webb et al., 2005; Klinke, 2006). The capacity of the lung's DCs to influence specific CD-4 and CD-8 T-lymphocytes makes them suitable candidates for vaccine development strategies for treating and preventing conditions and diseases such as allograft rejection responses, allergy, and asthma, as well as autoimmune diseases and cancers (Fong and Engelman, 2000; Syme and Gluck, 2001; Sharma et al., 2003; Schott and Seissler, 2003; Decker et al., 2006; Sbiera et al., 2008).

6. Pleural macrophages (PlMs)

The PlMs are one of the pulmonary macrophage cell lineages that have been least studied (e.g. Brain 1992). Lehnert (1992) suggested that PlMs originate from peripheral blood monocytes that migrate across the mesothelial lining of the pleura. Meuret et al. (1980), Zlotnik et al. (1982) and Sestini et al. (1984) observed that PlMs were more morphologically similar to the peritoneal macrophages than to the PSMs. This may be attributed to the prevailing similarities and differences in the prevailing microenvironments (Brain, 1992) like the variation in the PO_2 (Brain 1988). Frankenberger et al. (2000) noted that PlMs are a unique kind of tissue macrophage. Under normal physiological conditions, the pleural cavity is in a state of negative (subatmospheric) pressure: low oxygen (O_2) tension (PO_2) prevails in it. Pleural O_2 exposure induces oxidative injury and aggravates latent systemic inflammatory response (Tsukioka et al., 2007). Resident PlMs sense perturbations in the local environment and initiate neutrophil infiltration (Cailheir et al., 2006). The drugs carrageenan and tetracycline prompt dramatic increase in PlMs (e.g. Sahn and Potts, 1978; Ackerman et al., 1980; Strange et al., 1989; Baumann et al., 1993) by recruiting monocytes from the peripheral circulation (Antony et al., 1985). *In vivo* experiments have demonstrated tumoricidal- (Basic et al., 1979; Nagashima et al., 1987), phagocytic- (Meuret et al., 1980; Zlotnik et al., 1982; Zlotnik and Crowle, 1982), and antimicrobial activities of the PlMs (Meuret et al., 1980; Hammerstrom, 1980; Zlotnik and Crowle, 1982). Compared to PSMs, the cells (PlMs) release prostaglandins E-1 and E-2 and respond differently to various cytokines (Sestini et al., 1984; Nagashima et al., 1987).

Agostini et al. (1972) suggested that PlMs may function as roller bearings that allow smooth movement between the parietal- and the visceral pleura. The PlMs seem to be functionally important in both health and disease (Zlotnik et al., 1982; Zlotnik and Crowle, 1982).

Morphologically, a normal resident PlM has prominent intermediate intracytoplasmic filaments and numerous microvilli that may be involved in the adherence to the pleural surfaces (Baumann et al., 1993). From assessment of the uptake of latex beads, the phagocytic capacity of the PlMs is lower than that of the bronchoalveolar mononuclear phagocytes (BAMP) (that comprise of the BMs and the PSMs) and when cultured together with autologous pulmonary interstitial DCs, PlMs exert a more potent ability to stimulate T-cell proliferation than the BAMPs (Gjomarkaj et al., 1999). Compared to the BAMPs, PlMs are less portent bactericidal and fungicidal cells (Gjomarkaj et al., 1999): functionally and phenotypically PlMs are different from the BAMPs and are similar to the peritoneal macrophages. PlMs play an important role in cell-mediated immune reactions in the pleural space (Gjomarkaj et al., 1999). Compared to the blood monocytes, PlMs seem to represent a cell-type intermediate between the regular CD-14(++) monocytes and the CD-14(+)CD-16(+) subset (Frankenberger et al., 2000). PlMs perform efficient Fc-receptor-mediated phagocytosis of antibody-coated sheep red blood cells and can inhibit apoptosis of malignant cells (Kaczmarek et al., 2008).

7. Pulmonary intravascular macrophages (PIVMs)

For the reasons that the PIMs are lacking in the lungs of most laboratory animals (e.g. Warner and Brain 1990; Warner, 1996; Brain et al., 1999) and since they are relatively less accessible for experimentation, the cells have not been as well-studied as the PSMs. Regarding their secretory, endolytic, and functional properties, PIVMs are a relatively newly identified constituent of the mononuclear phagocyte system. To date, for still unclear reasons, PIVMs have been reported mainly in the domestic mammals, especially in ruminant species like cattle, horse, goat, sheep, and pigs (e.g. Rybicka et al., 1974; Warner and Brain, 1984; Atwal and Saldanha, 1985; Wheeldon and Hansen-Flaschen, 1986; Warner et al., 1986; Winkler, 1988, 1989; Atwal et al., 1989, 1992; Warner and Brain, 1990; Longworth et al., 1994; Warner, 1996; Parbhakar et al., 2005; Molina and Brain, 2007) and in birds (Maina and Cowley, 1998) (Fig. 36). It is uncertain whether PIVMs occur in the human lung: while the cells were reported by Dehring and Wismar (1989), a comprehensive morphometric study of the human lung by Zeltner et al. (1987) didn't report macrophage or macrophage-like cells in the pulmonary capillaries. Particle uptake studies suggested that PIVMs may not exist in the human lung (e.g. Brain et al., 1999).

The PIVMs have distinctive morphological features of differentiated macrophages like irregular shape, a bean-shaped nucleus, abundant lysosomal bodies, numerous mitochondria, profuse rough endoplasmic reticulum, fuzzy glycocalyx, phagosomes, and pseudopods (e.g. Wheeldon and Hansen-Flaschen, 1986; Warner et al., 1986; Winkler and Cheville, 1985, 1987). They have an electron dense coat that appears to be predominantly lipoproteinaceous in nature (Atwal et al., 1989). PIVMs form membrane adhesion complexes with the endothelial cells (Warner et al., 1986; Winkler and Cheville, 1987) and tend to attach onto the thicker parts of the BGB (Winkler, 1988; Winkler and Cheville, 1987), probably minimizing interference with gas exchange (by thickening the BGB) which occurs mostly across the thin parts. Moreover, it is possible that the thicker parts of the BGB provide better support than the thinner ones, preventing the cells from being easily dislodged by flowing blood. PIVMs are large in size (20 to 80 μm in diameter), are closely apposed to the endothelium of the pulmonary blood capillaries (Wheeldon and Hansen-Flaschen, 1986;

Brain et al., 1999), and are abundantly endowed with organelles like vesicles, endosomes, and Golgi apparatus (e.g. Atwal et al., 1992) (Fig. 36). The PIVMs form an important part of the defence of the vertebrate lung. In the pig, perinatally, in a process that is completed by the 7th day of birth, blood monocytes colonize the lung, replicate within the blood capillaries, and attach to the endothelium by intercellular junctions as they differentiate (Winkler and Cheville, 1985). By actively synthesizing, storing, and secreting vasoactive substances, PIVMs stimulate biosynthetic pathways that lead to secretion of inflammatory mediators which compound certain disease processes (e.g. Brain, 1986; Kelly, 1990). They actively remove particles, bacteria, and endotoxins from circulating blood (Wheeldon and Hansen-Flaschen, 1986; Warner and Brain, 1986; Warner et al., 1986; Winkler, 1989; Brain et al., 1999). While in dogs, laboratory animals, and human beings, clearance of bacteria and particulates from blood occurs mainly in the Kupffer cells of the liver and the splenic macrophages, in calves, sheep, goats, cats, and pigs, the process is performed by the PIVMs (e.g. Warner et al., 1987; Winkler, 1988; Brain et al., 1999). In the sheep lung, PIVMs form 15.3% of the intravascular volume, attach onto 7.1% of the endothelial surface, and have 15.9 m^2 of their free surface available for contact with blood (Warner et al., 1986). Even in normal (steady-state) sheep lungs, there are more macrophages in their vast pulmonary blood vessels than on their alveolar surface and compared to the PSMs the PIVMs are relatively more actively phagocytic (Warner et al., 1986). In the deer, PIVMs are more than twice the number of PSMs but PIVMs are much smaller (47.625m^2) than the PSMs (101.260m^2) (Carrasco et al., 1996).

The PIVMs have been implicated in the vascular inflammation that results in lipopolysaccharide (LPS)-induced lung inflammation and endotoxemia in the horse (Aharonson-Raz and Singh, 2010), rat (Gill et al., 2008), and sheep (Warner et al., 1986, 1987) and with the oedema that occurs in the horse after infection with the African horse sickness virus (Carrasco et al., 1999). While in the newborn pig clearance of blood-borne bacteria (as well as carbon) is only ~10% of the injected dose (Mouton et al., 1963), in pigs of 15 to 20 kg body mass (~20-month old), 75% of intravenously infused bacteria (depending on species of bacteria) are cleared in the lungs (Wismar et al., 1984; Dehring et al., 1983). PIVMs play a significant role in regulating pulmonary blood flow, i.e., hemodynamics (e.g. Winkler 1989): stimulation of phagocytosis causes the PIVMs to increase in size thus narrowing or blocking the lumina of blood vessels (Winkler and Cheville, 1985). In pigs as well as calves and sheep, this increases resistance to blood flow, leading to pulmonary hypertension (Tucker et al., 1975; Atwal et al., 1989) and pulmonary oedema (Niehaus et al., 1980). Bovine PIVMs contain TNF-α (tumour necrotic factor) and their depletion significantly inhibits accumulation of inflammatory cells and pathology in acute lung disease in calves (Singh et al., 2004). In ruminants, PIVMs are involved in lipid metabolism and are the major source of vasoactive substances which significantly influence the dynamics of pulmonary circulation and surfactant turn over in the type-2 cells (Atwal et al., 1989).

8. Conclusion and future directions

Although substantial progress has been made in understanding the physical and functional phenotypes of macrophages in the lung, the knowledge remains scanty. This is evinced by lack of significant breakthroughs in the management and treatment of diseases like acute respiratory distress syndrome (ARDS). Furthermore, the specific functions performed by the different pulmonary macrophage lineages and the manner in which these cells communicate remain unclear.

Animals have evolved in close association with microorganisms some of which are harmful: intense selective pressure by the pathogens on the animal hosts and vice-versa has and continues to happen. In a critical encounter, when a pathogen contacts a host, a struggle between it and the host ensues. The outcome is infection and blatant disease or the pathogen is neutralized and eliminated. Successful microbial pathogens have been adept in developing means and strategies of evading the host defences while successful hosts have developed novel defence systems. Understanding the underpinnings behind the evolution of microbial pathogenicity and the intricate ways that animals counteract pathogens is vital in designing strategies of controlling microbial infection and stopping disease progression. Few other organs in the body are as well- and strategically protected as the lung: a cellular defence arsenal exists. From outside to inside are the pleural-, the intravascular, the interstitial-, and the surface (free) macrophages and along the airways (bronchi) are the bronchial macrophages, the dendritic cells, and the epithelial cells. This intricate level of protection has mainly developed because of the vast respiratory surface area that is constantly ventilated with air (which depending on locality contains harmful particulates and pathogenic microorganisms) and the fact that the lung is the only organ in the body which is perfused by the entire cardiac output, a feature that places it at greater risk from blood borne injurious agents. The biology of phagocytes and antigen presenting cells should provide insights on the pathogenesis of pulmonary diseases and may explain why some diseases, including the zoonotic ones, affect certain animal species and groups and not others. Important as it is, the area of comparative immunology offers much to be investigated.

9. Acknowledgment

I wish to thank the following colleagues who collaborated with me in the work that forms part of this contribution. These are: H. Cowley, L. Nganpiep, J. S. Adekunle, and S.G. Kiama. The National Research Foundation (NRF) funded this work.

10. References

Ackerman N, Tomolonis A, Miran L, Kheifets J, Martinez S, Carter A (1980) Three day pleural inflammation: a new model to detect drug effects on macrophage accumulation. *J. Pharmacol. Exp. Ther.* 215:588-595.

Adamson I, Bowden D (1981) Dose response of the pulmonary macrophagic system to various particulates and its relationship to transepithelial passage of free particles. *Exp. Lung Res.* 2:165-175.

Agostini E (1972) Mechanics of the pleural space. *Physiol. Rev.* 52:57-128.

Aharonson-Raz K, Singh B (2010) Pulmonary intravascular macrophages and endotoxin-induced pulmonary pathophysiology in horses. *Can. J. Vet. Res.* 74:45-49.

Alexis NE, Soukup J, Nierkens S, Becker S (2001) Association between airway hyperactivity and bronchial macrophage dysfunction in individuals with mild asthma. *Am. J. Physiol. Lung Cell Mol Physiol.* 280:L369-L375.

Alexis NE, Lay JC, Zeman KL, Geiser M, Kapp N, Bennett WD (2006) *In vivo* particle uptake by airway macrophages in healthy volunteers. *Am. J. Respir. Cell Mol. Biol.* 34:305-313.

Altraja S, Jaama J, Valk E, Altraja A (2009) Changes in the proteome of human bronchial epithelial cells following stimulation with leukotriene E4 and transforming growth factor-beta1. *Respirology* 14:39-45.

Antony VB, Sahn SA, Antony AC, Repine JE (1985) Bacillus-calmette-guerin-stimulated neutrophils release chemotaxins for monocytes in rabbit pleural spaces and *in vitro*. *Clin. Invest.* 76:1514-1521.

Apanius V, Penn D, Slev PR, Ruff LR, Potts WK (1997) The nature of selection on the major histocompatibility complex. *Crit. Rev. Immun.* 17:179-224.

Atwal O, Minhas K, Ferenczy B, Jassal D, Milton D, Mahadevappa V (1989) Morphology of pulmonary intravascular macrophages (PIMs) in ruminants: ultrastructural and cytochemical behaviour of dense surface coat. *Am. J. Anat.* 186:285-299.

Atwal OS, Saldanha KA (1985) Erythrophagocytosis in alveolar capillaries of goat lung: ultrastructural properties of blood monocytes. *Acta Anat.* 124:245-254.

Atwal OS, Singh B, Staempfli H, Minhas KJ (1992) Presence of pulmonary intravascular macrophages in the equine lung: some structural-functional properties. *Anat. Rec.* 234:530-540.

Austyn JM (1998) Dendritic cells. *Curr. Opin. Hematol.* 5:3-15.

Banchereau J, Steinman RM (1998) Dendritic cells and the control of immunity. *Nature* 392:245-252.

Bargmann W (1936) Die Lungenalveole. In: *Handbuch der mikroskopischen Anatomie des Menschen* (Möllendorf W ed). Springer, Berlin, pp. 799-859.

Baron S, Tyring ST, Fleischmann RW, Coppernhaver DH, Niesel DW et al. (1991) The interferons: mechanisms of action and clinical applications. *JAMA* 266:1375-1383.

Bartl S, Baltimore D, Weissman IL (1994) Molecular evolution of the vertebrate immune system. *Proc. Natl. Acad. Sci, USA* 91:10769-10770.

Basic I, Rode B, Kastelan A, Milas L (1979) Activation of pleural macrophages by intrapleural application of *Corynebacterium parvam*. In: *Advances in experimental medical biology, vol. 121(A)* (Escobar MR, Friedman H, eds). Plenum, New York, pp. 333-341.

Baumann MH, Heinrich K, Sahn SA, Green C, Harley R, Strange C (1993) Electron microscopic analysis of the normal and the activated pleural macrophage. *Exp. Lung Res.* 19:31-742.

Beck G, Habicht GS (1991) Primitive cytokines: harbingers of vertebrate defense. *Immun. Today* 3:180- 183.

Beck G, Habicht GS (1996) Immunity and the invertebrates. *Sci. Amer.* 1996:60-66.

Beck G, Cooper EL, Habicht GS, Marchalonis JJ (eds) (1994) Primordial immunity: foundations for the vertebrate immune system. *Ann. NY Acad. Sci.* 712:57-84.

Bedoret D, Wallemacq H, Marichal T, Desmet C, Calvo FQ, Henry E et al. (2009) Lung interstitial macrophages alter dendritic cell functions to prevent airway allergy in mice. *J. Clin. Invest.* 119:3723-3738.

Bellavite P, Dri P, Bisiachi B, Patricia P (1977) Catalase deficiency in myeloperoxidase deficient polymorphonuclear leukocytes from chicken. *Fed. Exp. Biol. Soc. Lets.* 81:73-76

Belz GT, Smith CM, Kleinert L, Reading P, Brooks A et al. (2004) Distinct migrating and nonmigrating dendritic cell populations are involved in MHC class 1-restricted antigen presentation after lung infection with virus. *PNAS* 101:8670-8675.

Bessa J, Jegerlehner A, Hinton HJ, Pumpens P, Saudan P et al. (2009) Alveolar macrophages and lungdendritic cells sense RNA and drive mucosal IgA responses. *J. Immun.* 183:3788-3799.

Bezuidenhout AJ, Groenewald HB, Soley JT (2000) An anatomical study of the respiratory air sacs in ostriches. *Onderstpoot J. Vet. Res.* 66:317-325.

Bilyk N, Mackenzie JS, Papadimitriou JM, Holt PG (1988) Functional studies on macrophage populations in the airways and the lung wall of SPF mice in the steady-state and during respiratory virus infection. *Immunology* 65:417-425.

Biswas SK, Sica A, Lewis CE (2008) Plasticity of macrophage function during tumour progression: regulation by distinct molecular mechanisms. *J. Immun.* 180:2011-2017.

Blum G, Falbo V, Caprioli A, Hacker J (1995) Gene clusters encoding the cytotoxic necrotizing factor type 1, Prs-fimbriae and alpha-hemolysin form the pathogenicity island II of the uropathogenic *Escherichia coli* strain 96. *FEMS Microbiol. Lett.* 126:189-195.

Blum G, Ott M, Lischewski A, Ritter A, Imrich H et al. (1994) Excision of large DNA regions termed pathogenicity islands from tRNA-specific loci in the chromosome of an *Escherichia coli* wild- type pathogen. *Infect. Immun.* 62:606-614.

Blussé van Oud Alblas A, Mattie H, van Furth R (1983) A quantitative evaluation of pulmonary macrophage kinetics. *Cell Tissue Res.* 16:211-219.

Blussé van Oud Alblas A, van Furth R (1979) Origin, kinetics, and characteristics of pulmonary macrophages in the normal steady state. *J. Exp. Med.* 149:1504-1527.

Boman HG, Hultmark D (1987) Cell-free immunity in insects. *Annu. Rev. Microbiol.* 41:103-126.

Bowden DH (1976) The pulmonary macrophage. *Environ. Health Perspect.* 16:55-60.

Bowden DH (1987) Macrophages, dust, and pulmonary disease. *Exp. Lung Res.* 12:89-107.

Bowden DH, Adamson IYR (1980) Role of monocytes and interstitial cells in the generation of alveolar macrophages, I: kinetic studies in normal mice. *Lab. Invest.* 42:511-517.

Brahmbhatt M (2005) Avian and human pandemic influenza: economic and social impacts. WHO Headquarters, Geneva, November Issue, pp. 7-9.

Brain JD (1971) The effects of increased particles on the number of alveolar macrophages. In: *Inhaled particles III, vol. 1* (Walton WH ed). Unwin Bros., Surrey, pp. 209-225.

Brain JD (1976) The pulmonary macrophage. *Environ. Health Perspect.* 16:55-60.

Brain JD (1980) Pulmonary macrophages and the pathogenesis of lung diseases. *Environ. Health Perspect.* 35:2-28.

Brain JD (1984) The alveolar macrophage. *Environ. Health Perspect.* 55:327-341.

Brain JD (1986) Toxicological aspects of alterations of pulmonary macrophage function. *Annu. Rev. Pharmacol. Toxicol.* 26:547-565.

Brain JD (1987) Macrophages, dust, and pulmonary diseases. *Exp. Lung Res.* 12:89-107.

Brain JD (1988) Lung macrophages: how many kinds are there? What do they do? *Am. Rev. Respir. Dis.* 137:507-509.

Brain JD (1992) Mechanisms, measurement, and significance of lung macrophage function. *Environ. Health Perspect.* 97:5-10.

Brain JD (1996) Environmental lung disease: exposure and mechanisms. *Chest* 109:74-78.

Brain JD, Gehr P, Kavet RI (1984) Airway macrophages: the importance of the fixation method. *Am. Rev. Respir. Dis.* 129:823-826.

Brain JD, Molina RM, DeCamp MM, Warner AE (1999) Pulmonary intravascular macrophages: their contribution to the mononuclear phagocyte system in 13 species. *Am. J. Physiol. (Lung Cell Mol. Physiol.)* 20:L146-L154.

Breeze RG, Wheeldon EB (1977) The cells of the pulmonary airways. *Am. Rev. Respir. Dis.* 116:705- 717.

Brook RD, Rajagopalan S, Pope CA, Brook JR, Bhatnagar A et al. (2010) Particulate matter air pollution and cardiovascular disease. *Circulation* 121:2331-2378.

Brown C (2004) Emerging zoonoses and pathogens of public health significance: an overview. *Rev. Sci. Tech. Off. Int. Epiz.* 23:435-442.

Brown RE, Brain JD, Wang N (1997) The avian respiratory system: a unique model for studies of respiratory toxicosis and for monitoring air quality. *Environ. Health Perspect.* 105:188-200.

Brownlie R, Allan B (2011) Avian toll-like receptors. *Cell Tissue Res.* 343:121-130.

Brunekreef B, Dockery DW, Krzyzanowski M (1995) Epidemiologic studies on short-term effects of low levels of major ambient air pollution components. *Environ. Health* Perspect. 103:3-13.

BTS (2006) (British Thoracic Society) *Burden of lung disease: a statistical report. http://ww.bts.com/libraries.*

Buckner MMC, Finlay B (2011) Innate immunity cues virulence. *Nature* 472:179-180.

Burri PH (1985) Morphology and respiratory function of the alveolar unit. *Int. Archs. Allergy Appl. Immun.* 76:2-12.

Burroughs T., Knobler, S., Lederberg, J. (eds) (2002) *The emergence of zoonotic diseases.* National Academy Press, Washington DC.

Caiheir JF, Sawatzky DA, Kipari T, Houlberg K, Walbaum D et al. (2006) Resident pleural macrophages are key orchestrators of neutrophil recruitment in pleural inflammation. *Am. J. Respir. Crit. Care Med.* 173:540-547.

Callaghan M, Voynov JA (2006) Respiratory tract mucin genes and mucin glycoproteins in health and disease. *Physiol. Rev.* 86:245-278.

Camner P, Lundborg M, Låstbom L, Gerde P, Gross N, Jarstrand C (2002) Experimantal and calculated parameters on particle phagocytosis by alveolar macrophages. *J. Appl. Physiol.* 92:2608- 2616.

Canning BJ (2008) The cough reflex in animals: relevance to human cough research. *Lung* 186:S23- S28.

Carrasco L, Gómez-Villamandos JC, Bautista MJ, Hervás J, Pulido B, Sierra MA (1996) Pulmonary intravascular macrophages in deer. *Vet. Res.* 27:71-77.

Carrasco L, Sanchez C, Gomez-Villamandos JC (1999) The role of pulmonary intravascular macrophages in the pathogenesis of African horse sickness. *J. Comp. Pathol.* 121:25-38.

Carter JD, Ghio AJ, Samet JM, Devlin RB (1997) Cytokine production by human airway epithelial cells after exposure to an air pollution particle is metal-dependent. *Toxicol. Appl. Pharmacol.* 46:180- 188.

Chandler DB, Bayles G, Fuller WC (1988) Prostaglandin synthesis and release by subpopulations of rat macrophages. *Am. Rev. Respir. Dis.* 138:901-907.

Chandler DB, Brannen AL (1990) Interstitial macrophage subpopulations: responsiveness to chemotactic stimuli. *Tissue Cell* 22:427-434.

Cheetham BF, Katz ME (1995) A role for bacteriophages in the evolution and transfer of bacterial virulence determinants. *Mol. Microbiol.* 18:201-208.

Chen H, Deng G, Li Z, Tian G, Li Y et al. (2004) The evolution of H5N1 influenza viruses in ducks in southern China. *Proc. Natl. Acad. Sci., USA* 101:10452-10457.

Chmiel JF, Davis PB (2003) State of art: why do the lungs of patients with cystic fibrosis become infected and why cant they clear the infection? *Respir. Res.* 4:8 *(http://respiratory- research.com/content/4/1/8).*

Chomel BB, Belotto A, Meslin FX (2007) Wildlife, exotic pets, and emerging zoonoses. *Emerg. Infect. Dis.* 13:6-11.

Cleaveland S, Laurenson MK, Taylor LH (2001) Diseases of humans and their domestic mammals: pathogen characteristics, host range and the risk of emergency. *Phil. Trans. R. Soc. B, Lond.* 356:991-999.

Conklin D (2011) Beware the air!: why particulate matter matters. *Circ. Res.* 108:644-647.

Conlon JM (2011) The contribution of skin antimicrobial peptides to the system of innate immunity in anurans. *Cell Tissue Res.* 343:201-212.

Crapo JD, Harmsen AG, Sherman MP, Musson RA (2000) Pulmonary immunobiology and inflammation in pulmonary diseases. *Am. J. Respir. Crit. Care Med.* 162:1983-1986.

Crowell RE, Heaphy E, Valdez YE, Mold C, Lehnert BE (1992) Alveolar and interstitial macrophage populations in the murine lung. *Exp. Lung Res.* 18:435-446.

Cuffs JHAJ, Meis JFGM, Hoogkamp-Korstanje JAA (1997) A primer on cytokines: sources, receptors, effects, and inducers. *Clin. Microbiol. Rev.* 10:742-780.

Currie RJW (1999) Ascites in poultry: recent investigations. *Avian Path.* 28:313-326.

Daszak P, Cunningham AA, Hyatt AD (2001) Anthropogenic environmental change and the emergence of infectious diseases in wildlife. *Acta Trop.* 78:103-116.

Decker WK, Xing D, Shepall EJ (2006) Dendritic cell immunotherapy for the treatment of neoplastic disease. *Biol. Blood Marrow Transplantation* 12:113-125.

Dehring DJ, Crocker SH, Wismar BL, Steinberg SM, Lowery BD, Cloutier CT (1983) Comparison of live bacteria infusions in a porcine model of acute respiratory failure. *J. Surg. Res.* 34:151-168.

Dehring DM, Wismar BL (1989) Intravascular macrophages in pulmonary capillaries of humans. *Am. Rev. Respir. Dis.* 139:1027-1029.

Dekich MA (1997) Broiler industry strategies for control of respiratory and enteric diseases. *Poult. Sci.* 77:1176-1180.

De Palma M, Lewis CE (2011) Macrophages limit chemotherapy. *Nature* 472:303-304.

Dethloff LA, Lehnert BE (1988) Pulmonary interstitial macrophages: isolation and flow cytometric comparisons with alveolar macrophages and blood monocytes. *J. Leukocyte Biol.* 43:80-90.

Devergne O (1996) A novel interleukin 12 p40-related protein induced by latent Epstein-Barr virus infection in B-lymphocytes. *J. Virol.* 157:1499-1507.

Dockery DW, Pope CA, Xu X, Spengler JD, Ware JH et al. (1993) An association between air pollution and mortality in six US cities. *N. Engl. J. Med.* 329:753-759.

Dougherty GJ, McBride WH (1984) Macrophage heterogeneity. *J. Clin. Lab. Immun.* 14:1-11.

Dreher D, Cochand L, Kok M, Kiama SG, Gehr P et al. (2001) Genetic background of attenuated *Salmonella typhimurium* has profound influence on infection and cytokine patterns in human dendritic cells. *J. Leukocyte Biol.* 69:583-589.

DuPasquier L (ed) (1993) *Evolution of the immune system, 3rd edtn.* Raven Press, New York.

Dzionek A, Fuchs A, Schmidt P, Cremer S, Sysk M et al. (2000) BDCA-2, BDCA-3, and BDCA-4: three markers for distinct subsets of dendritic cells in human peripheral blood. *J. Immun.* 165:6037- 6046.

Eckert DJ, Catcheside PG, Stadler DL, McDonald R, Hlavac MC, McEvoy RD (2006) Acute sustained hypoxia suppresses the cough reflex in healthy subjects. *Am. J. Respir.Crit. Care Med.* 173:506-511.

EPS (1996) *Environmental Protection Agency: Air quality criteria for particulate matter.* Res. Triangle Park, NC, US EPA (US EPA/600/P-95/00 1bF).

Fagerland JA, Arp LH (1990) A morphologic study of bronchus-associated lymphoid tissue in turkeys. *Am. J. Anat.* 189:4-34.

Fagerland JA, Arp LH (1993) Distribution and quantitation of plasma cells, T lymphocyte subsets, and B lymphocytes in bronchus-associated lymphoid tissue of chickens: age-related differences. *Reg. Immun.* 5:28-36.

Fan EO (2003) Economic impact and implications. Oxford University Press, Hong Kong.

Fathi M, Johansson A, Lundborg M, Orre L, Sköld MC, Canmer P (2001) Functional and morphological differences between human alveolar and interstitial macrophages. *Exp. Mol. Pathol.* 70:77-82.

Fawcett DW (1986) *A text book of histology, 11th edtn.* WB Saunders, Philadelphia.

Fedde MR (1980) The structure and gas flow pattern in the avian lung. *Poult. Sci.* 59:2642-2653.

Fedde MR (1997) Relationship of structure and function of the avian respiratory system to disease susceptibility. *Poult. Sci.* 77:1130-1138.

Fedosenko G, Chernogoryk G, Roslyyyakova E, Kirillova N (2010) The improvement of the macrophages morphological characteristics in bronchial region in stable COPD patients under influence of tiotropium bromide. *Eur. Respir. J.* P4007 *(www.erscongress2012.com/pages/default.aspx?id=1045...80607).*

Fels AOS, Cohn ZA (1986) The alveolar macrophage. *J. Appl. Physiol* 60:353-371.

Ficken MD, Edwards JF, Lay JC (1986) Induction, collection, and partial characterization of induced respiratory macrophages of the turkey. *Avian Dis.* 30:766-771.

Field H, Young P, Yob JM, Mills J, Hall L, Mackenzie J (2001) The natural history of Hendra and Nipah viruses. *Microbes and Infection* 3:307–314.

Finley BB, Falkow S (1997) Common themes in microbial pathogenicity revisited. *Microbiol. Mol. Biol.* 61:136-169.

Finley BB, Buckner MMC (2011) Innate immunity cues virulence. *Nature* 472:179-180.

Fireman E, Onn A, Levo Y, Bugolovov E, Kivity S (1999) Suppressive activity of bronchial macrophages recovered by induced sputum. *Allergy* 54:111-118.

Fong L, Engelman EG (2000) Dendritic cells in cancer immunotherapy. *Annu. Rev. Immun.* 18:245-273.

Frankenberger M, Passlick B, Hofer T, Siebeck M, Maier KL, Ziegler-Heitbrock LHW (2000) Immunologic characterization of normal human pleural macrophages. *Am. J. Respir. Cell Mol. Biol.* 23:419-426.

Franke-Ullmann G, Pförtner C, Walter P, Steinmüller C, Lohmann-Mathes ML, Kobzik L (1996) Characterization of murine lung interstitial macrophages in comparison with alveolar macrophages *in vitro*. *J. Immun.* 157:3097-3104.

Fries PN, Griebel PJ (2011) Mucosal dendritic cell diversity in the gastrointestinal tract. *Cell Tissue Res.* 343:33-41.

Fujii T, Hayashi S, Hogg JC, Mukae H, Suwa Y et al. (2002) Interaction of alveolar macrophages and airway epithelial cells following exposure to particulate matter produces mediators that stimulate the bone marrow. *Am. J. Respir. Cell Mol. Biol.* 27:34-41.

Fujii T, Hayashi S, Hogg JC, Vincent R, van Eeden SF (2001) Particulate matter induces cytokine expression in human bronchial epithelial cells. *Am. J. Respir. Cell Mol. Biol.* 25:265-271.

Gant VA, Hamblin AS (1985) Human bronchoalveolar macrophage heterogeneity demonstrated by histochemistry, surface markers, and phagocytosis. *Clin. Exp. Immun.* 60:539-545.

Garn H, Siese A, Stumpf S, Wensing A, Renz H, Gemsa D (2006) Phenotypical and functional characterization of alveolar macrophage subpopulations in the lungs of NO-exposed rats. *Respir. Res.* 7:4 *(doi:10.1186/1465-9921-7-4).*

Gehr P, Bachofen M, Weibel ER (1978) The normal human lung: ultrastructure and morphometric estimation of diffusion capacity. *Respir. Physiol.* 32:121-140.

Gehr P, Fabian B, Rothen-Rutishauser BM (2006) Fate of inhaled particles after interaction with the lung surface. *Paediatr. Respir. Rev.* 7S:S73-S75.

Gehr P, Schürch S, Berthiaume Y, Im H, Geiser M (1990b) Particle retention in airways by surfactant. *J. Aerosol Sci.* 3:27-43.

Gehr P, Schürch S, Geiser M, Hof VI (1990a) Retention and clearance mechanisms of inhaled particles. *J. Aerosol. Sci.* 21:S491-S496.

Geiser M (2002) Morphological aspects of particle uptake by lung phagocytes. *Microsc. Res. Tech.* 57:512-522.

Geiser P (2010) Update on macrophage clearance of inhaled micro- and nanoparticles. *J. Aerosol Med. Pulm. Drug Deliv.* 23:207-217.

Geiser M, Cruz-Orive LM, Hof VI, Gehr P (1990) Assessment of particle retention and clearance in the intrapulmonary conducting airways of hamster lungs with fractionator. *J. Microsc.* 160:75-88.

Geiser M, Im H, Gehr P, Cruz-Orive LM (1988) Histological and stereological analysis of particle deposition in the conducting airways of hamster lungs. *J. Aerosol. Med.* 1:19-211.

Geiser M, Matter M, Maye I, Im Hof V, Gehr P, Schulz S (2003) Influence of air space geometry and surfactant on the retention of man-made vitreous fibers (MMVF 10a). *Environ. Health Perspect.* 111:895-901.

Geissmann F, Gordon S, Hume DA, Mowat AM, Randolph GJ (2010a) Unraveling mononuclear phagocyte heterogeneity. *Nat. Rev. Immunol.* 10:453-460.

Geissmann F, Manz MG, Jung S, Sieweke MH, Merad M, Ley K (2010b) Development of monocytes, macrophages, and dendritic cells. Science 327:656-661.

Gerlach B, Cordier SM, Schmukle AC, Emmerich CH, Rieser E, Hass TL (2011) Linear ubiquitination prevents inflammation and regulates immune signalling. *Nature* 471:591-596.

Geurtsvankessel CH, Lambrecht BN (2008) Division of labour between dendritic cell subsets of the lung. *Mucosal Immun.* 1:442-450.

Gil J, Weibel ER (1971) Extracellular lining of bronchioles after perfusion-fixation of rat lungs for electron microscopy. *Anat. Rec.* 169:131-145.

Gill SS, Suri SS, Janardhan KS, Caldwell S, Duke T, Singh B (2008) Role of pulmonary intravascular macrophages in endotoxin-induced lung inflammation and mortality in a rat model. *Respir. Res.* 9:69 (doi: 10.1186/1465-9921-9-69).

Gjomarkaj M, Pace E, Melis M, Spatafora M, Profita M et al. (1999) Phenotypic and functional characterization of normal rat pleural macrophages in comparison with autologous peritoneal and alveolar macrophages. *Am. J. Respir. Cell Mol. Biol.* 20:135-142.

Godfrey RW (1997) Human airway epithelial tight junctions. *Microsc. Res. Tech.* 38:488-499.

Goldstein E, Bartlema HC (1977) Role of the alveolar macrophage in pulmonary bacterial defense. *Bull. Eur. Physiol. Pathol. Respir.* 13:57-67.

Gonzalez-Juarrero M, Orme IM (2001). Characterization of murine lung dendritic cells infected with *Mycobacterium tuberculosis. Infection Immunity* 69:1127-1133.

Gordon S (2002) Pattern recognition receptors: doubling up for the innate immune response. *Cell* 111:927-930.

Gordon S,Taylor PR (2005) Monocyte and macrophage heterogeneity. *Nat. Rev. Immunol.* 5:953-864.

Grant MM, Brain JD, Vinegar A (1981) Pulmonary defense mechanisms in boa constrictor. *J. Appl. Physiol.* 50:979-983.

Green GM (1973) Alveolar-bronchiolar transport mechanisms. *Arch. Intern. Med.* 131:109-114.

Green GM (1984) Similarities of host defense mechanisms against pulmonary infectious diseases in animals and man. *J. Toxicol. Environ. Health* 13:471-478.

Green GM, Jakab GJ, Low RB, Davis GS (1977) Defense mechanisms of the respiratory membrane. *Am. Rev. Respir. Dis.* 115:479-514.

Green GM, Kass EH (1964) The role of the alveolar macrophage in the clearance of bacteria from the lung. *J. Exp. Med.* 119:167-182.

Greger M (2007) The human/animal interface: emergence and resurgence of zoonotic infectious diseases. *Crit. Rev. Microbiol.* 33:243-299.

Hammerstrom J (1980) Structure and function of human effusion macrophages from patients with malignant and benign disease. *Acta Pathol. Microbiol., Scand.* 88:191-200.

Harada H, Imamura M, Okunishi K, Nakagome K, Matsumoto T et al. (2009) Upregulation of lung dendritic cell functions in elastase-induced emphysema. *Int. Arch. Allergy Immun.* 149:25-30.

Harkema JR, Mariassy A, George J, Hyde DM, Plopper C (1991) Epithelial cells of the conducting airways: a species comparison. In: *Lung biology in health and disease: the airway epithelium* (Farmer SG, Hay DWP, eds). Marcel Dekker Inc., New York, pp. 3-39.

Hart DN (1997) Dendritic cells: unique leukocyte populations which control the primary immune response. *Blood* 90:3245-3287.

Hartwig, Davies WA, Stossel TP (1977) Evidence for contractile protein translocation in macrophage spreading, phagocytosis and phagolysosome formation. J. *Cell Biol.* 75:956-967.

Havenith CEG, van Miert PPMC, Breedjik AJ, Beelen RHJ, Hoefsmit ECM (1993) Migration of dendritic cells into the draining lymph nodes of the lung after intratracheal instillation. *Am. J. Respir. Cell Mol. Biol.* 9:484-488.

Hawley RJ, Beaman BK, Williams MC, Yeager H (1979) The ultrastructure of bronchial macrophages and lymphocytes in sarcoidosis. *Human Pathol.* 10:155-163.

Hazlett L, Wu M (2011) Defensins in innate immunity. *Cell Tissue Res.* 343:175-188.

Hess CM, Edwards SV (2002) The evolution of the major histocompartibility complex in birds. *Bioscience* 52:423-431.

Hirano S (1996) Interaction of rat alveolar macrophages with pulmonary epithelial cells following exposure to lipopolysaccharide. *Arch. Toxicol.* 70:3-4.

Hof IM, Klauser M, Gehr P (1990) Phagocytic properties and organelle motility of pulmonary macrophages from smokers and nonsmokers estimated *in vitro* by magnetometric means. *Eur. Respir. J.* 3:157-162.

Hoffman JA, Hetru C (1992) Insect defensins: inducible antibacterial peptides. *Immun. Today* 13:411- 415.

Holt PG (1979) Alveolar macrophage. I. A simple technique for the preparation of high numbers of viable alveolar macrophages from small laboratory animals. *J. Immun. Methods* 27:189-198.

Holt PG (2005) Pulmonary dendritic cells in local immunity to inert and pathogenic antigens in the respiratory tract. *Pro. Am. Thorac. Soc.* 2:116-120.

Holt PC, Degebrodt A, Venaille T, O'Leary C, Krska K et al. (1985) Preparation of interstitial lung cells by enzymatic digestion of tissue slice: preliminary characterization by morphology and performance in functional assays. *Immunology* 54:139-147.

Holt PC, Marner LA, Papadimitriou JM (1982) Alveolar macrophages: functional heterogeneity within macrophage populations from rat lung. *Austr. J. Exp. Biol. Sci.* 60:607-618.

Holt PG, Haining S, Nelson DJ, Sedgwick JD (1994) Origin and steady-state turnover of class II MHC- bearing dendritic cells in the epithelium of the conducting airways. *J. Immun.* 153:256-261.

Holt PG, Schon-Hegrad MA, Oliver J (1988) MHC class II antigen-bearing dendritic cells in pulmonary tissues of the rat (regulation of antigen presentation activity by endogenous macrophage populations). *J. Exp. Med.* 167:262-274.

Holt PG, Strickland DH, Wikstrom ME, Jahnsen FL 2008) Regulation of immunological homeostasis in respiratory tract. *Nat. Rev. Immun.* 8:142-152.

Hughes AL (1999) *Adaptive evolution of genes and genomes.* Oxford University Press, New York.

Hughes AL, Neil M (1989) Evolution of the major histocompatibility complex: independent origin of nonclassical class I genes in different groups of mammals. *Mol. Biol. Evol.* 6:559-579.

IPCC (2007) Intergovernmental Panel on Climate Change: UNEP/WMO) In: *Fourth assessment report: climate change* (Pachauri RK, Reisinger A eds). Switzerland, Geneva, pp. 104.

Ishii H, Hayashi S, Hogg JC, Fujii T, Goto Y et al. (2005) Alveolar macrophage-epithelial cell interaction following exposure to atmospheric particles induces the release of mediators involved in monocyte mobilization and recruitment. *Respir. Res.* 6:87 *(doi:10.1186/1465-9921- 6-87).*

Jahnsen FL, Strickland DH, Thomas JA, Tobagu IT, Napoli S, Zosky GR (2006) Accelerated antigen sampling and transport by airway mucosal dendritic cells following inhalation of bacterial stimulus. *J. Immun.* 177:5861-5867.

Janeway CA (1993) How the immune system recognizes invaders. *Sci. Amer.* 269:72-79.

Johansson A, Lundborg M, Sköld CM, Lundhl J, Tornling G et al. (1997) Functional, morphological, and phenotypical differences between rat alveolar and interstitial macrophages. *Am. J. Respir. Cell Biol.* 16:582-588.

Johnson JE, Philp JR (1977) The defense of the lung: studies of the role of cell-mediated immunity. *Johns Hopkins Med. J.* 141:126-134.

Kaczmarek M, Frydrychowicz M, Nowicka A, Kozlowska M, Batura-Gabryel H et al. (2008) Influence of pleural and apoptosis regulating proteins of malignant cells. *J. Physiol. Pharmacol.* 59:321-330.

Kampfrath T, Maiseyeu A, Ying Z, Shah Z, Deiuliis JA et al. (2011) Chronic fine particulate matter exposure induces systemic vascular dysfunction via NADPH oxidase and TLR4 pathways. *Circ. Res.* 108:716-726.

Kapur V, Chauhan S, D'Cruz, Sachdev (2009) Kartagener's syndrome. *Lancet* 373:1973 *(doi:10.1016/S0140-6736(09)60306).*

Kaufman JD (2010) Does air pollution accelerate progression of atherosclerosis? *J. Am. Coll. Cardiol.* 56:1809-1811.

Kelly J (1990) Cytokines of the lung. *Am. Rev. Respir. Dis.* 141:765-788.

Kiama SK, Adekunle JS, Maina JN (2008) Comparative *in vitro* study of interactions between particles and respiratory surface macrophages, erythrocytes and epithelial cells of the chicken and the
rat. *J. Anat.* 213:452-463.

Kiama SG, Cochand L, Karlsson LM, Nicod LP, Gehr P (2001) Evaluation of phagocytic activity in human monocyte-derived dendritic cells. *J. Aerosol Med.* 14:289-299.

Kiama SG, Dreher D, Cochand L, Kok M, Obregon C et al. ehr P (2006) Host cell responces of *Salmonella typhimurium* infected human dendritic cells. *Immun. Cell Biol.* 84:475-481.

Kilburn H (1968) A hypothesis for pulmonary clearance and its implications. *Am. Rev. Respir. Dis.* 98:449-463.

Klein J (1986) *Natural history of the major histocompatibility complex.* Wiley, New York.

Klika E, Scheuermann DW, de Groodt-Lasseel MHA, Bazantova I, Switka A. (1996) Pulmonary macrophages in birds (barn owl, *Tyto tyto alba*), domestic fowl (*Gallus domestica*), quail (*Coturnix coturnix*), and pigeons (*Columba livia*). *Anat. Rec.* 256:87-97.

Klinke DJ (2006) An age related model of dendritic trafficking in the lung. *Am. J. Physiol.* 291:L1038- L1049.

Kobzik L, Godleski JJ, Barry BE, Brain JD (1988) Isolation and antigenic identification of hamster lung interstitial macrophages. *Am. Rev. Resp. Dis.* 138:908-914.

Kobzik L, Hancock WW, O'Hara C, Todd R, Godleski JJ (1986) Antigenic profile of human lung interstitial and alveolar macrophages. *Lab. Invest.* 54:32A.

Krauss H, Weber A, Appel M, Enders B, Isenberg D et al. (2003) *Zoonoses: infectious diseases transmissible from animals to humans, 3rd edtn.* ASM Press, American Society for Microbiology, Washington DC.

Krombach F, Münzing S, Allmeling AM, Gerlach JT, Behr J, Dörger M (1977) Cell size of alveolar macrophages: an interspecies comparison. *Envriron. Health Perspect.* 105:1261-1263.

Lambrecht BN, Prins JB, Hoogsteden HC (2001) Lung dendritic cells and host immunity to infection. *Eur. Respir. J.* 18:692-704.

Lambrecht BN, Salomon B, Klatzmann D, Pauwels RA (1998) Dendritic cells are required for the development of chronic eosinophilic airway inflammation in response to inhaled antigen in sensitized mice. *J. Immun.* 160:4090-4097.

Laskin DL, Weinberger B, Laskin JD (2001) Functional heterogeneity in liver and lung macrophages. *J. Leukocyte Biol.* 70:163-170.

Laurenzi GA, Berman L, First M, Kass EH (1964) A quantitative study of the deposition and clearance of bacteria in the murine lung. *J. Clin. Invest.* 43:759-768.

Lavnikova N, Prokhorova S, Helyar L, Laskin DL (1993) Isolation and partial characterization of subpopulations of alveolar macrophages, granulocytes, and highly enriched interstitial macrophages from rat lung. *Am. J. Respir Cell Mol. Biol.* 8:384-392.

Lee CA (1996) Pathogenicity islands and the evolution of bacterial pathogens. *Infect. Agents Dis.* 5:1-7.

Lee JW, McKibbin W (2003) *Globalization and disease: the case of SARS: working paper No. 2003/16.* The Brookings Institution, Research School of Pacific and Asian Studies, Australian National University (Canberra) and Washington DC.

Lehnert BE (1992) Pulmonary and thoracic macrophage subpopulations and clearance of particles from the lung. *Environ. Health Perspect.* 97:17-46.

Lehnert BE, Ortiz JB, London JE, Valdez YE, Cline AF et al. (1990) Migratory behaviours of alveolar macrophages during the alveolar clearance of light to heavy burdens of particles. *Exp. Lung Res.* 16:451-479.

Lehnert BE, Valdez Y, Holland L (1985) Pulmonary macrophages: alveolar and interstitial populations. *Exp. Lung Res.* 9:177-197.

Li N, Wang M, Oberley TD, Sempf JM, Nel AE (2002) Comparison of the pro-oxidative and proinflammatory effects of organic diesel exhaust particle chemicals in bronchial epithelial cells and macrophages. *J. Immun.* 169:4531-4541.

Lippmann M, Schlesinger RB (1984) Interspecies comparison of particle deposition and mucociliary clearance in tracheobronchial airways. *J. Toxicol. Environ. Health* 13:441-469.

Lipscomb MF, Masten BJ (2002) Dendritic cells: immune regulators in health and disease. *Physiol Rev* 82:97-130.

Litman GW (1996) Sharks and the origins of vertebrate immunity. *Sci. Amer.*1996:67-71.

Litman GW, Rast JP, Shamblott MJ, Haire RN, Hurst M et al. (1993) Phylogenetic diversification of immunoglobulin genes and the antibody repertoire. *Mol. Biol. Evol.* 10:60-72.

Liu YJ (2005) IPC: professional type 1 interferon-producing cells and plasmacytoid dendritic cell precursors. *Annu. Rev. Immun.* 23:275-306.

Lohmann-Matthes ML, Steinmüller C, Franke-Ullmann G (1994) Pulmonary macrophages. In: *Pulmonary immune cells* (Costael U, Kroegel C eds). *Eur. Resp. J.* 7:1678-1689.

Lommatzsch M, Bratke K, Bier A, Julius P, Kuepper M et al. (2007) Airway dendritic cell phenotypes in inflammatory diseases of the human lung. *Eur. Respir. J.* 30:878-886.

Lommatzsch M, Bratke K, Knappe T, Bier A, Dreschler K et al. (2010) Acute effects of tobacco smoke on human airway dendritic cells *in vivo*. *Eur. Respir. J.* 35:1130-1136.

Longworth KE, Jarvis KA, Tyler WS, Steffey EP, Staub NC (1994) Pulmonary intravascular macrophages in horses and ponies. *Am. J. Vet. Res.* 55:382-388.

Lorz C, López J (1997) Incidence of air pollution in the pulmonary surfactant system of the pigeon (*Columba livia*). *Anat. Rec.* 249:206-212.

Lundborg M, Johansson A, Låstbom L, Camner P (1999) Ingested aggregates of ultrafine carbon particles and interferon-γ impair rat alveolar macrophage function. *Environ. Res. 81:309-315.*

Lundborg M, Johard U, Låstbom L, Gerde P, Camner P (2001) Human alveolar macrophage function is impaired by aggregates of ultrafine carbon particles. *Environ. Res.* 86:244-253.

Mahsud I-U, Din S-U (2006) Kartagener's syndrome: case report. *Gomal J. Med. Sci.* 4:79-81.

Maina JN (1989) The morphology of the lung of the East African tree frog *Chiromantis petersi* with observations on the skin and the buccal cavity as secondary gas exchange organs: A TEM and SEM study. *J. Anat.* 165:29-43.

Maina JN (2005) *The lung air-sac system of birds: development, structure, and function.* Springer-Verlag, Berlin.

Maina JN, Cowley HM (1998) Ultrastructural characterization of the pulmonary cellular defences in the lung of a bird, the rock dove, *Columba livia. Proc R. Soc. B, Lond* 265:1567-1572.

Maina JN, King AS (1982) The thickness of the avian blood-gas barrier: qualitative and quantitative observations. *J. Anat.* 134:553-562.

Maina JN, King AS, Settle G (1989) An allometric study of the pulmonary morphometric parameters in birds, with mammalian comparison. *Phil. Trans. R. Soc. B, Lond* 326: 1-57.

Maina JN, Maloiy GMO (1988) A scanning and transmission electron microscopic study of the lung of a caecilian *Boulengerula taitanus*. *J. Zool., Lond* 215:739-751.

Maina JN, West JB (2005) Thin and strong! The bioengineering dilemma in the structural and functional design of the blood-gas barrier. *Physiol. Rev.* 85:811-844.

Maldonado CA, Sundblad V, Salatino M, Elia J, Garcia LN et al. (2011) Cell-type specific regulation of galectin-3 expression by glucocorticoids in lung Clara cells and macrophages. *Histol. Histopath.* 6:747-759.

Mateen FJ, Brook RD (2011) Air pollution as an emerging global risk factor for stroke. *JAMA* 305:1240- 1241.

McClung, CR (2011) Defence at dawn. *Nature* 470:44-45.

McKenna K, Beignon A, Bhardwaj N (2005). Plasmacytoid dendritic cells: linking innate and adaptive immunity. *J. Virol.* 79:17-27.

Mckibbin WJ, Sidorenko AA (2006) *Globalization macroeconomic consequences of pandemic influenza.* Lowy Institute for International Policy, Sydney (Australia).

McShane D, Davies JC, Wodehouse T, Bush A, Geddes D, Alton EWFW (2004) Normal nasal mucociliary clearance in CF children: evidence against a CFTR-related defect. *Eur. Respir. J.* 24:95-100.

Meban C (1980) Thicknesses of the air-blood barriers in vertebrate lungs. *J. Anat.* 131:299-307.

Mensah GA, Brain JD (1982) Deposition and clearance of inhaled aerosol in the respiratory tract of chickens. *J. Appl. Physiol.* 53:1423-1428.

Meuret G, Schildknecht O, Joder P, Senn H (1980) Proliferation activity and bacteriostatic potential of human blood monocytes, macrophages in pleural effusions, ascites, and of alveolar macrophages. *Blut* 40:17-25.

Meyer D, Mack SJ (2003) Major histocompatibility complex (MHC) genes: polymorphism. In: *Nature Encyclopedia of Human Genome.* Macmillan Publishers Ltd, Nature Publishing Group, London. *group/www.ehgoline.net.*

Meyer D, Thompson G (2001) How selection shapes variation of the human major histocompatibility complex: a review. *Ann. Hum. Genet.* 65:1-26.

Mills JN, Gage KL, Khan AS (2010) Potential influence of climate change on vector-borne and zoonotic diseases: a review and proposed research plan. *Environ. Health Perspect.* 118:1507-1514.

Molina RM, Brain JD (2007) *In vivo* comparison of cat alveolar and pulmonary intravascular macrophages: phagocytosis, particle clearance, and cytoplasmic motility. *Exp. Lung Res.* 33:53-70.

Moniuszko M, Bodzenta-Łukaszyk A, Kowal K (2007) Bronchial macrophages in asthmatics reveal decreased CD16 expression and substantial levels of receptors for IL-10 but not IL-4 and IL-7. *Folia Histochem.* 45:181-189.

Morrissette N, Gold E, Aderem A (1999) The macrophage - a cell for all seasons. *Trends Cell Biol.* 9:199-201.

Morrow PE (1988) Possible mechanisms to explain dust overloading of the lungs. *Fundam. Appl. Toxicol.* 10:369-384.

Mouton D, Bouthillier Y, Biozzi G, Stiffel C (1963) Phagocytosis of Salmonellae by reticuloendothelial cells of new-born piglets lacking natural antibody. *Nature* 197:706-712.

Mulnix AB, Dunn PE (1995) Molecular biology of the immune response. In: *Molecular model systems in the Lepidoptera* (Goldsmith MR, Wilkins AS, eds). Cambridge University Press, New York, pp. 369-395.

Myers RK, Arp LH (1987) Pulmonary clearance and lesions of lung and air sac in passively immunized and unimmunized turkeys following exposure to aerosolized *Escherichia coli. Avian Dis.* 31:622-628.

Nagashima A, Yasumoto K, Nakahashi H, Takeo S, Yano T, Nomoto K (1987) Antitumour activity of pleural cavity macrophages and its regulation by pleural cavity lymphocytes in patients with lung cancer. *Cancer Res.* 47:5497-5500.

Nagdeve DA (2004) Environmental pollution and control: a case study of Delhi Mega City. *Population Environ.* 25:461-473.

Nemmar A, Vanquickenborne B, Dinsdale D, Thomeer M, Hoylaerts MF et al. (2002) Passage of inhaled particles into the blood circulation in humans. *Circulation* 105:411-414.

Nganpiep L, Maina JN (2002) Composite cellular defense stratagem in the avian respiratory system: functional morphology of the free (surface) macrophages and specialized pulmonary epithelia. *J. Anat.* 200:499-516.

Nguyen BT, Peterson PK, Verbrugh HA, Quie PG, Hoidal JR (1982) Difference in phagocytosis and killing by alveolar macrophages from humans, rabbits, rats, and hamsters. *Infect. Immun.* 36:504-509.

Nicod LP (1997) Function of human lung dendritic cells. In: *Lung health and disease* (Lipscomb MF, Russels SW, eds). Marcel Dekker Inc., New York, pp. 311-334.

Nicod LP (2005) Lung defences: an overview. *Europ. Respir. Rev.* 95:45-50.

Niehaus GD, Schumacker PR, Saba TM (1980) Reticuloendothelial clearance of blood-borne particulates. *Ann. Surg.* 191:479-489.

Ochs DL, Toth TE, Pyle RH, Siegel PB (1988) Cellular defense of the avian lung respiratory system: effects of *Pasteurella multocida* on respiratory burst activity of avian respiratory tract phagocytes. *Am. J. Vet. Res.* 49:2081-2084.

Ooi H, Arakawa M, Ozawa H (1994) A morphological study of acute respiratory tract lesions in a lipopolysaccharide instilled rat model. *Arch. Histol. Cytol.* 57:87-105.

Pabst R, Tschernig T (2002) Perivascular capillaries in the lung: an important but neglected vascular bed in immune reactions? *J. Allergy Clin. Immun.* 110:209-214.

Parbhakar OP, Duke T, Twonsend HGG, Singh B (2005) Depletion of pulmonary intravascular macrophages partially inhibits lipopolysaccharide-induced lung inflammation in horses. *Vet. Res.* 36:557-569.

Patz JA, Daszak P, Tabor GM, Aguirre AA, Pearl M et al. (2004) Unhealthy landscapes: policy recommendations on land use change and infectious disease emergence. *Environ. Health Perspect.* 112:1092-1098.

Patz JA, Wolfe ND (2002) Global ecological change and human health. In: *Conservation medicine: ecological health and practice* (Aguirre AA, Osfeld RS, Tabor GM, House C, Pearl MC, eds). Oxford University Press, New York, pp. 167-181.

Peão MND, Águas AP, Grande NR (1993) Morphological evidence for migration of particle-laden macrophages through the interalveolar pores of Kohn in the murine lung. *Acta Anat.* 147:227- 232.

Pennial R, Spitznagel JK (1975) Chicken neutrophils: oxidative metabolism in phagocytic cells devoid of myeloperoxidase. *Proc. Natl. Acad Sci., USA* 72:5012-5015.

Peters A, Wichmann HE, Tuch T, Heinrich J, Heyder J (1997) Respiratory effects are associated with the number of ultrafine particles. *Am. J. Respir. Crit. Care Med.* 155:1376-1383.

Pope CA (2000) Epidemiology of fine particle air pollution and human health: biologic mechanisms and who's at risk? *Environ. Health Perspect.* 108:713-723.

Pope CA, Burnett RT, Thun MJ, Calle EE, Krewski D, Ito K, Thurston GD (2002) Lung cancer, cardiopulmonary mortality, and long-term exposure to fine particulate air pollution. *J. Am. Med. Assoc.* 287:1132-1141.

Poth CM, Matfin G (2010) *Essentials of pathophysiology.* Lippincott Williams, New York.

Power CK, Burke CM, Sreenan S, Hurson B, Poulter LW (1994) T-cell and macrophage subsets in the bronchial wall of clinically healthy subjects. *Eur. Respir. J.* 7:437-441.

Prokhorova S, Lavnikova N, Laskin DL (1994) Functional characterization of interstitial macrophages and subpopulations of alveolar macrophages from rat lung. *J. Leukocyte Biol.* 55:141-146.

Rawlins EL (2011) The building blocks of mammalian lung development. *Dev. Dyn.* 240:463-476.

Reaven EP, Axline SG (1973) Subplasmalemmal microfilaments and microtubules in resting and phagocytosing cultivated macrophages. *J. Cell Biol.* 59:12-27.

Reese S, Dalamani G, Kaspers B (2006) The avian lung-associated immune system: a review. *Vet. Res.* 37:311-324.

Reid CD (1997) The dendritic cell lineage in hemopoiesis. *Br. J. Hematol.* 96:217-223.

Rehman, D. A. 1998. Detection and identification of previously unrecognized microbial pathogens. *Emerg. Infect. Dis.* 4:382-389.

Rohmann K, Tschernig T, Pabst R, Goldmann T, Drömann D (2011) Innate immunity in the human lung: pathogen recognition and lung disease. *Cell Tissue Res.* 343:167-174.

Rubovitch V, Gershnabel S, Kalina M (2007) Lung epithelial cells modulate the inflammatory response of alveolar macrophages. *Inflammation* 30:236-243.

Rybicka K, Daly BDT, Migliore JJ, Norman JC (1974) Intravascular macrophages in normal calf lung. an electron microscopic study. *Am. J. Anat.* 139:353-368.

Sachan N, Singh VP (2010) Effects of climatic changes on the prevalence of zoonotic diseases. *Vet. World* 3:519-522.

Saetta M, Di Stefano A, Maestrelli P, Ferraresso A, Drigo R et al. (1993) Activated T-lymphocytes and macrophages in bronchial mucosa of subjects with chronic bronchitis. *Am. Rev. Respir. Dis.* 147:301-306.

Sahn SA, Potts DE (1978) The effect of tetracycline on rabbit pleura. *Am. Rev. Respir. Dis.* 117:493- 499.

Said IS, Foda HD (1989) Pharmacological modulation of lung injury. *Amer. Rev. Respir. Dis.* 139:1553- 1564.

Sallusto F, Lanzavecchia A (2002) The instructive role of dendritic cells on T-cell responses. *Arthritis Res. 4 Suppl.* 3:S127-S132.

Sanders CJ, Doherty PC, Thomas PG (2011) Respiratory epithelial cells in innate immunity to influenza virus infection. *Cell Tissue Res.* 343:13-21.

Satthaporn S, Eremin O (2001) Dendritic cells (I): biological functions. *J. R. Coll. Surg. Edinb.* 46:9-20.

Sbiera S, Wortmann S, Fassnacht M (2008) Dendritic cell based immunotherapy - a promising therapeutic approach for endocrine malignancies. *Hormone Metab. Res.* 40:89-98.

Schaumann F, Borm PJ, Herbrich A, Knoch J, Pitz M et al. (2004) Metal-rich ambient particles ($PM_{2.5}$) cause airway inflammation in healthy subjects. *Am. J. Crit. Care Med.* 170:898-903.

SchnebergerD, Raz-Aharonson K, Singh B (2011) Monocyte and macrophage heterogeneity and Toll- like receptors in the lung. *Cell Tissue Res.* 343:97-106.

Schon-Hegrad MA, Oliver J, McMenamin PG, Holt PG (1991) Studies on the density, distribution and surface phenotype of intraepithelial class II major histocompatibility complex antigen (Ia)- bearing dendritic cells (DC) in the conducting airways. *J. Exp. Med.* 173:1345-1356.

Schott M, Seissler J (2003) Dendritic cell vaccination: new hope for the treatment of metastasized endocrine malignancies. *Trends Endocrinol. Metab.* 14:156-162.

Schulz H, Harder N, Ibald-Mulli A, Khandoga A, Koenig W et al. (2005) Cardiovascular effects of fine and ultrafine particles. *J. Aerosol. Med.* 18:1-22.

Schürch S, Gehr P, Hof Im, Geiser M, Green F (1990) Surfactant displaces particles toward the epithelium in airways and alveoli. *Respir. Physiol.* 80:17-32.

Schwartz J (1994) Why are people dying of high air pollution? *Environ. Res.* 64:26-35.

Sebring RJ, Lehnert BE (1992) Morphometric comparisons of rat alveolar macrophages, pulmonary interstitial macrophages, and blood monocytes. *Exp. Lung. Res.* 18:479-496.

Sestini P, Tagliabue A, Boraschi D (1984) Modulation of macrophage suppressive activity and prostaglandin release by lymphokines and interferon: comparison of alveolar, pleural and peritoneal macrophages. *Clin. Exp. Immun.* 58:573-580.

Sharma S, Yang SC, Batra RK, Dubinett SM (2003) Intratumoral therapy with cytokine gene-modified dendritic cells in murine lung cancer models. *Methods Mol. Med.* 5:711-722.

Shellito J, Esparza C, Armstrong C (1987) Maintenance of the normal rat alveolar macrophage population: the roles of monocyte influx and alveolar macrophage proliferation *in situ*. *Am. Rev. Respir. Dis.* 135:78-82.

Shimotakahara A, Kuebler JF, Vieten G, Metzelder MI, Petersen C, Ure BM (2007) Pleural macrophages are the dominant cell population in the thoracic cavity with an inflammatory cytokine profile similar to peritoneal macrophages. *Pediatr. Surg. Int.* 23:447-451.

Sibile Y, Reynolds HY (1990) Macrophages and polymorphonuclear neutrophils in lung defense and injury. *Am. Rev. Respir. Dis.* 141:471-501.

Sica A, Bronte V (2007) Altered macrophage differentiation and immune dysfunction in tumour development. *J. Clin. Invest.* 117:1155-1166.

Sichletidis L, Tsiotsios I, Gavriilidis A, Chloros D, Gioulekas D et al. (2005) The effects of environmental pollution on the respiratory system of children in Western Macedonia, Greece. *J. Invest. Allergol. Clin. Immun.* 15:117-123.

Singh B, Pearce JW, Gamage LNA, Janardhan K, Cadwell S (2004) Depletion of pulmonary intravascular macrophages inhibits acute lung inflammation. *Am. J. Physiol.* 286:L363-L372.

Sorokin SP, Brain JD (1975) Pathways of clearance in mouse lungs exposed to iron oxide aerosols. *Anat. Rec.* 181:581-626.

Sorokin SP, Hoyt RF, Grant MM (1984) Development of macrophage in the lungs of fetal rabbits, rats, and hamsters. *Anat. Rec.* 208:103-121.

Spira A (1996) Disorders of the respiratory system. In: *Diseases of cage and aviary birds* (Rosskopf W, Woerpel R, eds). Lea and Febiger, Baltimore, pp. 415-428.

Spiteri MA, Clarke SW, Poulter LW (1992) Isolation of phenotypically and functionally distinct macrophage subpopulations from human bronchoalveolar lavage. *Eur. Resp. J.* 5:717-726.

Spritzer AA, Watson JA, Auld JA, Guetthoff MA (1968) Pulmonary macrophage clearance. The hourly rates of transfer of pulmonary macrophages to the oropharynx in the rat. *Arch. Environ. Health* 17:726-730.

Spurgin LG, Richardson DS (2010) How pathogens drive genetic diversity: MHC, mechanisms and misunderstandings. *Proc. R. Soc. B, Lond.* 277:979-988.

Stearns RC, Barnas GM, Walski M, Brain JD (1986) Phagocytosis in the gas exchange region of avian lungs. *Fed. Proc.* 45:959.

Steinman RM (1991) The dendritic cell system and its role in immunogenicity. *Annu. Rev. Immun.* 9:271-296.
Steinman RM, Cohn ZA (1973) Identification of a novel cell type in peripheral lymphoid organs of mice: I. Morphology, quantitation, tissue distribution. *J. Exp. Med.* 137:1142-1162.
Steinmüller C, Franke-Ullmann G, Lohman-Matthes ML, Emmendörffer A (2000) Local activation of non- specific defense against a respiratory model infection by application of interferon-γ: comparison between rat alveolar- and interstitial lung macrophages. *Am. J. Respir. Cell Mol. Biol.* 22:481- 490.
Stossel TP (1978) Contractile proteins in cell structure and function. *Ann. Rev. Med.* 29:427-457.
Stossel TP, Hartwig JH (1976) Interactions of actin, myosin and new actin-binding protein of rabbit pulmonary macrophages. II. Role of cytoplasmic movement and phagocytosis. *J. Cell Biol.* 68:602-619.
Strange C, Tomlinson JR, Wilson C, Harley R, Miller KS, Sahn SA (1989) The histology of experimental pleural injury with tetracycline, empyema, and carrageenan. *Exp. Mol. Pathol.* 51:205-219.
Suwa T, Hogg JC, Quinlan KB, Ohgami A, Vincent R, van Eeden SF (2002) Particulate air pollution induces progression of atherosclerosis. *J. Am. Coll. Cardiol.* 39:935-942.
Syme R, Gluck S (2001) Generation of dendritic cells: role of cytokines and potential clinical applications. *Trans. Apheres Sci.* 24:117-124.
Takizawa H, Beckmann JD, Shoji S, Claassen LR, Ertl RF et al. (1990) Pulmonary macrophages can stimulate cell growth of bovine bronchial epithelial cells. *Am. J. Respir. Cell Mol. Biol.* 2:233- 244.
Thet LA, Wrobel DJ, Crapo JD (1983) Morphologic aspects of the protection by endotoxin against acute and chronic oxygen-induced lung injury in adult rats. *Lab. Invest.* 48:448-457.
Tilman D, Fargione J, Wolff B, D'Antonio C, Dobson A et al. (2001) Forecasting agriculturally driven global environmental change. *Science* 292:281-284.
Toth TE, Siegel PB (1986) Cellular defence for the avian respiratory tract: paucity of free-residing macrophages in the normal chicken. *Avian Dis.* 30:67-75.
Toth TE, Siegel PB, Veit H (1987) Cellular defense of the avian respiratory system - influx of phagocytes: elicition versus activation. *Avian Dis.* 31:67-75.
Toth TE, Pyle RH, Caceci T, Siegel PB, Ochs D (1988) Cellular defense of the avian respiratory system: influx and nonopsonic phagocytosis by respiratory phagocytes activated by *Pasteurella multocida. Infect. Immun.* 56:1171-1179.
Tschernig T, Pabst R (2009) What is the clinical relevance of different lung compartments? *BMC Pulm. Med.* 9:39 *(doi:10.1186/1471-2466-9-39).*
Tschernig T, de Vries VC, Debertin AS, Braun A, Wallers T et al. (2006) Density of dendritic cells in the human tracheal mucosa is age dependent and site specific. *Thorax* 61:986-991.
Tsukioka T, Takemura S, Minamiyama Y, Nishiyama N, Mizuguchi S et al. (2007) Local and systemic impacts of pleural oxygen exposure in thoracotomy. *BioFactors* 30:117-128.
Tucker A, McMurtry IF, Reeves JT, Alexander AF, Will DH, Grover RF (1975) Lung vascular smooth muscle as a determinant of pulmonary hypertension at high altitude. *Am. J. Physiol.* 228:762- 778.

UNEP-WHO (1994) U.N. Environment Program and WHO Report: air pollution in the world's megacities. *Environment* 36:5-37.

Vanbervliet B, Bendriss-Vermare N, Massacrier C, Homey B, Boutillier O et al. (2003) The inducible CXCR3 ligands control plasmacytoid dendritic cell responsiveness to the constitutive chemokine stromal cell-derived factor-1 (SDF-1)/CXCL12. *J. Exp. Med.* 198:823-830.

van den Hooven EH, de Kluizenaar Y, Pierik FH, Hofman A, van Ratingen SW et al. (2011) Air pollution, blood pressure, and the risk of hypertensive complications during pregnancy: The generation R study. *Hypertension* 57:406-412.

van Furth R (1970) The origin and turnover of promonocytes, monocytes and macrophages in normal mice. In: *Mononuclear phagocytes* (van Furth R, ed). Blackwell, Oxford, pp. 151-165.

van Furth R (1982) Current view on the mononuclear phagocyte system. *Immunobiology* 161:178-185.

van Haarst JMV, Hoogsteden HC, de Wit HJ, Verhoeven, GT, Havenith CEG, Drexhage HA (1994) Dendritic cells and their precursors isolated from human bronchoalveolar lavage: immunocytologic and functional properties. *Am. J. Respir. Cell Mol. Biol.* 11:344-350.

Vassallo R, Walters PR, Lamont J, Kottom TJ, Yi ES, Limper AH (2010) Cigarette smoke promotes dendritic cell accumulation in COPD; a lung tissue research consortium study. *Respir. Res.* 11:45 *(http://respiratory-research.com/content/11/1/45).*

von Garnier C, Nicod LP (2009) Immunology taught by lung dendritic cells. *Swiss Med. Wkly Online Publ. 8th Jan, 2009,* pp. 9.

von Garnier C, Filgueira L, Wikstrom M, Smith M, Thomas JA, Strickland DH (2005) Anatomical location determines the distribution and function of dendritic cells and other APCs in the respiratory tract. *J. Immun.* 175:1609-1618.

Walter E, Dreher D, Kok M, Thiele L, Kiama SG et al. (2001) Hydrophilic poly (DL-lactide-co-glycolide) microspheres for the delivery of DNA to human-derived macrophages and dendritic cells. *J. Controlled Release* 76:149-168.

Wang, W., Barnaby, J.Y., Tada, Y., Li, H., Tör, H. et al. (2011) Timing of plant immune responses by a central circardian regulator. *Nature* 470:110-114.

Ware JH (2000) Particulate air pollution and mortality: clearing the air. *N. Engl. J. Med.* 343:1798-1799.

Warheit DB, Hartsky MA (1993) Role of alveolar macrophages chemotaxis and phagocytosis in pulmonary clearance responses to inhaled particles: comparisons among rodent species. *Microsc. Res. Tech.* 26:412-422.

Warheit DB, Hartsky MA, Stefaniak MS (1988) Comparative physiology of rodent pulmonary macrophages: *in vitro* functional responses. *J. Appl. Physiol* 64:1953-1959.

Warheit DB, Hill LH, Brody AR (1984) Surface morphology and correlated phagocytic capacity of pulmonary macrophages lavaged from the lungs of rats. *Exp. Lung Res.* 6:71-82.

Warheit DB, Hill LH, George G, Brody AR (1986) Time course of chemotactic factor generation and the corresponding macrophage response to asbestors inhalation. *Am. Rev. Respir. Dis.* 134:128- 138.

Warheit DB, Reed KL, Sayes CM (2009). A role for nanoparticle surface reactivity in facilitating pulmonary toxicology and development of a base set of hazard assays as a component of nanoparticle risk management. *Inhal. Toxicol.* 21:61-67.

Warner AE (1996) Pulmonary intravascular macrophages: role in acute lung injury. *Clin. Chest Med.* 17:125-135.

Warner AE, Barry BA, Brain JD (1986) Pulmonary intravascular macrophages in sheep: morphology and function of a novel constituent of the mononuclear phagocyte system. *Lab. Invest.* 55:276-288.

Warner AE, Brain JD (1984) Intravascular pulmonary macrophages in ruminants actively participate in reticuloendothelial clearance of particles. *Fed. Proc.* 43:1001.

Warner AE, Brain JD (1986) Intravascular macrophages: a novel cell removes particles from blood. *Am. J. Physiol.* 19:R728-732.

Warner AE, Brain JD (1990) The cell biology and pathogenic role of pulmonary intravascular macrophages. *Amer. J. Physiol.* 258:L1-L12.

Warner AE, Barry BE, Brain JD (1986) Pulmonary intravascular macrophages in sheep: morphology and function of a novel constituent of the mononuclear phagocyte system. *Lab. Invest.* 55:276-288.

Warner AE, Molina RM, Brain JD (1987) Uptake of bloodborne bacteria by pulmonary intravascular macrophages and consequent inflammatory responses in sheep. *Am. Rev. Respir. Dis.* 136:683-690.

Webb TJ, Sumpter TL, Thiele AT, Swanson KA, Wilkes DS (2005) The phenotype and function of lung dendritic cells. *Crit. Rev Immun.* 25:465-492.

Weibel ER (1984) *The pathways for oxygen: structure and function in the mammalian respiratory system.* Harvard University Press. Harvard (MA).

Weibel ER (1985) Lung cell biology. In: *Handbook of physiology: respiration, vol. 3, sect 2.* (Fishman AP, ed). American Physiological Society, Bethesda, pp. 47-91.

Weissler JC, Lyons CR, Lipscomb MF, Toews GB (1986) Human pulmonary macrophages: functional comparison of cells obtained from whole lung by bronchoalveolar lavage. *Am. Rev. Respir. Dis.* 133:473-477.

Welsch U (1981) Fine structural and enzyme histochemical observations on the respiratory epithelium of the caecilian lungs and gills, a contribution to the understanding of the evolution of the vertebrate respiratory epithelium. *Arch. Histol jap.* 44:117-133.

Welsch U (1983) Phagocytosis in the amphibian lung. *Anat. Anz.* 154:323-327.

Welsch U, Müller W (1980) Feinstrukturelle Beobachtungen am Alveolarepithel von Reptilien ubterschiedlicher Lebensweise. *Z. microsk.-anat. Forsch.* 94:333-348.

Wheeldon EB, Hansen-Flaschen JH (1986) Intravascular macrophages in the sheep lung. *J. Leukocyte Biol.* 40:657-661.

Whitsett JA (2002) Intrinsic and innate defenses in the lung: intersection of pathways regulating lung morphogenesis, host defense, and repair. *J. Clin. Invest.* 109:565-522.

Wichman HE, Peters A (2000) Epidemiological evidence of the effects of ultrafine particle exposure. *Philos. Trans. R. Soc., Lond. A* 358:2751-2769.

Wideman RE (2005) Pathophysiology of heart/lung disorders: pulmonary hypertension syndrome in broiler chickens. *World's Poult. Sci. J.* 57:289-307.

Winkler GC (1988) Pulmonary intravascular macrophages in domestic animal species: review of structural and functional properties. *Am. J. Anat.* 181:217-234.

Winkler GC (1989) Review of the significance of pulmonary intravascular macrophages with respect to animal species and age. *Exp. Cell Biol.* 57:281-286.

Winkler GC, Cheville N (1985) Monocytic origin and postnatal mitosis of intravascular macrophages in the porcine lung. *J. Leukocyte Biol.* 38:471-480.

Winkler GC, Cheville N (1987) Postnatal colonization of porcine lung capillaries by intravascular macrophages: an ultrastructural, morphometric analysis. *Microvasc. Res.* 33:223-232.

Wismar BL, Dehring DJ, Lowery BD, Cloutier CT, Carey LC (1984) Electron microscopic evidence of intravascular phagocytosis in the lungs of a porcine model of septic acute respiratory failure. *Am. Rev. Respir. Dis.* 129:A290.

Wizeman TM, Laskin DL (1994) Enhanced phagocytosis, chemotaxis, and production of reactive oxygen intermediates by interstitial lung macrophages following acute endotoxemia. *Am. J. Respir. Cell Miol. Biol.* 11:358-365.

Wu L, Liu YJ (2007) Development of dendritic-cell lineages. *Immunity* 26:741-750.

Xia WJ, Pinto CE, Kradin RL (1995) The antigen-presenting activities of Ia^+ dendritic cells shift dynamically from lung to lymph node after an airway challenge with soluble antigen. *J. Exp. Med.* 181:1275-1283.

Yamaya M, Fukushima T, Sekisawa K, Ohrui T, Sasaki H (1995) Cytoplasmic motility reflects phagocytic activity in alveolar macrophages from dog lungs. *Respir. Physiol.* 101:199-205.

Yamaya M, Sayasu K, Sekisawa K, Yamauchi K, Shimura S et al. (1989) Acute effect of cigarrette smoke on cytoplasmic motility of alveolar macrophages in dogs. *J. Appl. Physiol.* 66:1172- 1178.

Yamaya M, Sayasu K, Sekisawa K, Yamauchi K, Shimura H et al. (1990) Mechanisms of decrease in cytoplasmic motility of alveolar macrophages during immediate asthmatic response in dogs. *Am. J. Physiol.* 258:L220-L226.

Yanagawa H, Yano S, Haku T, Ohmoto Y, Sone S (1996) Interleukin-1 receptor antagonist in pleural effusion due to inflammatory and malignant lung disease. *Eur. Respir. J.* 9:1211-1216.

Yewdell JW, Dolan BP (2011) Cross-dressers turn on T-cells. *Nature* 471:581-582.

Yoshikawa T, Hill TE, Yoshikawa N, Popov VL, Galindo CL et al. (2010) Dynamic innate immune responses of human bronchial epithelial cells to severe acute respiratory syndrome-associated coronavirus infection. *PLoS ONE 5(1):e8729 (doi:10.1371/journal.pone.0008729).*

Yu CP, Chen YK, Morrow PE (1989) An analysis of alveolar macrophage mobility kinetics at dust overloading of the lungs. *Fundam. Appl. Toxicol.* 13:452-459.

Zeltner T, Caduff J, Gehr P, Pfenninger J, Burri P (1987) The postnatal development and growth of the human lung. I. Morphometry. *Respir. Physiol.* 67:247-267.

Zetterberg G, Johansson A, Lundahl J, Lundoborg M, Sköld CM et al. (1998) Differences between rat alveolar and interstitial macrophages 5 weeks after quartz exposure. *Am. J. Physiol.* 274:L226- L234.

Zhou LJ, Tedder TF (1995) A distinct pattern of cytokine gene expression by human $CD83^+$ blood dendritic cells. *Blood* 86:3295-3301.

Zigmond SH, Hirsch JG (1979) Effects of cytochalasin B on polymorphonuclear leukocyte locomotion, phagocytosis and glycolysis. *Exp. Cell Res.* 73:383-393.

Zlotnik A, Crowle AJ (1992) Lymphokine-induced mycobacteriostatic activity in mouse pleural macrophages. *Infect. Immun.* 37:786-793.

Zlotnik A, Vatter A, Hayes RL, Blumentahl E, Crowle AJ (1982) Mouse pleural macrophages: characterization and comparison with mouse alveolar and peritoneal macrophages. *J Reticuloendothel. Soc.* 31:207-220.

Zwilling BS, Campolito LB, Reiches NA (1982) Alveolar macrophage subpopulations identified by differential centrifugation on discontinuous albumin density gradient. *Am. Rev. Respir. Dis.* 125:448-452.

Part 2

Lung Pathology and Inflammation

3

The Contrasting Roles of T Regulatory Cells in Bacterial Lung Diseases

Adam N. Odeh and Jerry W. Simecka
Department of Molecular Biology and Immunology
University of North Texas Health Science Center, Fort Worth, TX
USA

1. Introduction

The respiratory environment is exposed to a variety of different pathogens and irritants from the environment. We breathe in about 10,000 liters of air per day. As such, the immune cells along the respiratory tract constantly come into contact with pathogens and potential immunogens within the air. Since development of inflammatory responses to all these stimuli could result in persistent host responses and inflammation that could eventually be damaging to the lungs, the responses to potential respiratory pathogens, antigens and irritants must be tightly regulated and in some cases tolerated. Ideally, inflammatory responses should only occur when other initial mechanisms of protection, e.g. mucus, mucociliary clearance and phagocytes, are insufficient. Thus, in addition to the ability to differentiate between self and foreign antigens, as is done throughout the rest of the body, respiratory immune responses must also have the capacity to differentiate between harmful and innocuous antigens.

Regulatory mechanisms throughout the body have evolved to control these immune and inflammatory responses, normally allowing for an immune response strong enough to deal with dangerous pathogens, but not so aggressive as to result in harmful immunopathology. Strong suppression by these regulatory mechanisms has been implicated in the pathogenesis of cancer, while weak suppression has been suggested to contribute to autoimmunity. In the lungs, mechanisms have evolved to similarly modulate host responses. This includes surfactants and alveolar macrophages that dampen host immune responses. Lymphocyte populations can also regulate pulmonary immune responses. The lymphocyte population most commonly associated with regulation of host immune and inflammatory responses, including tolerance to innocuous antigens, is the regulatory T (T_{reg}) cell. Although much research has been done in the role of T_{reg} cells in the pathogenesis of asthma, relatively little work has been performed examining these mechanisms in the context of bacterial infections, but the limited studies demonstrate that they can have a significant impact on these diseases. In this article, we will first briefly review the immune environment of the lung and the T_{reg} cells and their function. We then focus on some bacterial lung diseases and what is known about the impact of T_{reg} cells. Specifically, we will examine the potential for T_{reg} cells to have both positive and negative effects on disease progression, depending upon the pathogen.

2. The pulmonary immune environment

The lung is exposed to a variety of different pathogens and irritants from the environment. It would be harmful to the host if immune and inflammatory responses were generated in response to these agents, as it could result in constant inflammation and tissue destruction. Therefore, immune responses must be tolerant of these organisms so as not to upset the equilibrium that exists in the mucosal environment (Sansonetti, 2011). This requires a delicate balance between T_{reg} cells and proinflammatory cells (Sansonetti, 2011).

Research suggests that the lung environment tends to preferentially mount T helper type 2 responses (Th2), though this is not absolute (Constant et al., 2000). The type of immune response elicited during bacterial infection is somewhat dependent on the site of infection, and the size of the antigen dose (Constant et al., 2000; Morokata et al., 2000). In addition, the type of antigen encountered by toll-like receptor-expressing cells can also determine the nature of the resultant immune response (Pulendran, 2004; Wissinger et al., 2009). Toll-like receptors are traditionally associated with antigen presenting cells, such as dendritic cells, macrophages, and B cells, though toll-like receptor stimulation on T helper cells has also been demonstrated to play an important role (Kawai & S. Akira, 2011; Palusinska-Szysz & Janczarek, 2010; Wissinger et al., 2009).

3. Regulatory T cells

T_{reg} cells are a heterogeneous T cell population thought to maintain immunologic balance and prevent or minimize tissue damaging immune responses (Fehervari & Sakaguchi, 2004a; Fehervari & Sakaguchi, 2004b; Sakaguchi, 2000, 2002, 2003). T_{reg} cells are a subset of $CD4^+$ T cells that make up anywhere from 1-10% of all $CD4^+$ cells in the thymus, blood, and lymph (McHugh & Shevach, 2002). Unlike traditional T helper (Th) cells, T_{reg} cells act to suppress or dampen the immune response. While evidence indicates that other cell populations may also have suppressive capabilities, such as natural killer T cells, gamma-delta ($\gamma\delta$) T cells, and $CD8^+$ suppressor cells, classical T_{reg} cells are by far the most highly studied, the best understood, and, as far as the current evidence indicates, the most important in controlling the body's immune responses (Bach, 2003; Born et al., 2000; Oh et al., 2008; Wang & Alexander, 2009).

Very early on, T_{reg} cells were implicated in autoimmune disorders. A lack of T_{reg} cells was thought to be at least related to the onset of autoimmunity, if not the principal cause of it (Ellner, 1981). To date, T_{reg} cell numbers have been found to be either abnormally low or poorly functioning in patients suffering from diseases such as lupus, rheumatoid arthritis, and myasthenia gravis (Flores-Borja et al., 2008; Mudd et al., 2006; Wang et al., 2008). Laboratory experiments have shown that adoptive transfer of T_{reg} cells into lab animals prone to type I diabetes results in improved prognosis and delay of disease onset (Sakaguchi et al., 2006). Overall, these cells inhibit a wide range of autoimmune and inflammatory reactions, such as gastritis, oophoritis, orchitis, thryoiditis, inflammatory bowel disease (IBD), and spontaneous autoimmune diabetes.

However, in some situations, T_{reg} cells may restrict the actions of the immune system too much. The presence of T_{reg} cells has been suggested to contribute to the progression of cancer. Again, laboratory experiments have shown that depletion of T_{reg} cells can result in enhanced killing of tumor cells by the immune response (Nomura & Sakaguchi, 2005). Similarly, T_{reg} cells were also shown to contribute to the persistence of *Leishmania major* infection (Belkaid, 2003; Mendez et al., 2004). It is thought that T_{reg} cells suppress the protective immune responses against cancer and some pathogens, resulting in prolonged disease. Furthermore T_{reg} cells can suppress the cytokine production and proliferation of conventional Th cells (Jonuleit et al., 2001; Thornton & Shevach, 1998), but the T_{reg} cells' effects on Th cell subsets are conflicting with some studies (Stassen et al., 2004) suggesting dampening of Th2 responses and others (Suto et al., 2001) indicating promotion of Th2 cell responses. As a result, Treg cells may in some circumstances promote immune responses with varied results. Thus, Treg cells can have both positive and negative impacts on host responses in disease, highlighting the potential dual nature of T_{reg} cells.

First studied in the 1970's, T_{reg} cells, known then as suppressor T cells, were identified based on their ability to suppress antigen-specific immune responses. At that time, it was very difficult to study T_{reg} cells due to the lack of any known markers specific to the cell type. As a result, the existence of T_{reg} cells remained a very controversial idea for a long time. In 1995, it was shown by Sakaguchi et al. that T_{reg} cells constitutively express the interleukin (IL)-2 receptor alpha chain, CD25, at a high level (Nomura & Sakaguchi, 2005). The expression of the IL-2 receptor chain which is normally associated with activated T cells was theorized to be due to the continued T cell receptor engagement of self-antigens by these T_{reg} cells, resulting in a perpetually active state. Thus, the characterization of T_{reg} cells as $CD4^{+}CD25^{hi}$ cells became widely accepted. Still, it remained somewhat difficult to distinguish T_{reg} cells from activated Th cells, which also can express CD25, albeit at lower levels. Recently, the association of the intracellular transcription factor forkhead P3 (FoxP3) with T_{reg} cells has led to the most accurate characterization of these cells to date: $CD4^{+}CD25^{hi}FoxP3^{+}$ (Hori et al., 2003). $CD4^{+}CD25^{hi}FoxP3^{+}$ T_{reg} cells also have other distinguishing surface markers such as GITR, CTLA-4, CD103, CCR4, CD62L, and $CD127^{lo}$; however, the evidence that these markers are useful to phenotype T_{reg} cells has yet to be established (Bayer et al., 2008; Fu et al., 2004; Liu et al., 2006; Sather et al., 2007; Shimizu et al., 2002; Wing et al., 2008; Zhao et al., 2008).

The mechanisms through which T_{reg} cells exert their suppressive effects throughout the host appear to be numerous, and are likely dependent on the same factors that affect the typical immune response, such as the antigen dose, the nature of the pathogen or allergen, and the route of entry. The most common mechanism observed in both *in vitro* and *in vivo* experiments is secretion of cytokines, particularly IL-10 and transforming growth factor (TGF)-β (Bluestone & A. K. Abbas, 2003; Vignali et al., 2008; von Boehmer, 2005). Both of these cytokines are associated with Th2 responses, and, as such, are at odds with the more common Th1 response. Therefore, secretion of these cytokines by T_{reg} cells reduces or dampens Th1 inflammatory responses. However, these are not the only cytokines that have been associated with T_{reg} cells. IL-35, a member of the IL-12 family of cytokines, has recently been shown to play a role in T_{reg} cell-mediated suppression (Chaturvedi et al., 2011; Collison et al., 2007; Collison et al., 2010). IL-35 is thought to be secreted only by T_{reg} cells, and, while it is known to have a potent anti-inflammatory effect, the mechanism through which it exerts this effect is still poorly understood (Chaturvedi et al., 2011; Collison et al., 2007; Collison et al., 2010). In addition, recent experiments have suggested that T_{reg} cells may also be able to suppress Th2 immune responses through the secretion of interferon (IFN)- γ and

IL-17, though this is still being studied (Ayyoub et al., 2009; Beriou et al., 2009; Esposito et al., 2010; Fang et al., 2009; Voo et al., 2009).

Recent research has also shown that T_{reg} cells may be able to exert suppression through galectin-1, which may be secreted or membrane-bound (Garin et al., 2007; Shevach, 2009). Galectin-1 has been implicated in cell cycle arrest, inhibition of proinflammatory cytokines, and even apoptosis of responder cells, though the mechanism remains unclear (Garin et al., 2007; Shevach, 2009). Blockade of galectin-1 has been shown to abrogate suppression in both human and murine suppressive assays (Garin et al., 2007; Shevach, 2009).

Direct killing of responder cells has also been proposed as a mechanism through which T_{reg} cells can suppress immune responses (Cao et al., 2007; Shevach, 2009). T_{reg} cells have been shown to express perforin, granzyme A, and granzyme B under certain conditions (Cao et al., 2007; Shevach, 2009). T_{reg} cells that express this phenotype have been implicated in cytolysis of natural killer cells, T cells, and B cells (Cao et al., 2007; Shevach, 2009). Fas-FasL interaction has also been observed as a suppressive mechanism of T_{reg} cells (Gorbachev & Fairchild, 2010; Strauss et al., 2009). Specifically, stimulation through Fas-FasL coupling has been shown to result in apoptosis of B cells and CD8 T cells in humans (Janssens et al., 2003; Strauss et al., 2009). In addition, there is evidence suggesting that T_{reg} cells can interfere with priming of dendritic cells through Fas-FasL interaction, though it is not clear whether or not this involves cytotoxicity (Gorbachev & Fairchild, 2010).

Other mechanisms that involve T_{reg} cell interference with antigen-presenting cells have also been observed. T_{reg} cells constitutively express CTLA-4, which binds the costimulatory molecules CD80 and CD86 (Shevach, 2009). The role of CTLA-4 is not clear, but there are a number of theories as to how it may function. First, CTLA-4 engagement of CD80 and CD86 may restrict the further expression of costimulatory molecules by antigen-presenting cells (Onishi et al., 2008). Second, CTLA-4 may actually signal antigen-presenting cells to downregulate the expression of CD80 and CD86 (Onishi et al., 2008; Shevach, 2009). Third, the binding of CTLA-4 may simply block CD80 and CD86 from interacting with other cells, thus preventing the delivery of costimulatory signals (Shevach, 2009).

The expression of LAG-3, a homolog of CD4 that binds MHC class II (Liang et al., 2008), by T_{reg} cells may also be a mechanism through which these cells exert their influences. LAG-3 produced by T_{reg} cells has been demonstrated to suppress the maturation of antigen-presenting cells (Liang et al., 2008). T_{reg} cell expression of CD39 and CD73 may also prevent activation of antigen-presenting cells (Deaglio et al., 2007). These two surface molecules function together to break down extracellular ATP, which is released in large concentrations from damaged cells (Deaglio et al., 2007). Antigen-presenting cells can sense this extracellular ATP and undergo maturation and activation (Deaglio et al., 2007; Shevach, 2009). By breaking down this ATP, T_{reg} cells may be able to prevent activation of these antigen-presenting cells (Deaglio et al., 2007). Other mechanisms have also been suggested, such as secretion of fibrinogen-like protein 2 (fgl2), which may also depress the function of antigen-presenting cells, or surface expression of neurolipin-1 (Nrp-1), which may increase the strength of T_{reg} cell binding to antigen-presenting cells (Sarris et al., 2008; Shalev et al., 2008).

Finally, there is evidence to suggest that T_{reg} cells can prevent the activation of other cells by selective uptake of IL-2 (Chen et al., 2011; de la Rosa et al., 2004; Pandiyan et al., 2007).

Without IL-2, responder cells may never become activated, or they may become anergic or undergo apoptosis in the absence of costimulatory IL-2 (Chen et al., 2011; de la Rosa et al., 2004; Pandiyan et al., 2007). These potential mechanisms are summarized in Table 1.

Within the respiratory environment, most T_{reg} cell research has focused on the role of these cells in the suppression of asthma. Asthma is a chronic inflammatory disease that afflicts the airways, resulting in airway hyperreactivity and spontaneous airway obstruction (Lloyd &. Hawrylowicz, 2009). It currently affects an estimated 300 million people worldwide, most of whom control the symptoms with glucocorticoid treatment (Lloyd & Hawrylowicz, 2009). Asthma is generally associated with a Th2 response, involving release of inflammatory mediators by T cells, mast cells and eosinophils (Lloyd & Hawrylowicz, 2009; Ray et al., 2010).

T_{reg} cells have long been implicated in the control of asthma, though the mechanisms through which they accomplish this control are still being studied (Lloyd & Hawrylowicz, 2009; McGuirk et al., 2010; Ray et al., 2010). Depletion of T_{reg} cells in murine models of asthma has been shown to greatly exacerbate symptoms (Lewkowich et al., 2005). This has been connected to a decrease in the Th1-promoting cytokine IL-12 and a concurrent increase in the Th2-associated cytokine IL-13 (Lewkowich et al., 2005). In addition, adoptive transfer of T_{reg} cells has been shown to prevent airway inflammation and hyperreactivity, or even to suppress symptoms when transferred after the onset of disease (Kearley et al., 2008).

Importantly, humans with mutations that impair T_{reg} cell function tend to have a higher incidence of asthma (Caudy et al., 2007; Lloyd & Hawrylowicz, 2009). Asthmatic children have been observed to have lower levels of T_{reg} cells in their lungs as compared with non-asthmatics (Hartl et al., 2007). Another study suggests that asthmatics have lower overall expression of FoxP3 compared to healthy donors (Lloyd & Hawrylowicz, 2009). Furthermore, glucocorticoid treatment has been shown to transiently increase T_{reg} cell numbers in asthmatic patients (Ryanna et al., 2009). A number of strategies have been proposed to increase T_{reg} cells in asthmatics, including isolation and *in vitro* expansion of T_{reg} cells, followed by their transfer back into the host (Ryanna et al., 2009). However, this would be an expensive and lengthy process. Thus, other therapies designed to promote *in vivo* T_{reg} cell expansion are currently being explored.

Recently, T_{reg} cells have also been shown to express toll-like receptors, and experiments have demonstrated that toll-like receptors have an impact on T_{reg} cell function (Dai et al., 2009; van Maren et al., 2008). However, depending on the type of toll-like receptor that is stimulated, T_{reg} cell function may be either enhanced or depressed (Dai et al., 2009; van Maren et al., 2008). This suggests, of course, that T_{reg} cells may have different responses to pathogens depending on the type of antigen encountered and the type of toll-like receptor signal that is received. Thus, the role of T_{reg} cells in different bacterial infections may vary widely depending on the nature of the bacteria. As such, the effect of T_{reg} cells in respiratory infections can be complex and difficult to predict.

4. Bacterial Respiratory Pathogens

4.1 Mycoplasma

As an infectious disease, mycoplasmas are probably the most under recognized pathogens known today. Often misconceived as a common cross-contaminate (Homberger &

Associated Protein/s	Potential Mechanism	Target Cell
Interleukin-10, TGF-β	Interference with T helper type 1 development and with secretion of proinflammatory cytokines	T cells, B cells, antigen-presenting cells (Bluestone & Abbas, 2003; Vignali et al., 2008; von Boehmer, 2005)
Interleukin-35	Unknown	Unknown (Chaturvedi et al., 2011; Collison et al., 2007; Collison et al., 2010)
Interferon-γ, Interleukin-17	Interference with T helper type 2 responses	Unknown
Galectin-1	Cell cycle arrest, inhibition of proinflammatory cytokine secretion, apoptosis	T cells, B cells (Garin et al., 2007; Shevach, 2009)
Perforin, Granzyme A, Granzyme B	Direct cytotoxicity	T cells, B cells, NK cells (Cao et al., 2007; Shevach, 2009)
Fas-FasL	Direct cytotoxicity, interference with antigen priming (dendritic cells)	B cells, CD8 T cells, Dendritic cells (Gorbachev & Fairchild, 2010; Strauss et al., 2009)
CTLA-4	Inhibition of antigen-presenting cell maturation, induced downregulation of CD80 and CD86 expression, blockade of CD80 and CD86	Antigen-presenting cells (Onishi et al., 2008; Shevach, 2009)
LAG-3	Inhibition of antigen-presenting cell maturation	Antigen-presenting cells (Liang et al., 2008)
CD39, CD73	Inhibition of antigen-presenting cell activation through breakdown of extracellular ATP	Antigen-presenting cells (Deaglio et al., 2007; Shevach, 2009)
Fgl2	Inhibition of antigen-presenting cells	Antigen-presenting cells (Sarris et al., 2008; Shalev et al., 2008)
Nrp-1	Strengthening of interaction with antigen-presenting cells	Antigen-presenting cells (Sarris et al., 2008; Shalev et al., 2008)
Interleukin-2	Uptake of exogenous interleukin-2, prevention of responder cell activation	T cells, B cells, Antigen-presenting cells (Chen et al., 2011; de la Rosa et al., 2004; Pandiyan et al., 2007)

Table 1. Mechanisms of Regulatory T Cell-Mediated Suppression

Thomann, 1994), mycoplasmas are in fact the etiological agent of a wide range of diseases in both animals and humans (Krause & Taylor-Robinson, 1992; Simecka et al., 1992). Because of their small size, mycoplasmas were first believed to be of viral origin. First isolated in 1898, *Mycoplasma mycoides* subsp. *mycoides*, was reported as the agent of contagious bovine pleuropneumonia in cattle (Nocard & Roux, 1990). Since, Mycoplasma species have been isolated from almost every domestic and laboratory animal.

Mycoplasma is commonly found as a respiratory pathogen. For example, *Mycoplasma pneumoniae*, the most common Mycoplasma in humans, causes up to 30% of all cases of community-acquired pneumonia. One study detected *M. pneumoniae* in over half of children above the age of five. This would make Mycoplasma the single most common pathogen in humans. While most cases of Mycoplasma infection are not life threatening, some do require hospitalization (more than 100,000 people per year). Mycoplasmas have also been suggested to have a role in the exacerbation of chronic asthma and certain autoimmune conditions (Atkinson et al., 2008; Dobbs et al., 2010; Woolard et al., 2004).

There exists an interesting interplay between Mycoplasma and the host immune response. Most of the information in this regard is due to studies using the natural murine pathogen *Mycoplasma pulmonis*, which causes acute and chronic diseases of the respiratory tract in rats and mice (Hardy et al., 2002). Several studies demonstrated that immune responses against mycoplasma can be immunopathologic, contributing to disease severity. However, immune responses are also important in restricting infection to the lungs, preventing dissemination to other sites. Severe combined immunodeficient mice (T and B cell deficient) and athymic mice (T cell-deficient) develop less severe pulmonary lesions due to *M. pulmonis* infection than similarly infected wild type mice (Evengard et al., 1994; Keystone et al., 1980). Adoptive transfer of lymphocytes into severe combined immunodeficient mice prior to *M. pulmonis* infection restored the level of mycoplasma disease (Cartner et al., 1998). Importantly, no difference in lung colony forming units was observed in these studies, providing further evidence that the development of disease is due to immunopathologic immune responses. Depletion of T cells from hamsters showed a similar reduction in lesions after infection with *M. pneumoniae* (Taylor et al., 1974). Studies utilizing *M. pulmonis* have shown that disease severity is directly related to Th cells. Depletion of these cells prior to infection led to significant decreases in disease severity, as measured by weight loss and lesion incidence (Jones et al., 2002). Since Th cell responses can be separated into Th1 or Th2 lineages, further studies were performed using IFN-γ-deficient mice and IL-4-deficient mice. Mice lacking IFN-γ (which preferentially mounted a Th2 cell response) developed more severe disease upon infection with *Mycoplasma pulmonis* at an early time point (Woolard et al., 2004). In contrast, mice lacking IL-4 (which preferentially mounted a Th1 cell response) did not demonstrate any exacerbation of disease (Woolard et al., 2004). Furthermore, immunization with mycoplasma antigen results in resistance to infection in IL-4-deficient mice, but not IFN-γ– deficient mice (Bodhankar et al., 2010). Overall, these studies suggest that Th2 responses contribute to mycoplasma-associated immunopathology, while Th1 responses promote resistance to infection.

$CD8^+$ cytotoxic T cells also play a role in mycoplasma disease, though their role may be regulatory in nature. When $CD8^+$ T cells were depleted from mice prior to infection with *M. pulmonis*, disease severity increased (Jones et al., 2002). Similar results were observed in studies involving rats. F344 rats developed less severe disease after infection with *M. pulmonis* as compared to LEW rats (Davis & Cassell, 1982; Davis et al., 1982, 1985). This was connected to higher levels of $CD8^+$ T cells in the lungs and draining lymph nodes of F344 rats compared to LEW rats. This effect may be due to the secretion of IFN-γ by $CD8^+$ T cells, which could dampen immunopathologic Th2 cell responses.

Recent studies from our lab showed that T_{reg} cells clearly control the severity of disease in mycoplasma respiratory infection. Depletion of T_{reg} cells using anti-CD25 antibody prior to infection with *M. pulmonis* resulted in significant increases in clinical disease severity. The T_{reg} cell-depleted mice lost significantly more weight over the course of the study and displayed a significantly higher incidence of gross lung lesions. In addition, T_{reg} cell-depleted mice had more severe histological lung lesions, which included increased peribronchial infiltration of inflammatory cells, airway exudate, epithelial hyperplasia, and alveolitis. This effect was clearly related to a decrease in the level of T_{reg} cells, as the anti-CD25 antibody was shown to specifically deplete $CD4^+CD25^+FoxP3^+$ cells without affecting other cell populations. Increased disease in T_{reg} cell-depleted mice was also concurrent not only with increases in lung cell infiltration but also with increases in the levels of mycoplasma-specific serum antibodies. Significantly, depletion of T_{reg} cells had no effect on mycoplasma numbers (Odeh & Simecka, in preparation). Thus, T_{reg} cells dampen the severity of inflammatory disease due to mycoplasma respiratory infection most likely through regulation of immune responses, in an apparent attempt to limit damage within the lung, but T_{reg} cell activity does not contribute to persistence of mycoplasma infections, in contrast to other studies such as those discussed above with Leishmania infection.

The mechanisms of how T_{reg} cells regulate the development of inflammatory lesions is under investigation, but our results suggest that it is a result of activities of a novel population of T_{reg} cells. Our studies demonstrated that there was an increase in total cell numbers in the lung of infected mice after T_{reg} cell depletion, with almost all populations being affected. Most interestingly, there was a preferential increase in the percentage of IL-13$^+$ cells in the lower respiratory lymph nodes due to T_{reg} cell depletion prior to infection, suggesting T_{reg} cells suppressed Th2 cell responses and perhaps promoted Th1 cell responses. Interestingly, there were increases in T_{reg} cells in lower respiratory tract lymph nodes during mycoplasma disease pathogenesis, but neither IL-10 nor TGF-β production by these T_{reg} cells in response to mycoplasma could be demonstrated. Further characterization found that these T_{reg} cells included two subpopulations that expressed either intracellular IFN-γ or IL-17, suggesting that mycoplasma-specific T_{reg} cells may act through novel mechanisms. In fact, *in vitro* cultures containing T_{reg} cells and Th cells from infected mice secreted significantly higher levels of IFN-γ and IL-17 when stimulated with mycoplasma antigen as compared to Th cells alone. These data provided evidence that T_{reg} cells might stimulate the secretion of IFN-γ and IL-17 cytokines by Th cells. In support, depletion of T_{reg} cells from infected mice led to a decrease in the *in vivo* secretion of IFN-γ and IL-17 by T helper cells (Odeh & Simecka, in preparation). These data suggest that two unique populations of T_{reg} cells, IFN-γ$^+$ or IL-17$^+$, develop in mycoplasma-infected mice, and that these novel populations of T_{reg} cells participate in control of the disease. Furthermore, these data suggest that IFN-γ$^+$ and IL-17$^+$ T_{reg} cells promote the secretion of these cytokines by Th cells. Thus, the activation of this unique population of T_{reg} cells in mycoplasma infections may be beneficial, as the stimulation of IFN-γ and IL-17 production by Th cells would suppress the development of immunopathologic Th2 cell responses.

4.2 Mycobacterium

Current estimates are that one-third of the world population is infected with *Mycobacterium tuberculosis* (Bloom & Small, 1998; Dai et al., 2009; Urdahl et al., 2011). *M. tuberculosis* is responsible for 1.7 million deaths worldwide each year, though most of these deaths occur in developing countries, and/or in immunocompromised individuals (Kwan & Ernst, 2011;

Lawn & Zumla, 2011). The pathogenesis of tuberculosis is interesting. The disease is characterized by the persistence of infection and the formation of granulomas by the host to prevent the spread of the infection. Upon initial exposure, mycobacteria are phagocytosed by alveolar macrophages (Redford et al., 2011). However, through mechanisms that involve altered production of reactive nitrogen intermediates and prevention of phagosome maturation, *M. tuberculosis* bacteria are able to survive within the host cells (Flynn & Chan, 2003; Redford et al., 2011). The persistence of Mycobacteria leads to granuloma formation, which not only prevents spread of the infection, but also benefits the bacteria by masking them from the immune response (Flynn & Chan, 2003). This results in a latent infection that never progresses to symptomatic tuberculosis (Flynn & Chan, 2003). Studies have demonstrated that control of tuberculosis is dependent on IL-12 and Th1 cell responses (Altare et al., 1998; Newport et al., 2003; Redford et al., 2011; Urdahl et al., 2011). Th1 cell responses are critical in macrophage activation and the formation and maintenance of the granuloma (Saunders & Britton, 2007). Thus, like Mycoplasma and other infectious diseases, the host response to *M. tuberculosis* infection is critical in determining the extent of lesions and outcome of infection, and, in the case of *M. tuberculosis*, impairment of Th1 responses against the pathogen leads to spread of infection and more severe disease.

A small percentage of infected individuals, for reasons that are still not well understood, will develop symptoms, which include fever, cough, chest pain, and night sweats (Bark et al., 2011; Redford et al., 2011), but this is likely linked to a breakdown in Th1 responses meant to isolate the infection. One of the common findings in individuals with symptomatic tuberculosis, either from primary exposure or from reactivation of latent infection, is a high concentration of IL-10 in the blood (Boussiotis et al., 2000; Redford et al., 2011). In support of a critical role for IL-10 production in the pathogenesis of tuberculosis, IL-10 production was associated with the reactivation of tuberculosis in a mouse model of this disease (Turner et al., 2002). IL-10 can dampen macrophage activation and help stimulate the development of Th2 cell responses and alternatively activated macrophages (Kahnert et al., 2006). Taken together, IL-10 production in patients with active tuberculosis likely impairs the development or maintenance of a Th1 proinflammatory response, leading to a breakdown of the granulomas that are critical in limiting the spread of infection and damage to the host.

Since populations of T_{reg} cells are often a source of IL-10, studies were performed examining the role of T_{reg} cells in *M. tuberculosis* respiratory infection. T_{reg} cells in mice were indeed found to proliferate in response to mycobacteria infection (Shafiani et al., 2010) and were observed to localize to sites of Th cell responses in the lungs (Kahnert et al., 2006). By adoptively transferring *M. tuberculosis* specific T_{reg} cells, it was found that T_{reg} cells delayed the infiltration of effector T cells into the lung environment, and led to higher bacterial counts in the lungs of recipient mice (Shafiani et al., 2010). This delay in cell infiltration due to T_{reg} cells likely impaired host responses that effectively control mycobacteria infection, disrupting protective granuloma formation. In fact, depletion of T_{reg} cells results in higher numbers of mycobacteria (Kahnert et al., 2006). Thus, the production of T_{reg} cell responses in tuberculosis can impair host resistance to infection, and in fact, the overactivity of T_{reg} cells could participate in the transition of quiescent forms of tuberculosis to active disease. This represents a case where the attempt of T_{reg} cells to dampen inflammatory responses may actually have a negative effect on disease outcome.

4.3 Bordetella

Bordetella pertussis is the bacterium responsible for whooping cough, a disease that can afflict all age groups, but which is especially predominant and dangerous in children (Dunne et al., 2009; Marzouqi et al., 2010). In addition to the cough itself, other symptoms can include fever, nausea, convulsions, pneumonia, and, in severe cases, encephalopathy (Marzouqi et al., 2010). Even with the use of pertussis vaccines, the incidence of Bordetella infections is very high, with 40-50 million cases reported worldwide each year (Marzouqi et al., 2010). Of these, 300,000-400,000 result in death, mostly in children living in developing countries (Marzouqi et al., 2010). This makes whooping cough the most common vaccine-preventable disease in the world (Marzouqi et al., 2010).

Upon initial exposure, *B. pertussis* adheres to the mucosal epithelium along the respiratory tract (de Gouw et al., 2011). It can then form a protective biofilm that allows it to mask itself from immune cells (de Gouw et al., 2011). There is even evidence that certain strains of Bordetella can invade host cells, thus avoiding many host responses (de Gouw et al., 2011). To promote its longevity and survival within the host, *B. pertussis* produces a number of toxins and virulence factors (de Gouw et al., 2011). It is well established at this point that clearance of Bordetella from the host requires a Th1 response, mediated by IFN-γ (de Gouw et al., 2011). Experiments with vaccines have shown that augmentation of the IFN-γ-mediated Th1 cell response leads to increased clearance of Bordetella (Marzouqi et al., 2010). To interfere with this, Bordetella can induce the production of IL-10, and, most interestingly, can stimulate the proliferation of IL-10-producing T_{reg} cells (de Gouw et al., 2011; Higgins et al., 2003). T_{reg} cells and IL-10 production can then dampen the Th1 cell response against the pathogen, delaying clearance of the organism and increasing its chances of transmission to another host (de Gouw et al., 2011). In mice depleted of T_{reg} cells, there was an increase in the infiltration of immune cells into the lung environment (Higgins et al., 2003). This corresponded with a significant increase in the incidence of lung lesions, indicating a strong inflammatory response against the infection (Higgins et al., 2003). Thus, it appears that *B. pertussis* harnesses the host's own mechanisms to modulate inflammatory responses by stimulating T_{reg} cells to dampen these responses, thus preventing efficient elimination of the pathogen.

However, the role of T_{reg} cells in Bordetella infections is more complex. The cascade of events through which *B. pertussis* stimulates T_{reg} cell activity is mediated by toll-like receptors. Studies demonstrated that Bordetella infection results in the production of IL-10 by dendritic cells (Higgins et al., 2003). The stimulation of dendritic cells to produce IL-10 is driven by engagement of toll-like receptor 4 (TLR4). The IL-10 released by Bordetella-stimulated dendritic cells, in turn, helps to promote the expansion of the IL-10-secreting T_{reg} cell population (Higgins et al., 2003). This is supported by studies showing that *B. pertussis* infection of TLR4-deficient mice results in a significantly lower number of antigen-specific T_{reg} cells than is found in wild-type mice. Furthermore, there was a concurrent decrease in the IL-10 levels (Higgins et al., 2003). The absence of IL-10-secreting T_{reg} cells resulted in an increase in the infiltration of immune cells into the lung environment (Higgins et al., 2003). This corresponded with a significant increase in the incidence of lung lesions, indicating a strong immunopathologic response (Higgins et al., 2003). Thus, *B. pertussis* utilizes a pathway mediated by TLR4 recognition of the organisms to stimulate T_{reg} cell-mediated suppression of inflammatory responses that prevents both efficient clearance of the organism and damaging immunopathologic responses.

4.4 Chlamydia and streptococcus

There has been little additional work done on the role of T_{reg} cells in other types of respiratory infections. However, there are some interesting studies on Chlamydia and Streptococcus respiratory infections that suggest an important role for T_{reg} cells in these diseases.

Chlamydia muridarum is a murine pathogen that causes disease similar to that of *Chlamydia trachomatis* in humans (Carey et al., 2011). As such, it is commonly used as a murine model. Normally, *C. trachomatis* manifests in humans as a sexually-transmitted disease, infecting the genital tract (Carey et al., 2011). However, it can infect other sites as well, including the respiratory tract, and, as a result, experiments have been performed using experimental *C. muridarum* lung infections (He et al., 2011). TLR2-deficient mice infected intranasally with *C. muridarum* developed more severe lung inflammation and more severe overall disease as compared to chlamydia-infected wild type mice (He et al., 2011). This was associated with an increase in the concentrations of the profinflammatory cytokines IFN-γ, IL-12, and IL-17, and a concurrent increase in the infiltration of immune cells in lung tissue (He et al., 2011). However, the lack of TLR2 had no effect on the clearance of the organism, as no differences in bacterial counts were found between wild type mice and TLR2-deficient mice (He et al., 2011). Recently, engagement of TLR2 was shown to promote the development of T_{reg} cells (Chen et al., 2009). Thus, it has been theorized that the increased immunopathology in *C. muridarum*-infected, TLR2-deficient mice may be due to a deficiency of T_{reg} cells, though this has not yet been conclusively demonstrated (He et al., 2011). If so, the TLR-mediated mechanisms involved in promoting T_{reg} cell activity by *C. muridarum* infection may be similar to those described above for Bordetella, and this could be a common approach through which some bacteria harness the immunosuppressive activity of T_{reg} cells.

One of the most common respiratory bacteria, and the one most often responsible for severe cases of pneumonia, is *Streptococcus pneumoniae* (Jones et al., 2010). Despite its role as the quintessential pneumococcal pathogen, very little work has been performed in the area of *S. pneumoniae* and T_{reg} cells. In studies that examined the role of Streptococcus in asthma and airway hyperreactivity, it was shown that both intact *S. pneumoniae* and pneumococcal proteins can induce the development of T_{reg} cells (Preston et al., 2011; Thorburn et al., 2010). The role of T_{reg} cells in pneumococcal disease is unclear, but recent studies have begun examining the role of T_{reg} cells in the generation of humoral immune responses against *S. pneumoniae*. Mice were treated with T_{reg} cell-depleting antibodies and infected with live streptococcus. These mice develop similar levels of antibody responses as those in normal mice with intact T_{reg} cell activity (Lee et al., 2005). Similar results were obtained when mice were given heat-killed streptococcus or protein-polysaccharide conjugates (which are used in *S. pneumoniae* vaccines) (Lee et al., 2005). Thus, it appears that T_{reg} cells do not play a role in the development of anti-streptococcal humoral immunity. Further studies are needed to determine whether T_{reg} cells play a role in disease pathogenesis or modulating protective immunity against *S. pneumoniae*. However, the data do suggest that other bacterial species can promote the development of T_{reg} cell responses, which may play variable levels of importance depending upon the bacteria, the host, and the infection.

5. Conclusion

As discussed above, there has been limited work examining the role of T_{reg} cells in the pathogenesis of bacterial lung diseases. It is clear that modulation of T_{reg} cell activity is done in some cases to benefit the host and in other cases benefitting the pathogen. Because the lung is a critical organ and a common site for exposure to infection, T_{reg} cell activity is probably most important in dampening inflammatory responses to infections in order to minimize damage to the lung tissue. As indicated earlier, there are multiple mechanisms through which T_{reg} cells modulate these inflammatory responses and lesions. Although one of the most common mechanisms is through the production of the anti-inflammatory cytokine IL-10, T_{reg} cells, as shown in Mycoplasma pneumonia, may also prevent the development of potentially damaging immune responses by promoting other types of immunity. Interestingly, some respiratory pathogens, as well as other bacteria, have devised mechanisms to promote T_{reg} cell development in an apparent attempt to interfere with host resistance and delay their clearance. Thus, T_{reg} cells likely have varied activities in pulmonary bacterial diseases, which are probably host and bacterial species specific.

Research on T_{reg} cells and bacterial infections may also benefit treatment of other respiratory diseases. In recent years, a large amount of research has examined the role of T_{reg} cells in asthma and other allergic diseases. Specifically, research indicates that stimulating the development and activation of regulatory T cells may suppress allergic reactions and asthma (Ray et al., 2010). Suggested methods for how to stimulate the development of T_{reg} cell responses vary. Interestingly, one possible approach involves treatment of patients with bacteria or bacterial products (Fonseca & Kline, 2009; Trujillo & Erb, 2003), and indeed, there are cases in which this type of therapy has been experimentally validated (Crother et al., 2011; Preston et al., 2011; Thorburn et al., 2010). This promising approach may have a broader utility since, as discussed in this article, different kinds of bacteria appear to be able to elicit different types of T_{reg} cell responses. This suggests that further studies into how bacteria activate T_{reg} cells are merited and could result in novel approaches to selectively and appropriately activate T_{reg} cells in the treatment of certain human diseases.

6. Acknowledgements

The authors wish to thank some of the individuals which contributed to and inspired the work described, Drs Nicole Dobbs, Harlan Jones, Matthew "Doc" Woolard, Xiangle Sun and Sheetal Bodhankar, as well as Leslie Tabor and others. Some of the work described in this report was supported by a grant from the National Institute of Allergy and Infectious Disease (NIAID, 5RO1AI042075) of the National Institutes of Health (NIH).

7. References

Altare, Durandy, Lammas, et al. (1998). Impairment of mycobacterial immunity in human interleukin-12 receptor deficiency. *Science,* 280, 5368, (May 29), pp. 1432-1435, 0036-8075; 0036-8075

Atkinson, Balish & Waites. (2008). Epidemiology, clinical manifestations, pathogenesis and laboratory detection of Mycoplasma pneumoniae infections. *FEMS Microbiol.Rev.,* 32, 6, (Nov), pp. 956-973, 0168-6445

Ayyoub, Deknuydt, Raimbaud, et al. (2009). Human memory FOXP3+ Tregs secrete IL-17 ex vivo and constitutively express the T (H)17 lineage-specific transcription factor RORgamma t. *Proc.Natl.Acad.Sci.U.S.A.*, 106, 21, (May 26), pp. 8635-8640, 1091-6490; 0027-8424

Bach. (2003). Regulatory T cells under scrutiny. *Nat.Rev.Immunol.*, 3, 3, (Mar), pp. 189-198, 1474-1733

Bark, Dietze, Okwera, Quelapio, Thiel & Johnson. (2011). Clinical symptoms and microbiological outcomes in tuberculosis treatment trials. *Tuberculosis (Edinb)*, (Aug 1), 1873-281X; 1472-9792

Bayer, Lee, de la Barrera, Surh & Malek. (2008). A function for IL-7R for CD4+CD25+Foxp3+ T regulatory cells. *J.Immunol.*, 181, 1, (Jul 1), pp. 225-234, 0022-1767

Belkaid. (2003). The role of CD4 (+)CD25 (+) regulatory T cells in Leishmania infection. *Expert Opin.Biol.Ther.*, 3, 6, (Sep), pp. 875-885, 1471-2598; 1471-2598

Beriou, Costantino, Ashley, et al. (2009). IL-17-producing human peripheral regulatory T cells retain suppressive function. *Blood*, 113, 18, (Apr 30), pp. 4240-4249, 1528-0020; 0006-4971

Bloom & Small. (1998). The evolving relation between humans and Mycobacterium tuberculosis. *N.Engl.J.Med.*, 338, 10, (Mar 5), pp. 677-678, 0028-4793; 0028-4793

Bluestone & Abbas. (2003). Natural versus adaptive regulatory T cells. *Nat.Rev.Immunol.*, 3, 3, (Mar), pp. 253-257, 1474-1733

Bodhankar, Sun, Woolard & Simecka. (2010). Interferon gamma and interleukin 4 have contrasting effects on immunopathology and the development of protective adaptive immunity against mycoplasma respiratory disease. *J.Infect.Dis.*, 202, 1, (Jul 1), pp. 39-51, 1537-6613; 0022-1899

Born, Lahn, Takeda, Kanehiro, O'Brien & Gelfand. (2000). Role of gammadelta T cells in protecting normal airway function. *Respir.Res.*, 1, 3, pp. 151-158, 1465-9921; 1465-9921

Boussiotis, Tsai, Yunis, et al. (2000). IL-10-producing T cells suppress immune responses in anergic tuberculosis patients. *J.Clin.Invest.*, 105, 9, (May), pp. 1317-1325, 0021-9738; 0021-9738

Cao, Cai, Fehniger, et al. (2007). Granzyme B and perforin are important for regulatory T cell-mediated suppression of tumor clearance. *Immunity*, 27, 4, (Oct), pp. 635-646, 1074-7613

Carey, Cunningham, Andrew, Hafner, Timms & Beagley. (2011). A comparison of the effects of a chlamydial vaccine administered during or after a C. muridarum urogenital infection of female mice. *Vaccine*, 29, 38, (Sep 2), pp. 6505-6513, 1873-2518; 0264-410X

Cartner, Lindsey, Gibbs-Erwin, Cassell & Simecka. (1998). Roles of innate and adaptive immunity in respiratory mycoplasmosis. *Infect.Immun.*, 66, 8, (Aug), pp. 3485-3491, 0019-9567; 0019-9567

Caudy, Reddy, Chatila, Atkinson & Verbsky. (2007). CD25 deficiency causes an immune dysregulation, polyendocrinopathy, enteropathy, X-linked-like syndrome, and defective IL-10 expression from CD4 lymphocytes. *J.Allergy Clin.Immunol.*, 119, 2, (Feb), pp. 482-487, 0091-6749; 0091-6749

Chaturvedi, Collison, Guy, Workman & Vignali. (2011). Cutting edge: Human regulatory T cells require IL-35 to mediate suppression and infectious tolerance. *J.Immunol.,* 186, 12, (Jun 15), pp. 6661-6666, 1550-6606; 0022-1767

Chen, Davidson, Huter & Shevach. (2009). Engagement of TLR2 does not reverse the suppressor function of mouse regulatory T cells, but promotes their survival. *J.Immunol.,* 183, 7, (Oct 1), pp. 4458-4466, 1550-6606; 0022-1767

Chen, Haines, Gutcher, et al. (2011). Foxp3 (+) Regulatory T Cells Promote T Helper 17 Cell Development In Vivo through Regulation of Interleukin-2. *Immunity,* 34, 3, (Mar 25), pp. 409-421, 1097-4180; 1074-7613

Collison, Chaturvedi, Henderson, et al. (2010). IL-35-mediated induction of a potent regulatory T cell population. *Nat.Immunol.,* 11, 12, (Dec), pp. 1093-1101, 1529-2916; 1529-2908

Collison, Workman, Kuo, et al. (2007). The inhibitory cytokine IL-35 contributes to regulatory T-cell function. *Nature,* 450, 7169, (Nov 22), pp. 566-569, 1476-4687; 0028-0836

Constant, Lee & Bottomly. (2000). Site of antigen delivery can influence T cell priming: pulmonary environment promotes preferential Th2-type differentiation. *Eur.J.Immunol.,* 30, 3, (Mar), pp. 840-847, 0014-2980; 0014-2980

Crother, Schroder, Karlin, et al. (2011). Chlamydia pneumoniae infection induced allergic airway sensitization is controlled by regulatory T-cells and plasmacytoid dendritic cells. *PLoS One,* 6, 6, pp. e20784, 1932-6203; 1932-6203

Dai, Liu & Li. (2009). Regulatory T cells and Toll-like receptors: what is the missing link? *Int.Immunopharmacol.,* 9, 5, (May), pp. 528-533, 1878-1705; 1567-5769

Davis, Simecka, Williamson, et al. (1985). Nonspecific lymphocyte responses in F344 and LEW rats: susceptibility to murine respiratory mycoplasmosis and examination of cellular basis for strain differences. *Infect.Immun.,* 49, 1, (Jul), pp. 152-158, 0019-9567; 0019-9567

Davis & Cassell. (1982). Murine respiratory mycoplasmosis in LEW and F344 rats: strain differences in lesion severity. *Vet.Pathol.,* 19, 3, (May), pp. 280-293, 0300-9858; 0300-9858

Davis, Thorp, Maddox, Brown & Cassell. (1982). Murine respiratory mycoplasmosis in F344 and LEW rats: evolution of lesions and lung lymphoid cell populations. *Infect.Immun.,* 36, 2, (May), pp. 720-729, 0019-9567; 0019-9567

de Gouw, Diavatopoulos, Bootsma, Hermans & Mooi. (2011). Pertussis: a matter of immune modulation. *FEMS Microbiol.Rev.,* 35, 3, (May), pp. 441-474, 1574-6976; 0168-6445

de la Rosa, Rutz, Dorninger & Scheffold. (2004). Interleukin-2 is essential for CD4+CD25+ regulatory T cell function. *Eur.J.Immunol.,* 34, 9, (Sep), pp. 2480-2488, 0014-2980; 0014-2980

Deaglio, Dwyer, Gao, et al. (2007). Adenosine generation catalyzed by CD39 and CD73 expressed on regulatory T cells mediates immune suppression. *J.Exp.Med.,* 204, 6, (Jun 11), pp. 1257-1265, 0022-1007; 0022-1007

Dobbs, Odeh, Sun & Simecka. (2010). The Multifaceted Role of T cell-mediated Immunity in Pathogenesis and Resistance to Mycoplasma Respiratory Disease, In: *Current Trends in Immunology,* Anonymous (Eds.), Research Trends, Kerala, India

Dunne, Moran, Cummins & Mills. (2009). CD11c+CD8alpha+ dendritic cells promote protective immunity to respiratory infection with Bordetella pertussis. *J.Immunol.*, 183, 1, (Jul 1), pp. 400-410, 1550-6606; 0022-1767

Ellner. (1981). Suppressor cells of man. *Clin.Immunol.Rev.*, 1, 1, pp. 119-214, 0277-9366

Esposito, Ruffini, Bergami, et al. (2010). IL-17- and IFN-gamma-secreting Foxp3+ T cells infiltrate the target tissue in experimental autoimmunity. *J.Immunol.*, 185, 12, (Dec 15), pp. 7467-7473, 1550-6606; 0022-1767

Evengard, Sandstedt, Bolske, Feinstein, Riesenfelt-Orn & Smith. (1994). Intranasal inoculation of Mycoplasma pulmonis in mice with severe combined immunodeficiency (SCID) causes a wasting disease with grave arthritis. *Clin.Exp.Immunol.*, 98, 3, (Dec), pp. 388-394, 0009-9104; 0009-9104

Fang, Ismail, Shelite & Walker. (2009). CD4+ CD25+ Foxp3- T-regulatory cells produce both gamma interferon and interleukin-10 during acute severe murine spotted fever rickettsiosis. *Infect.Immun.*, 77, 9, (Sep), pp. 3838-3849, 1098-5522

Fehervari & Sakaguchi. (2004a). Development and function of CD25+CD4+ regulatory T cells. *Curr.Opin.Immunol.*, 16, 2, (Apr), pp. 203-208, 0952-7915; 0952-7915

Fehervari & Sakaguchi. (2004b). A paragon of self-tolerance: CD25+CD4+ regulatory T cells and the control of immune responses. *Arthritis Res.Ther.*, 6, 1, pp. 19-25, 1478-6362; 1478-6354

Flores-Borja, Mauri & Ehrenstein. (2008). Restoring the balance: harnessing regulatory T cells for therapy in rheumatoid arthritis. *Eur.J.Immunol.*, 38, 4, (Apr), pp. 934-937, 0014-2980

Flynn & Chan. (2003). Immune evasion by Mycobacterium tuberculosis: living with the enemy. *Curr.Opin.Immunol.*, 15, 4, (Aug), pp. 450-455, 0952-7915; 0952-7915

Fonseca & Kline. (2009). Use of CpG oligonucleotides in treatment of asthma and allergic disease. *Adv.Drug Deliv.Rev.*, 61, 3, (Mar 28), pp. 256-262, 1872-8294; 0169-409X

Fu, Yopp, Mao, et al. (2004). CD4+ CD25+ CD62+ T-regulatory cell subset has optimal suppressive and proliferative potential. *Am.J.Transplant.*, 4, 1, (Jan), pp. 65-78, 1600-6135; 1600-6135

Garin, Chu, Golshayan, Cernuda-Morollon, Wait & Lechler. (2007). Galectin-1: a key effector of regulation mediated by CD4+CD25+ T cells. *Blood*, 109, 5, (Mar 1), pp. 2058-2065, 0006-4971; 0006-4971

Gorbachev & Fairchild. (2010). CD4+CD25+ regulatory T cells utilize FasL as a mechanism to restrict DC priming functions in cutaneous immune responses. *Eur.J.Immunol.*, 40, 7, (Jul), pp. 2006-2015, 1521-4141; 0014-2980

Hardy, Jafri, Olsen, et al. (2002). *Mycoplasma pneumoniae* induces chronic respiratory infection, airway hyperreactivity, and pulmonary inflammation: a murine model of infection-associated chronic reactive airway disease. *Infect.Immun.*, 70, 2, (Feb), pp. 649-654, 0019-9567; 0019-9567

Hartl, Koller, Mehlhorn, et al. (2007). Quantitative and functional impairment of pulmonary CD4+CD25hi regulatory T cells in pediatric asthma. *J.Allergy Clin.Immunol.*, 119, 5, (May), pp. 1258-1266, 0091-6749; 0091-6749

He, Nair, Mekasha, Alroy, O'Connell & Ingalls. (2011). Enhanced virulence of Chlamydia muridarum respiratory infections in the absence of TLR2 activation. *PLoS One*, 6, 6, pp. e20846, 1932-6203; 1932-6203

Higgins, Lavelle, McCann, et al. (2003). Toll-like receptor 4-mediated innate IL-10 activates antigen-specific regulatory T cells and confers resistance to Bordetella pertussis by inhibiting inflammatory pathology. *J.Immunol.,* 171, 6, (Sep 15), pp. 3119-3127, 0022-1767; 0022-1767

Homberger & Thomann. (1994). Transmission of murine viruses and mycoplasma in laboratory mouse colonies with respect to housing conditions. *Lab.Anim.,* 28, 2, (Apr), pp. 113-120, 0023-6772; 0023-6772

Hori, Nomura & Sakaguchi. (2003). Control of regulatory T cell development by the transcription factor Foxp3. *Science,* 299, 5609, (Feb 14), pp. 1057-1061,

Janssens, Carlier, Wu, VanderElst, Jacquemin & Saint-Remy. (2003). CD4+CD25+ T cells lyse antigen-presenting B cells by Fas-Fas ligand interaction in an epitope-specific manner. *J.Immunol.,* 171, 9, (Nov 1), pp. 4604-4612, 0022-1767; 0022-1767

Jones, Tabor, Sun, Woolard & Simecka. (2002). Depletion of CD8+ T cells exacerbates CD4+ Th cell-associated inflammatory lesions during murine mycoplasma respiratory disease. *J.Immunol.,* 168, 7, (Apr 1), pp. 3493-3501, 0022-1767

Jones, Jacobs & Sader. (2010). Evolving trends in Streptococcus pneumoniae resistance: implications for therapy of community-acquired bacterial pneumonia. *Int.J.Antimicrob.Agents,* 36, 3, (Sep), pp. 197-204, 1872-7913; 0924-8579

Jonuleit, Schmitt, Stassen, Tuettenberg, Knop & Enk. (2001). Identification and functional characterization of human CD4 (+)CD25 (+) T cells with regulatory properties isolated from peripheral blood. *J.Exp.Med.,* 193, 11, (Jun 4), pp. 1285-1294, 0022-1007; 0022-1007

Kahnert, Seiler, Stein, et al. (2006). Alternative activation deprives macrophages of a coordinated defense program to Mycobacterium tuberculosis. *Eur.J.Immunol.,* 36, 3, (Mar), pp. 631-647, 0014-2980; 0014-2980

Kawai & Akira. (2011). Toll-like receptors and their crosstalk with other innate receptors in infection and immunity. *Immunity,* 34, 5, (May 27), pp. 637-650, 1097-4180; 1074-7613

Kearley, Robinson & Lloyd. (2008). CD4+CD25+ regulatory T cells reverse established allergic airway inflammation and prevent airway remodeling. *J.Allergy Clin.Immunol.,* 122, 3, (Sep), pp. 617-24.e6, 1097-6825; 0091-6749

Keystone, Taylor-Robinson, Osborn, Ling, Pope & Fornasier. (1980). Effect of T-cell deficiency on the chronicity of arthritis induced in mice by Mycoplasma pulmonis. *Infect.Immun.,* 27, 1, (Jan), pp. 192-196, 0019-9567; 0019-9567

Krause & Taylor-Robinson. (1992). Mycoplasmas which infect humans In: *Mycoplasmas: molecular biology and pathogenesis,* Anonymous (Eds.), pp. 417, American Society for Microbiology, 1555810500, Washington, D.C.

Kwan & Ernst. (2011). HIV and tuberculosis: a deadly human syndemic. *Clin.Microbiol.Rev.,* 24, 2, (Apr), pp. 351-376, 1098-6618; 0893-8512

Lawn & Zumla. (2011). Tuberculosis. *Lancet,* 378, 9785, (Jul 2), pp. 57-72, 1474-547X; 0140-6736

Lee, Sen & Snapper. (2005). Endogenous CD4+ CD25+ regulatory T cells play no apparent role in the acute humoral response to intact Streptococcus pneumoniae. *Infect.Immun.,* 73, 7, (Jul), pp. 4427-4431, 0019-9567; 0019-9567

Lewkowich, Herman, Schleifer, et al. (2005). CD4+CD25+ T cells protect against experimentally induced asthma and alter pulmonary dendritic cell phenotype and function. *J.Exp.Med.*, 202, 11, (Dec 5), pp. 1549-1561, 0022-1007

Liang, Workman, Lee, et al. (2008). Regulatory T cells inhibit dendritic cells by lymphocyte activation gene-3 engagement of MHC class II. *J.Immunol.*, 180, 9, (May 1), pp. 5916-5926, 0022-1767; 0022-1767

Liu, Putnam, Xu-Yu, et al. (2006). CD127 expression inversely correlates with FoxP3 and suppressive function of human CD4+ T reg cells. *J.Exp.Med.*, 203, 7, (Jul 10), pp. 1701-1711, 0022-1007; 0022-1007

Lloyd & Hawrylowicz. (2009). Regulatory T cells in asthma. *Immunity*, 31, 3, (Sep 18), pp. 438-449, 1097-4180

Marzouqi, Richmond, Fry, Wetherall & Mukkur. (2010). Development of improved vaccines against whooping cough: current status. *Hum.Vaccin*, 6, 7, (Jul), pp. 543-553, 1554-8619; 1554-8600

McGuirk, Higgins & Mills. (2010). The role of regulatory T cells in respiratory infections and allergy and asthma. *Curr.Allergy Asthma Rep.*, 10, 1, (Jan), pp. 21-28, 1534-6315; 1529-7322

McHugh & Shevach. (2002). The role of suppressor T cells in regulation of immune responses. *J.Allergy Clin.Immunol.*, 110, 5, (Nov), pp. 693-702, 0091-6749

Mendez, Reckling, Piccirillo, Sacks & Belkaid. (2004). Role for CD4 (+) CD25 (+) regulatory T cells in reactivation of persistent leishmaniasis and control of concomitant immunity. *J.Exp.Med.*, 200, 2, (Jul 19), pp. 201-210, 0022-1007; 0022-1007

Morokata, Ishikawa & Yamada. (2000). Antigen dose defines T helper 1 and T helper 2 responses in the lungs of C57BL/6 and BALB/c mice independently of splenic responses. *Immunol.Lett.*, 72, 2, (May 1), pp. 119-126, 0165-2478; 0165-2478

Mudd, Teague & Farris. (2006). Regulatory T cells and systemic lupus erythematosus. *Scand.J.Immunol.*, 64, 3, (Sep), pp. 211-218, 0300-9475

Newport, Awomoyi & Blackwell. (2003). Polymorphism in the interferon-gamma receptor-1 gene and susceptibility to pulmonary tuberculosis in The Gambia. *Scand.J.Immunol.*, 58, 4, (Oct), pp. 383-385, 0300-9475; 0300-9475

Nocard & Roux. (1990). The microbe of pleuropneumonia. 1896. *Rev.Infect.Dis.*, 12, 2, (Mar-Apr), pp. 354-358, 0162-0886; 0162-0886

Nomura & Sakaguchi. (2005). Naturally arising CD25+CD4+ regulatory T cells in tumor immunity. *Curr.Top.Microbiol.Immunol.*, 293, pp. 287-302, 0070-217X

Oh, Kim, Min & Chung. (2008). Role of type II NKT cells in the suppression of graft-versus-host disease. *Crit.Rev.Immunol.*, 28, 3, pp. 249-267, 1040-8401; 1040-8401

Onishi, Fehervari, Yamaguchi & Sakaguchi. (2008). Foxp3+ natural regulatory T cells preferentially form aggregates on dendritic cells in vitro and actively inhibit their maturation. *Proc.Natl.Acad.Sci.U.S.A.*, 105, 29, (Jul 22), pp. 10113-10118, 1091-6490; 0027-8424

Palusinska-Szysz & Janczarek. (2010). Innate immunity to Legionella and toll-like receptors - review. *Folia Microbiol. (Praha)*, 55, 5, (Sep), pp. 508-514, 1874-9356; 0015-5632

Pandiyan, Zheng, Ishihara, Reed & Lenardo. (2007). CD4+CD25+Foxp3+ regulatory T cells induce cytokine deprivation-mediated apoptosis of effector CD4+ T cells. *Nat.Immunol.*, 8, 12, (Dec), pp. 1353-1362, 1529-2916

Preston, Thorburn, Starkey, et al. (2011). Streptococcus pneumoniae infection suppresses allergic airways disease by inducing regulatory T-cells. *Eur.Respir.J.*, 37, 1, (Jan), pp. 53-64, 1399-3003; 0903-1936

Pulendran. (2004). Modulating TH1/TH2 responses with microbes, dendritic cells, and pathogen recognition receptors. *Immunol.Res.*, 29, 1-3, pp. 187-196, 0257-277X; 0257-277X

Ray, Khare, Krishnamoorthy, Qi & Ray. (2010). Regulatory T cells in many flavors control asthma. *Mucosal Immunol.*, 3, 3, (May), pp. 216-229, 1935-3456; 1933-0219

Redford, Murray & O'Garra. (2011). The role of IL-10 in immune regulation during M. tuberculosis infection. *Mucosal Immunol.*, 4, 3, (May), pp. 261-270, 1935-3456; 1933-0219

Ryanna, Stratigou, Safinia & Hawrylowicz. (2009). Regulatory T cells in bronchial asthma. *Allergy*, 64, 3, (Mar), pp. 335-347, 1398-9995; 0105-4538

Sakaguchi, Setoguchi, Yagi & Nomura. (2006). Naturally arising Foxp3-expressing CD25+CD4+ regulatory T cells in self-tolerance and autoimmune disease. *Curr.Top.Microbiol.Immunol.*, 305, pp. 51-66, 0070-217X

Sakaguchi. (2003). Regulatory T cells: mediating compromises between host and parasite. *Nat.Immunol.*, 4, 1, (Jan), pp. 10-11, 1529-2908; 1529-2908

Sakaguchi. (2002). Immunologic tolerance maintained by regulatory T cells: implications for autoimmunity, tumor immunity and transplantation tolerance. *Vox Sang.*, 83 Suppl 1, (Aug), pp. 151-153, 0042-9007; 0042-9007

Sakaguchi. (2000). Regulatory T cells: key controllers of immunologic self-tolerance. *Cell*, 101, 5, (May 26), pp. 455-458, 0092-8674; 0092-8674

Sansonetti. (2011). To be or not to be a pathogen: that is the mucosally relevant question. *Mucosal Immunol.*, 4, 1, (Jan), pp. 8-14, 1935-3456; 1933-0219

Sarris, Andersen, Randow, Mayr & Betz. (2008). Neuropilin-1 expression on regulatory T cells enhances their interactions with dendritic cells during antigen recognition. *Immunity*, 28, 3, (Mar), pp. 402-413, 1097-4180; 1074-7613

Sather, Treuting, Perdue, et al. (2007). Altering the distribution of Foxp3 (+) regulatory T cells results in tissue-specific inflammatory disease. *J.Exp.Med.*, 204, 6, (Jun 11), pp. 1335-1347, 0022-1007; 0022-1007

Saunders & Britton. (2007). Life and death in the granuloma: immunopathology of tuberculosis. *Immunol.Cell Biol.*, 85, 2, (Feb-Mar), pp. 103-111, 0818-9641; 0818-9641

Shafiani, Tucker-Heard, Kariyone, Takatsu & Urdahl. (2010). Pathogen-specific regulatory T cells delay the arrival of effector T cells in the lung during early tuberculosis. *J.Exp.Med.*, 207, 7, (Jul 5), pp. 1409-1420, 1540-9538; 0022-1007

Shalev, Liu, Koscik, et al. (2008). Targeted deletion of fgl2 leads to impaired regulatory T cell activity and development of autoimmune glomerulonephritis. *J.Immunol.*, 180, 1, (Jan 1), pp. 249-260, 0022-1767; 0022-1767

Shevach. (2009). Mechanisms of foxp3+ T regulatory cell-mediated suppression. *Immunity*, 30, 5, (May), pp. 636-645, 1097-4180

Shimizu, Yamazaki, Takahashi, Ishida & Sakaguchi. (2002). Stimulation of CD25 (+)CD4 (+) regulatory T cells through GITR breaks immunological self-tolerance. *Nat.Immunol.*, 3, 2, (Feb), pp. 135-142, 1529-2908

Simecka, Davis, Davidson, Ross, Stadtlander & Cassell. (1992). Mycoplasma diseases of animals In: *Mycoplasmas: molecular biology and pathogenesis,* Anonymous (Eds.), pp. 391, American Society for Microbiology, 1555810500, Washington, D.C.

Stassen, Jonuleit, Muller, et al. (2004). Differential regulatory capacity of CD25+ T regulatory cells and preactivated CD25+ T regulatory cells on development, functional activation, and proliferation of Th2 cells. *J.Immunol.,* 173, 1, (Jul 1), pp. 267-274, 0022-1767; 0022-1767

Strauss, Bergmann & Whiteside. (2009). Human circulating CD4+CD25highFoxp3+ regulatory T cells kill autologous CD8+ but not CD4+ responder cells by Fas-mediated apoptosis. *J.Immunol.,* 182, 3, (Feb 1), pp. 1469-1480, 1550-6606

Suto, Nakajima, Kagami, Suzuki, Saito & Iwamoto. (2001). Role of CD4 (+) CD25 (+) regulatory T cells in T helper 2 cell-mediated allergic inflammation in the airways. *Am.J.Respir.Crit.Care Med.,* 164, 4, (Aug 15), pp. 680-687, 1073-449X; 1073-449X

Taylor, Taylor-Robinson & Fernald. (1974). Reduction in the severity of Mycoplasma pneumoniae-induced pneumonia in hamsters by immunosuppressive treatment with antithymocyte sera. *J.Med.Microbiol.,* 7, 3, (Aug), pp. 343-348, 0022-2615; 0022-2615

Thorburn, O'Sullivan, Thomas, et al. (2010). Pneumococcal conjugate vaccine-induced regulatory T cells suppress the development of allergic airways disease. *Thorax,* 65, 12, (Dec), pp. 1053-1060, 1468-3296; 0040-6376

Thornton & Shevach. (1998). CD4+CD25+ immunoregulatory T cells suppress polyclonal T cell activation in vitro by inhibiting interleukin 2 production. *J.Exp.Med.,* 188, 2, (Jul 20), pp. 287-296, 0022-1007; 0022-1007

Trujillo & Erb. (2003). Inhibition of allergic disorders by infection with bacteria or the exposure to bacterial products. *Int.J.Med.Microbiol.,* 293, 2-3, (Jun), pp. 123-131, 1438-4221; 1438-4221

Turner, Gonzalez-Juarrero, Ellis, et al. (2002). In vivo IL-10 production reactivates chronic pulmonary tuberculosis in C57BL/6 mice. *J.Immunol.,* 169, 11, (Dec 1), pp. 6343-6351, 0022-1767; 0022-1767

Urdahl, Shafiani & Ernst. (2011). Initiation and regulation of T-cell responses in tuberculosis. *Mucosal Immunol.,* 4, 3, (May), pp. 288-293, 1935-3456; 1933-0219

van Maren, Jacobs, de Vries, Nierkens & Adema. (2008). Toll-like receptor signalling on Tregs: to suppress or not to suppress? *Immunology,* 124, 4, (Aug), pp. 445-452, 1365-2567; 0019-2805

Vignali, Collison & Workman. (2008). How regulatory T cells work. *Nat.Rev.Immunol.,* 8, 7, (Jul), pp. 523-532, 1474-1741

von Boehmer. (2005). Mechanisms of suppression by suppressor T cells. *Nat.Immunol.,* 6, 4, (Apr), pp. 338-344, 1529-2908

Voo, Wang, Santori, et al. (2009). Identification of IL-17-producing FOXP3+ regulatory T cells in humans. *Proc.Natl.Acad.Sci.U.S.A.,* 106, 12, (Mar 24), pp. 4793-4798, 1091-6490; 0027-8424

Wang, Zhang & Chui. (2008). Identification of correlations between numbers of CD4+ CD25+ Treg cells, levels of sera anti-AChR antibodies and transfer growth factor-beta in patients with myasthenia gravis. *Zhonghua Yi Xue Za Zhi,* 88, 15, (Apr 15), pp. 1036-1040, 0376-2491

Wang & Alexander. (2009). CD8 regulatory T cells: what's old is now new. *Immunol.Cell Biol.*, 87, 3, (Mar-Apr), pp. 192-193, 0818-9641; 0818-9641

Wing, Onishi, Prieto-Martin, et al. (2008). CTLA-4 control over Foxp3+ regulatory T cell function. *Science*, 322, 5899, (Oct 10), pp. 271-275, 1095-9203

Wissinger, Goulding & Hussell. (2009). Immune homeostasis in the respiratory tract and its impact on heterologous infection. *Semin.Immunol.*, 21, 3, (Jun), pp. 147-155, 1096-3618; 1044-5323

Woolard, Hodge, Jones, Schoeb & Simecka. (2004). The upper and lower respiratory tracts differ in their requirement of IFN-gamma and IL-4 in controlling respiratory mycoplasma infection and disease. *J.Immunol.*, 172, 11, (Jun 1), pp. 6875-6883, 0022-1767

Zhao, Zhang, Yi, et al. (2008). In vivo-activated CD103+CD4+ regulatory T cells ameliorate ongoing chronic graft-versus-host disease. *Blood*, 112, 5, (Sep 1), pp. 2129-2138, 1528-0020; 1528-0020

Part 3

Obstructive Lung Diseases

4

Special Consideration in Treating Patients of Overlap Between Asthma and COPD

So Ri Kim[1,2] and Yang Keun Rhee[1]
[1]*Department of Internal Medicine,*
[2]*Research Center for Pulmonary Disorders,*
Chonbuk National University Medical School, Jeonju,
South Korea

1. Introduction

Asthma and chronic obstructive pulmonary disease (COPD) are distinct in pathobiological characteristics. Asthma is a disease with its origins in child hood, is related to allergies and eosinophils, and is best treated by targeting inflammation, whereas COPD is related to adults who smoke and to neutrophils, and is best treated with bronchodilators and the removal of risk factors. However, this distinction is not always clear-cut and there is a considerable overlap in pathogenesis and clinical features; patients with severe asthma may present with fixed airway obstruction while patients with COPD may have hyperresponsiveness and eosinophilia (Kim & Rhee, 2010). In fact, the classification of patients having asthma or COPD may vary day-to-day based on established diagnostic criteria, due to their overlap and inherent variability in bronchodilator responsiveness (Calverley et al., 2003). Moreover, several hypotheses/theories have been proposed to explain whether they are in a single disease entity.

In accord with this concept for the two diseases, recent diagnostic approaches appear to be concentrated on various and specific phenotypes because of their different therapeutic responses to the standard treatment for each disorder depending on the phenotypes. The refractory asthmatic patients share several characteristics of patients with COPD, suggesting that drugs in discovery for COPD might also be effective in treating severe asthma (Barnes, Mar 2008, Dec 2008). In fact, many new drugs under pre- or clinical trials are expected to be effective in both diseases and overlapping situations. However, there remains still a need to extend novel drug development and to investigate the mechanisms and treatment of overlapping asthma and COPD. In this chapter, we will review these special therapeutic considerations for severe or refractory entity, i.e., overlap of two major airway obstructive disorders, asthma and COPD.

2. The overlap between asthma and COPD

Asthma and COPD are pulmonary disorders characterized by various degrees of airflow limitation, inflammation, and tissue remodeling. Classical definition of two disorders describes the physiological and anatomic extremes of asthma and COPD and allows them to be recognized as distinct disease entities. Actually, asthma has been differentiated from pure COPD through several condition described as follows; i) youthful onset, ii) non-smokers, iii) episodic and completely reversible airway obstruction and airway hyperresponsiveness, and iv) allergic history including the association with rhinitis. In addition, a dysregulated T helper cell (Th) type 2 inflammatory response is responsible for the eosinophilic and mononuclear cell infiltration, mucous metaplasia, airway remodeling are seen in asthma patients and characterize asthma. However, each disorder has a very wide spectrum of clinical and pathobiological phenotypes thereby in considerable patients the diagnosis becomes vague, confusing, and being overlapped (Kim & Rhee, 2010). Thus, the current classification of obstructive airway diseases is not adequate to precisely treat COPD and asthma. Recently, different statistical techniques have been used to better understand and describe the multiple dimensions of airway diseases with the ultimate goal being identification of distinct subgroups of patients with different prognosis or response to treatment (Shirtcliffe et al., 2011).

Asthma and COPD are representative chronic inflammatory lung diseases. In both conditions, inflammation is associated with episodic exacerbation and/or structural alteration at large and small airway levels (Guerra, 2005; Jeffery, 2004). These can result in a transient phenotypic overlap or a combined syndrome with characteristics of both diseases.

Exacerbation of asthma and COPD is a clinically significant event and frequently associated with a decline in lung function and symptomatic aggravation (Gibson & Simpson, 2009). During exacerbation, airway inflammation becomes more exaggerated than in the mild and stable disease states, thereby the inflammation pattern changes (Mauad & Dolhnikoff, 2008). Neutrophil recruitment is a prominent feature of acute exacerbation of chronic asthma (Lamblin et al., 1998), probably owing to respiratory tract infection by viruses (Fahy et al., 1995; Wark et al., 2002). Furthermore, neutrophilic inflammation in the absence of eosinophils is largely present in sudden-onset fatal asthma, and neutrophil numbers are highly elevated in status asthmaticus (Lamblin et al., 1998; Tsokos & Paulsen, 2002). Thus, severe and fatal asthma may be mediated by neutrophils, which is quite different from the classical Th2-driven eosinophilic form. In COPD patients, an allergic profile of inflammation can occur, particularly during exacerbation. Airway eosinophilia is observed in chronic bronchitic patients with exacerbation and is associated with the upregulation of RANTES in the airway epithelium (Saet et al., 1994; Zhu et al., 2001). These observations indicate that inflammatory characteristics of asthma and COPD are interchangeable during exacerbation and infection.

The cytokine profile is also affected by disease severity. During exacerbation, Th1/Th2 patterns are reversed to some degree in each disease. Several studies have demonstrated that the level of IL-17 is elevated in asthma and COPD and is correlated with the presence of neutrophils and the decrease of lung function (Bullens et al., 2006; Matsunaga et al., 2006; Molet et al., 2001; Wong et al., 2001). The elevation of IL-17 level is associated with increased neutrophilic inflammation during severe asthma or acute exacerbation (Wong et al., 2001). In COPD, the role of IL-17 remains unclear, although the importance of IL-17 in stimulating chemokine production and the involvement of neutrophils and macrophages in promoting COPD pathogenesis suggest a potential connection (Curtis et al., 2007).

Disease exacerbation in both asthma and COPD can lead to an accelerated decline in lung function (Stein et al., 1999; Stern et al., 2007). Previous reports have shown an association between severe asthma exacerbation and an accelerated decline in forced expiratory volume in 1 s (FEV1), to a degree similar to that seen in patients with smoking and COPD (Vonk et al., 2003). Another important observation is that the decline in FEV1 seen in patients with infrequent exacerbation is similar to that in a population without asthma. These findings suggest that repetitive episodes of exacerbation may result in fixed airflow obstruction in asthma and contribute to the phenotypic overlap between asthma and COPD.

Decreased distensibility and increased collapsibility of small airways including alveoli are prominent in asthmatic emphysema, whereas loss of elastic recoil is an important factor in the dynamic collapse of the airway in COPD (James & Wenzel, 2007). Currently, there are at least two major pathophysiological mechanisms responsible for the development of emphysema: protease–antiprotease imbalance and apoptosis of structural cells (Spurzem & Rennard, 2005). Increased elastin degradation and enhanced expression of proteases have been documented in asthma patients (Bousquet et al., 1996; James & Wenzel, 2007). In IL-13-overexpressing transgenic mice, emphysema and the increased expression of a variety of matrix metalloproteinases (MMPs) and cathepsins have been observed (Zheng et al., 2000). Intervention that neutralize MMPs or cathepsins has been shown to dramatically ameliorate IL-13-induced emphysematous responses. These findings suggest that IL-13 has the ability to induce alveolar remodeling responses in asthmatics. Moreover, in human asthma patients, the numbers of eosinophils, $CD4^+$ T-cells, and macrophages are increased in alveolar tissue at the time symptoms appeared (Kraft et al., 1996, 1999). Furthermore, the degree of eosinophilic inflammation correlates positively with lung volume in asthma patients (Sutherland et al., 2004). These data indicate that destruction of distal airways is a consequence of a chronic, long-lasting injury, which affects lung function in both COPD and asthma.

In addition, in COPD, there is evidence for remodeling, fibrosis, and inflammation in epithelium, reticular basement membrane, airway smooth muscles (ASM), and mucous glands, albeit with patterns different from those seen in asthmatics (Bosken et al., 1990; Nagai et al., 1985; Wright et al., 1983). Furthermore, bronchodilator reversibility and AHR may be present in a significant proportion of COPD patients (Kerstjens et al., 1993). Poorer pulmonary function is associated with a greater magnitude of AHR, and increasing severity of airway hyperresponsiveness is associated with faster rates of decline in lung function in continuing smokers (Tashkin et al., 1996).

Taken together, both states of transient overlapping with exacerbation and permanent/chronic structural changes between asthma and COPD may exhibit severe phenotype and respond poorly to standard treatment for each disease.

3. Need for new therapeutic concept for overlap between asthma and COPD

There is now sufficient evidence to suggest that both asthma and COPD are complex heterogeneous disorders including overlapped features each other with distinct risk factors, pathophysiological processes, natural history, and treatment responses. However, current treatment guidelines for COPD and asthma are based on randomized trials of highly selected subgroups of patients, especially the very typical phenotypic group, i.e., Th2-

predominant asthma and pure COPD (Shirtcliffe et al., 2011). Therefore, the major unmet needs of current therapies include better treatment of severe and refractory disease entities such as overlap between asthma and COPD. In addition, considering the poor and different responses to current therapy in patients with overlap, the ultimate goal of treatment targeted to this group can be achieved when the interrelationship between overlapping situation and its cellular and molecular basis is understood. In fact, there are enormous efforts to find the pharmacological therapeutic ways to control these specific phenotypic conditions worldwide.

4. New therapeutic approaches for overlap between asthma and COPD

4.1 Bronchodilators

Bronchodilators are an important component for pharmacologic approaches preventing and relieving bronchoconstriction. Recent popular bronchodilators are β_2-agonists with long action duration (long acting β_2-agonist, LABA) such as salmeterol and formoterol, which last for over 12 hours. There are now several even longer-acting β_2-agonists (ultra-LABA) in development, including indacaterol, carmoterol, GW-642444, and BI-1744, which have a duration of action >24 hours and are suitable for once daily use (Cazzola & Matera, 2009). A once daily muscarinic antagonist, tiotropium bromide, is less effective as a bronchodilator in asthma than the β_2-agonists and is used predominantly in COPD, but might be a useful add-on therapy in some patients with severe asthma (H.W. Park et al., 2009). Several new classes of bronchodilators including other once daily muscarinic antagonists are also in development. However, there are lots of challenges and hurdles to overcome bronchodilators' weaknesses as a single therapeutic agent.

4.2 Novel corticosteroids

Inhaled corticosteroids (ICS) are the most effective anti-inflammatory therapy for asthma and COPD. In addition, in case of asthma, corticosteroids are used as fixed combination inhalers, i.e., LABA plus corticosteroid, and to date, this combination therapy is known to be the most effective available therapy based on their synergistic effects. However, all currently available ICS are absorbed from the lung and thus have the potential for systemic side effect. This has led to a concerted effort to find safer ICS, with reduced oral bioavailability, reduced absorption from the lung or inactivation in the circulation. Moreover, airway inflammation in COPD responds poorly to corticosteroid administration (Barnes & Stockley, 2005; Culpitt et al., 1999; Keatings et al., 1997), presumably because it is associated with neutrophils, CD8+T lymphocytes, and CD68+ macrophages, cells that are minimally inhibited by corticosteroids. Since asthma exacerbation exhibits mixed inflammatory pattern of asthma and COPD, in the case of overlap between asthma and COPD, the therapeutic efficacy of current corticosteroid to asthma is attenuated. To achieve disease modification, reductions in the frequency and severity of acute exacerbations and effective suppression of asthmatic and COPD-type airway inflammation, new corticosteroids and/or anti-inflammatory strategies are required. Actually, dissociated steroids designed to separate the side effect mechanisms from the anti-inflammatory mechanisms are expected to have a greater effect on enhancement of transcription for anti-inflammatory genes, and thus might have a better therapeutic efficacy with the reduction of side effects (Schaecke et al., 2004). On the other hand, nonsteroidal selective glucocorticoid receptor activators (SEGRA), such as AL-438 and

ZK-216438, are in development, although the effect of these drugs may not be efficacious as pre-existing corticosteroids.

4.3 Modulation of cytokines; IL-17

Several cytokines act as important players in pathogenesis of asthma and COPD (Barnes, 2008). As for asthma, Th2 cytokines have been thought to play a major role in its pathobiology traditionally. Inhibition of Th2 cytokine, IL-4 is proven to be disappointing, but there is a continuing interest in blocking IL-13, a related cytokine that regulates IgE formation, particularly in severe asthma. In fact, several IL-13 and IL-4Rα blocking antibodies are now in clinical trials but to date, clinical studies in severe asthma have also been disappointing (Chiba et al., 2009; Wenzel et al., 2007). Therefore, recent therapeutic approach for asthma and COPD is deviated to develop the drugs for these severe and mixed phenotypic groups. As one of hopeful candidates, mepolizumab is shown to reduce exacerbation in a particular subset of patients who have persistent sputum eosinophilia (Haldar et al., 2009; Nair et al., 2009).

IL-17, the cytokine being studied most actively nowadays, has attracted interest as a target in severe asthma as it might be a mediator of neutrophilic inflammation in severe asthma (James & Wenzel, 2007). Given the role of IL-17 in the regulation of growth factors that promote granulopoiesis and production of chemokines that are involved in recruitment neutrophils, IL-17 plays a pivotal role in the neutrophil responses in the lung. In addition to severe asthma, steroid-resistant asthma may also feature a neutrophil-dependent component (Louis & Djukanovic, 2006). In fact, neutrophils are largely steroid insensitive, and corticosteroids inhibit neutrophil apoptosis (Cox, 1995; Schleimer et al., 1989), perhaps explaining the increase in neutrophilia in severe and steroid resistant asthmatics. Another key neutrophil protease, MMP-9, is a primary MMP enhanced in asthmatics, and the level of MMP-9 correlates with asthma severity (Cundall et al., 2003; Wenzel et al., 2003). Furthermore, IL-17 increases MMP-9 level via recruitment of neutrophils to the lung (Prause et al., 2004).

Yet, the role of IL-17 and Th17 cells in COPD remains largely speculative, although the importance of IL-17 in stimulating chemokine production and the role of neutrophils and macrophages in promoting COPD pathogenesis have led to great deal of interest on their interrelationship (Curtis, 2007). In addition, another possible link derives from IL-17's ability to drive MMP-9 production, which may directly link to tissue destruction observed in COPD (Prause et al., 2004).

Taken together, these observations suggest a role of neutrophils in mediating severe and steroid-resistant asthma (Foley & Hamid, 2007; Kamath et al., 2005; Louis & Djukanovic, 2006), indicating the therapeutic potential of blockade of IL-17 for the control of severe and steroid resistant asthma such as overlap with COPD.

4.4 Regulation of lipid mediators

To date, the only mediator antagonists currently used in therapy for airway inflammatory disorders are anti-leukotrienes, which block cysteinyl leukotriene (cysLT) type 1-receptors. Although these drugs are much less effective than ICS, a recent study has revealed that cysLTs are implicated in sub-epithelial fibrosis, one of structural changes in airway remodeling, in asthmatic airways through the induction of IL-11 expression (Lee et al., 2007). Several other drugs that inhibit receptors or synthesis of lipid mediators are currently in development. Among them, some novel 5′-LO and 5′-LO-activating protein (FLAP) inhibitors are more effective in patients with neutrophilic inflammation because they block the production of leukotriene (LT)B4. However, an LTB4 receptor (BLT1) antagonist had no effect in mild asthma (Evans et al., 1996).

4.5 Phosphodiesterase (PDE) inhibitors; targeting PDE4

PDE4 inhibitors have been in development for many years. Interest in this class of compound arose in the 1980s when it became clear that methylxanthines such as theophylline, which had been widely used for its bronchodilator action since the 1930s, were difficult to use and could be dangerous because of its side effects. As a consequence, safer substitutes have been sought. At the same time, it was discovered that theophylline is an nonselective inhibitor of PDEs. There are multiple families of PDEs; one of these families, PDE4, is expressed in ASM and in immune and pro-inflammatory cells (Torphy, 1988, 1990, 1991, 1998). PDE4 inhibitors have a wide spectrum of anti-inflammatory effects, inhibiting T cells, eosinophils, mast cells, ASM cells, epithelial cells, and nerve cells, and are very effective in animal models of asthma (Chung, 2006). In accordance with these findings, an oral PDE4 inhibitor, roflumilast, has an inhibitory effect on allergen-induced responses in asthma and also reduces symptoms of asthma and lung function, similar to low doses of ICS (Bousquet et al., 2006). In addition to asthma, COPD is also the target airway disorder of PDE4 inhibitors with improving FEV1 and preventing the acute exacerbation (Calverley et al., 2007, 2009; Rabe et al., 2005). Therefore, PDE4 inhibitors are expected to use for treating COPD associated with asthma or patients at risk of transient overlapping situation such as acute exacerbation.

4.6 Adenosine receptor inhibitors

One inflammatory mediator common to both airway diseases is adenosine, making its receptor signaling pathway to be a therapeutic target for asthma and COPD. Adenosine levels have been shown to increase in patients with asthma and COPD and in animal models having features of chronic airway disease (Zhou et al., 2009). Moreover, inhalation of adenosine induces bronchoconstriction in patients with asthma and COPD (Caruso et al, 2007). A non-selective adenosine receptor antagonist, theophylline, improves lung function and symptoms in asthma and COPD (Caruso et al, 2007; Zhou et al., 2009). Furthermore, adenosine receptors are expressed on most, if not all, inflammatory and stromal cell types involved in the pathogenesis of asthma and COPD. Extracellular adenosine elicits its effects by interacting with four adenosine receptors: A1R, A2AR, A2BR, and A3R (Polosa & Blackburn, 2009). Adenosine receptor signaling systems are complex, displaying different and specific actions in various inflammatory responses. Studies with animal models of airway disease have suggested that A1, A3, and A2B antagonists may be useful for the treatment of asthma and COPD, although their therapeutic efficacy remains to be fully evaluated. Various selective adenosine receptor antagonists are under preclinical or clinical studies with patients of asthma and/or COPD.

4.7 Kinase inhibitors: Nuclear factor (NF)-κB, mitogen-activated protein kinase (MAPK), and phosphoinositide-3 kinase (PI3K) signaling pathways

Generally, kinases are a pivotal component of biological actions in living things. In airway inflammation, a tremendous number of kinases are implicated and play critical roles. NF-κB regulates expression of various inflammatory genes that are involved in airway diseases (Adcock et al., 2006). Indeed, small molecule inhibitors of the key enzyme IKK2/IKKb (inhibitor of κB kinase) block inflammation induced by NF-κB activation and are now in preclinical test (Karin et al., 2004). In addition, p38 MAPK activates similar inflammatory genes to NF-κB, and is activated in cells from patients with severe asthma (Bhavsar et al., 2008). Several small molecule inhibitors are now in clinical study for the treatment of inflammatory diseases (Cuenda & Rousseau, 2007). Most of all, PI3K signaling is the most anticipated target of future drugs for asthma and COPD. In particular, the major focus of interest has been PI3Kγ and δ isoforms in respiratory disorders including asthma. PI3Kγ is important for chemotactic responses, and selective inhibitors are in development, whereas PI3Kδ activation results in reduced steroid responsiveness through reducing histone deacetylase (HDAC)2 activity, thus PI3Kδ inhibitors could potentially reverse corticosteroid resistance in severe asthma (To et al., 2010). In addition, selective inhibition of the PI3Kδ signaling pathway suppresses IL-17 expression through regulation of NF-κB activity in asthma (Park et al, 2010). These findings suggest that PI3Kγ/δ targeting agent can be a promising therapeutic tool for the treatment and prevention of severe asthma having COPD natures and acute exacerbation.

4.8 Targeting regulatory T cells

Regulatory T cells in patients with corticosteroid resistance produce less IL-10 but this can be restored with vitamin D3 supplementation *in vitro* (Xystrakis et al., 2006). Additionally, in corticosteroid-resistant patients with asthma, intake of vitamin D3 enhances IL-10 secretion from regulatory T cells in response to dexamethasone (Xystrakis et al., 2006). However, the therapeutic effects of vitamin D3 and its analogue 1a,25-vitamin D3 (calcitriol) on refractory or steroid resistant asthma remains unclear and need to test in large-scaled clinical trials.

5. Conclusion

Despite the distinct clinical phenotypic features of asthma and COPD, there is considerable overlap of symptoms and pathogenesis, and several hypotheses have been proposed regarding the status of asthma and COPD as a single disease entity. Overlapping features may occur not only in a permanent form but also as a transient symptom, as in exacerbation. In accordance with this, recent therapeutic approaches have concentrated on a target common to the pathogenesis of both asthma and COPD. Classic pharmacologic agents are innovating as new drugs to avoid significant side effects and to cover the patients at risk frequent exacerbation and refractory severe disease status in asthma and COPD. Novel candidate targets include various kinase pathways, adenosine receptors, lipid mediators, and PDE4, and almost of them are under preclinical or clinical trials. However, it still requires enormous efforts to develop novel classes of drugs overcoming the limitations of pre-existing medicines and to investigate the mechanisms and treatment of overlapping asthma and COPD.

6. Acknowledgment

We thank Professor Yong Chul Lee (Chonbuk National University Medical School, Jeonju, South Korea) for the helpful discussion throughout the preparation of this work and Professor Mie-Jae Im (Chonbuk National University Hospital, Jeonju, South Korea) for critically reading this manuscript. This work was supported by a grant from the Korea Healthcare Technology R&D Project, Ministry for Health, Welfare, and Family Affairs, Republic of Korea (A084144) (to S.R.K).

7. References

Adcock, I.M., Chung, K.F., Caramori, G., & Ito, K. (2006). Kinase inhibitors and airway inflammation. *European Journal of Pharmacology*, Vol.533, No.1-3, (March 2006), pp. 118-132, ISSN 0014-2999

Barnes, P.J. & Stockley, R.A. (2005). COPD: current therapeutic interventions and future approaches. *European Respiratory Journal*, Vol.25, No.6, (June 2005), pp. 1084–1106, ISSN 0903-1936

Barnes, P.J. (2008). Immunology of asthma and chronic obstructive pulmonary disease. *Nature Review Immunology*, Vol.8, No.3, (March 2008), pp. 183–192, ISSN 1474-1733

Barnes, P.J. (2008). The cytokine networks in asthma and chronic obstructive pulmonary disease. *Journal of Clinical Investigation*, Vol.118, No.11, (November 2008), pp. 3546–3556, ISSN 0021-9738

Barnes, P.J. (2008) Emerging pharmacotherapies for COPD. *Chest*, Vol. 134, No. 6, (December 2008), pp. 1278–1286, ISSN 0012-3692

Bhavsar, P., Hew, M., Khorasani, N., Torrego, A., Barnes, P.J., Adcock, I., & Chung, K.F. (2008). Relative corticosteroid insensitivity of alveolar macrophages in severe asthma compared to non-severe asthma. *Thorax*, Vol.63, No.9, (September 2008), pp. 784–790, ISSN 0040-6376

Bosken, C.H., Wiggs, B.R., Pare, P.D., & Hogg, J.C. (1990). Small airway dimensions in smokers with obstruction to airflow. *American Review of Respiratory Disease*, Vol.142, No.3, (September 1990), pp. 563-570, ISSN 0003-0805

Bousquet, J., Lacoste, J.Y., Chanez, P., Vic, P., Godard, P., & Michel, F.B. (1996). Bronchial elastic fibers in normal subjects and asthmatic patients. *American Journal of Respiratory and Critical Care Medicine*, Vol.153, No.5, (May 1996), pp. 1648-1654, ISSN 1073-449X

Bousquet, J., Aubier, M., Sastre, J., Izquierdo, J.L., Adler, L.M., Hofbauer, P., Rost K,D., Harnest, U., Kroemer, B., Albrecht, A., & Bredenbröker, D. (2006). Comparison of roflumilast, an oral antiinflammatory, with beclomethasone dipropionate in the treatment of persistent asthma. *Allergy*, Vol.61, No.1, (January 2006), pp. 72–78, ISSN 0105-4538

Bullens, D.M., Truyen, E., Coteur, L., Dilissen, E., Hellings, P.W., Dupont, L.J., & Ceuppens, J.L. (2006). IL-17 mRNA in sputum of asthmatic patients: linking T cell driven inflammation and granulocytic influx? *Respiratory Research*, Vol.7, (November 2006), pp. 135, ISSN 1465-9921

Calverley, P,M., Burge, P,S., Spencer, S., Anderson, J,A., & Jones, P,W. (2003). Bronchodilator reversibility testing in chronic obstructive pulmonary disease. *Thorax*, Vol.58, No.8, (August 2003), pp. 659–664, ISSN 0040-6376

Calverley, P.M., Sanchez-Toril, F., McIvor, A., Teichmann, P., Bredenbroeker, D., & Fabbri, L.M. (2007). Effect of 1-year treatment with roflumilast in severe chronic obstructive pulmonary disease. *American Journal of Respiratory and Critical Care Medicine*, Vol.176, No.2, (July 2007), pp. 154–161, ISSN 1073-449X

Calverley, P.M., Rabe, K.F., Goehring, U.M., Kristiansen, S., Fabbri, L.M., & Martinez F,J.; M2-124 and M2-125 study groups. (2009). Roflumilast in symptomatic chronic obstructive pulmonary disease: two randomised clinical trials. *Lancet*, Vol.374, No.9691, (August 2009), pp. 685–694, ISSN 0140-6736

Caruso, M., Tringali, G., & Polosa, R. (2007). Evidence for a functional contribution of adenosine signalling in inflammatory airway diseases. *Current Medicinal Chemistry - Immunology, Endocrine & Metabolic Agents*, Vol.7, No.4 (August 2007), pp. 286-297, ISSN 1568-0134

Cazzola, M. & Matera. M.G. (2009). Emerging inhaled bronchodilators: an update. *European Respiratory Journal*, Vol.34, No.3, (September 2009), pp. 757–769, ISSN 0903-1936

Chiba, Y., Todoroki. M., Nishida, Y., Tanabe, M., & Misawa M. (2009). A novel STAT6 inhibitor AS1517499 ameliorates antigen-induced bronchial hypercontractility in mice. *American Journal of Respiratory Cell and Molecular Biology*, Vol.41, No.5, (November 2009), pp. 516–524, ISSN 1044-1549

Chung. K.F. (2006). Phosphodiesterase inhibitors in airways disease. *European Journal of Pharmacology*, Vol.533, No.1-3, (March 2006), pp. 110–117, ISSN 0014-2999

Cox, G. (1995). Glucocorticoid treatment inhibits apoptosis in human neutrophils. Separation of survival and activation outcomes. *Journal of Immunology*, Vol.154, No.9, (May 1995), pp. 4719–4725, ISSN 0022-1767

Cuenda, A. & Rousseau, S. (2007). p38 MAP-kinases pathway regulation, function and role in human diseases. *Biochimica et Biophysica Acta*, Vol.1773, No.8, (August 2007), pp. 1358–1375, ISSN 0006-3002

Culpitt, S.V., Maziak, W., Loukidis, S., Nightingale, J.A., Matthews, J.L., & Barnes, P.J. (1999). Effect of high dose inhaled steroid on cells, cytokines, and proteases in induced sputum in chronic obstructive pulmonary disease. *American Journal of Respiratory and Critical Care Medicine*, Vol.160, No.5 Pt 1, (November 1999), pp. 1635–1639, ISSN 1073-449X

Cundall, M., Sun, Y., Miranda, C., Trudeau, J.B., Barnes, S., & Wenzel, S.E. (2003). Neutrophil-derived matrix metalloproteinase-9 is increased in severe asthma and poorly inhibited by glucocorticoids. *Journal of Allergy and Clinical Immunology*, Vol.112, No.6, (December 2003), pp. 1064–1071, ISSN 0091-6749

Curtis, J.L., Freeman, C.M., & Hogg, J.C. (2007). The immunopathogenesis of chronic obstructive pulmonary disease: insights from recent research. *Proceedings of the American Thoracic Society*, Vol.4, No.7, (October 2007), pp. 512-521, ISSN 1546-3222

Evans, D.J., Barnes, P.J., Spaethe, S.M., van Alstyne, E.L., Mitchell, M.I., & O'Connor, B.J. (1996). The effect of a leukotriene B4 antagonist LY293111 on allergen- induced responses in asthma. *Thorax*, Vol.51, No.12, (December 1996), pp. 1178–1184, ISSN 0040-6376

Fahy, J.V., Kim, K.W., Liu, J., & Boushey, H.A. (1995). Prominent neutrophilic inflammation in sputum from subjects with asthma exacerbation. *Journal of Allergy and Clinical Immunology*, Vol.95, No.4, (April 1995), pp. 843-852, ISSN 0091-6749

Foley, S.C. & Hamid, Q. (2007). Images in allergy and immunology: neutrophils in asthma. *Journal of Allergy and Clinical Immunology*, Vol.119, No.5, (May 2007), pp. 1282–1286, ISSN 0091-6749

Gibson, P.G. & Simpson, J.L. (2009). The overlap syndrome of asthma and COPD: what are its features and how important is it? *Thorax*, Vol.64, No.8, (August 2009), pp. 728-735, ISSN 0040-6376

Guerra, S. (2005). The overlap of asthma and chronic obstructive pulmonary disease. *Current Opinion in Pulmonary Medicine*, Vol.11, No.1, (January 2005), pp. 7-13, ISSN 1070-5287

Haldar, P., Brightling, C.E., Hargadon, B., Gupta, S., Monteiro, W., Sousa, A., Marshall, R.P., Bradding, P., Green, R.H., Wardlaw, A.J., & Pavord, I.D. (2009). Mepolizumab and exacerbations of refractory eosinophilic asthma. *New England Journal of Medicine*, Vol.360, No.10, (March 2009), pp. 973–984, ISSN 0028-4793

James, A.L., & Wenzel, S. (2007). Clinical relevance of airway remodelling in airway diseases. *European Respiratory Journal*, Vol.30, No.1, (July 2007), pp. 134-155, ISSN 0903-1936

Jeffery, P.K. (2004). Remodeling and inflammation of bronchi in asthma and chronic obstructive pulmonary disease. *Proceedings of the American Thoracic Society*, Vol.1, No.3, (November 2004), pp. 176-183, ISSN 1546-3222

Kamath, A.V., Pavord, I.D., Ruparelia, P.R., & Chilvers, E.R. (2005). Is the neutrophil the key effector cell in severe asthma? *Thorax*, Vol.60, No.7, (July 2005), pp. 529–530, ISSN 0040-6376

Karin, M. Yamamoto, Y., & Wang, QM. (2004). The IKK NF-kappa B system: a treasure trove for drug development. *Nat Reviews Drug Discovery*, Vol.3, No.1, (January 2004), pp. 17–26, ISSN 1474-1776

Keatings, V.M., Jatakanon, A., Worsdell, Y.M., & Barnes, P.J. (1997). Effects of inhaled and oral glucocorticoids on inflammatory indices in asthma and COPD. *American Journal of Respiratory and Critical Care Medicine*, Vol.155, No.2, (Febuary1997), pp. 542–548, ISSN 1073-449X

Kerstjens, H.A., Brand, P.L., Quanjer, P.H., van der Bruggen-Bogaarts, B.A., Koëter, G.H., & Postma, D.S. (1993). Variability of bronchodilator response and effects of inhaled corticosteroid treatment in obstructive airways disease. Dutch CNSLD Study Group. *Thorax*, Vol.48, No.7, (July 1993), pp. 722-729, ISSN 0040-6376

Kim, S.R. & Rhee, Y.K. (2010). Overlap Between Asthma and COPD: Where the Two Diseases Converge. *Allergy, Asthma & Immunology Research*, Vol.2, No.4, (October 2010), pp. 209-214, ISSN 2092-7355

Kraft, M., Djukanovic, R., Wilson, S., Holgate, S.T., & Martin, R.J. (1996). Alveolar tissue inflammation in asthma. *American Journal of Respiratory and Critical Care Medicine*, Vol.154, No.5, (November 1996), pp. 1505-1510, ISSN 1073-449X

Kraft, M., Martin, R.J., Wilson, S., Djukanovic, R., & Holgate, S.T. (1999). Lymphocyte and eosinophil influx into alveolar tissue in nocturnal asthma. *American Journal of Respiratory and Critical Care Medicine*, Vol.159, No.1, (January 1999), pp. 228-234, ISSN 1073-449X

Lamblin, C., Gosset, P., Tillie-Leblond, I., Saulnier, F., Marquette, C.H., Wallaert, B., & Tonnel, A.B. (1998). Bronchial neutrophilia in patients with noninfectious status asthmaticus. *American Journal of Respiratory and Critical Care Medicine*, Vol.157, No.2, (Febuary 1998), pp. 394-402, ISSN 1073-449X

Lee, K.S., Kim, S.R., Park, H.S., Park, S.J., Min, K.H., Lee, K.Y., Jin, S.M., & Lee, Y.C. (2007). Cysteinyl leukotriene upregulates IL-11 expression in allergic airway disease of mice. *Journal of Allergy and Clinical Immunology*, Vol.119, No.1, (January 2007), pp. 141-149, ISSN 0091-6749

Louis, R. & Djukanovic, R. (2006). Is the neutrophil a worthy target in severe asthma and chronic obstructive pulmonary disease? *Clinical & Experimental Allergy*, Vol.36, No.5, (February 2006), pp. 563-567, ISSN 0954-7894

Matsunaga, K., Yanagisawa, S., Ichikawa, T., Ueshima, K., Akamatsu, K., Hirano, T., Nakanishi, M., Yamagata, T., Minakata, Y., & Ichinose, M. (2006). Airway cytokine expression measured by means of protein array in exhaled breath condensate: correlation with physiologic properties in asthmatic patients. *Journal of Allergy and Clinical Immunology*, Vol.118, No.1, (July 2006), pp. 84-90, ISSN 0091-6749

Mauad, T. & Dolhnikoff, M. (2008). Pathologic similarities and differences between asthma and chronic obstructive pulmonary disease. *Current Opinion in Pulmonary Medicine*, Vol.14, No.1, (January 2008), pp. 31-38, ISSN 1070-5287

Molet, S., Hamid, Q., Davoine, F., Nutku, E., Taha, R., Pagé, N., Olivenstein, R., Elias, J., & Chakir, J. (2001). IL-17 is increased in asthmatic airways and induces human bronchial fibroblasts to produce cytokines. *Journal of Allergy and Clinical Immunology*, Vol.108, No.3, (September 2001), pp. 430-438, ISSN 0091-6749

Nagai, A., West, W.W., & Thurlbeck, W.M. (1985). The National Institutes of Health Intermittent Positive-Pressure Breathing trial: pathology studies. II. Correlation between morphologic findings, clinical findings, and evidence of expiratory air-flow obstruction. *American Review of Respiratory Disease*, Vol.132, No.5, (November 1985), pp. 946-953, ISSN 0003-0805

Nair, P., Pizzichini, M.M., Kjarsgaard, M., Inman, M.D., Efthimiadis, A., Pizzichini, E., Hargreave, F.E., & O'Byrne, P.M. (2009). Mepolizumab for prednisone-dependent asthma with sputum eosinophilia. *New England Journal of Medicine*, Vol.360, No.10, (March 2009), pp. 985-993, ISSN 0028-4793

Park, H.W., Yang, M.S., Park, C.S., Kim, T.B., Moon, H.B., Min, K.U., Kim, Y.Y., & Cho, S.H. (2009). Additive role of tiotropium in severe asthmatics and Arg16Gly in ADRB2 as a potential marker to predict response. *Allergy*, Vol.64, No.5, (May 2009), pp. 778-783, ISSN 0954-7894

Park, S.J., Lee, K.S., Kim, S.R., Min, K.H., Moon, H., Lee, M.H., Chung, C.R., Han, H.J., Puri, K.D., & Lee, Y.C. (2010). Phosphoinositide 3-kinase δ inhibitor suppresses interleukin-17 expression in a murine asthma model. *European Respiratory Journal*, Vol.36, No.6, (December 2010), pp. 1448-1459, ISSN 0903-1936

Polosa, R. & Blackburn, M.R. (2009). Adenosine receptors as targets for therapeutic intervention in asthma and chronic obstructive pulmonary disease. *Trends in Pharmacological Sciences*, Vol.30, No.10, (October 2009), pp. 528-535, ISSN 0165-6147

Prause, O., Bozinovski, S., Anderson, G.P., & Linden, A. (2004). Increased matrix metalloproteinase-9 concentration and activity after stimulation with interleukin-17 in mouse airways. *Thorax*, Vol.59, No.4, (April 2004), pp. 313-317, ISSN 0040-6376

Rabe, K.F., Bateman. E.D., O'Donnell. D., Witte. S., Bredenbroker, D., & Bethke, T.D. (2005). Roflumilast—an oral anti-inflammatory treatment for chronic obstructive pulmonary disease: a randomised controlled trial. *Lancet*, Vol.366, No.9485, (August 2005), pp. 563–571, ISSN 0140-6736

Saet, M., Di Stefano, A., Maestrelli, P., Turato, G., Ruggieri, M,P., Roggeri, A., Calcagni, P., Mapp, C.E., Ciaccia, A., & Fabbri, L.M. (1994). Airway eosinophilia in chronic bronchitis during exacerbations. *American Journal of Respiratory and Critical Care Medicine*, Vol.150, No.6 Pt 1, (December 1994), pp. 1646-1652, ISSN 1073-449X

Schaecke, H., Schottelius, A., Döcke, W.D., Strehlke, P., Jaroch, S., Schmees, N., Rehwinkel, H., Hennekes, H., & Asadullah, K. (2004). Dissociation of transactivation from transrepression by a selective glucocorticoid receptor agonist leads to separation of therapeutic effects from side effects. *Proceedings of the National Academy of Sciences of the United States of America*, Vol.101, No.1, (Junuary 2004), pp. 227–232, ISSN 0027-8424

Schleimer, R.P., Freeland, H.S., Peters, S.P., Brown, K.E., & Derse, C.P. (1989). An assessment of the effects of glucocorticoids on degranulation, chemotaxis, binding to vascular endothelium and formation of leukotriene B4 by purified human neutrophils. *Journal of Pharmacology and Experimental Therapeutics*, Vol.250, No.2, (August 1989), pp. 598–605, ISSN 0022-3565

Shirtcliffe, P., Weatherall, M., Travers, J., & Beasley, R. (2011). The multiple dimensions of airways disease: targeting treatment to clinical phenotypes. *Current Opinion in Pulmonary Medicine*, Vol.11, No.17, (March 2011), pp. 272–278, ISSN 1070-5287

Spurzem, J.R., & Rennard, S.I. (2005). Pathogenesis of COPD. *Seminars in Respiratory and Critical Care Medicine*, Vol.26, No.2, (April 2005), pp. 142-153, ISSN 1069-3424

Stein, R.T., Holberg, C.J., Sherrill, D., Wright, A.L., Morgan, W.J., Taussig, L., & Martinez, F.D. (1999). Influence of parental smoking on respiratory symptoms during the first decade of life: the Tucson Children's Respiratory Study. *American Journal of Epidemiology*, Vol.149, No.11, (June 1999), pp. 1030-1037, ISSN 0002-9262

Stern, D.A., Morgan, W.J., & Wright, A.L. (2007). Poor airwayin early infancy and lung function by age 22 years: a non-selective longitudinal cohort study. *Lancet*, Vol.370, No.9589, (September 2007), pp. 758-764, ISSN 0140-6736

Sutherland, E.R., Martin, R.J., Bowler, R.P., Zhang, Y., Rex, M.D., & Kraft, M. (2004). Physiologic correlates of distal lung inflammation in asthma. *Journal of Allergy and Clinical Immunology*, Vol.113, No.6, (June 2004), pp. 1046-1050, ISSN 0091-6749

Tashkin, D.P., Altose, M.D., Connett, J.E., Kanner, R.E., Lee, W.W., & Wise, R.A. (1996). Methacholine reactivity predicts changes in lung function over time in smokers with early chronic obstructive pulmonary disease. The Lung Health Study Research Group. *American Journal of Respiratory and Critical Care Medicine*, Vol.153, No.6 Pt 1, (Jun 1996), pp. (1802-1811), ISSN 1073-449X

To, Y., Ito, K., Kizawa, Y., Failla, M., Ito, M., Kusama, T., Elliott, W.M., Hogg, J.C., Adcock, I.M., & Barnes, P.J. (2010). Targeting phosphoinositide-3-kinase-d with theophylline reverses corticosteroid insensitivity in COPD. *American Journal of Respiratory and Critical Care Medicine*, Vol.182, No.7, (October 2010), pp. 897-904. ISSN 1073-449X

Torphy, T.J. (1988). Action of mediators on airway smooth muscle: functional antagonism as a mechanism for bronchodilator drugs. *Agents and Actions Supplments*, Vol.23, (1988), pp. 37–53, ISSN 0379-0363

Torphy, T.J. (1998). Phosphodiesterase isozymes: molecular targets for novel antiasthma agents. *American Journal of Respiratory and Critical Care Medicine,* Vol.157, No.2, (February 1998), pp. 351–370, ISSN 1073-449X

Torphy, T.J. & Cieslinski, L.B. (1990). Characterization and selective inhibition of cyclic nucleotide phosphodiesterase isozymes in canine tracheal smooth muscle. *Molecular Pharmacology,* Vol.37, No.2, (February 1990), pp. 206–214, ISSN 0026-895X

Torphy, T.J. & Undem, B.J. (1991). Phosphodiesterase inhibitors: new opportunities for the treatment of asthma. *Thorax,* Vol.46, No.7, (July 1991), pp. 512–523, ISSN 0040-6376

Tsokos, M. & Paulsen, F. (2002). Expression of pulmonary lactoferrin in sudden-onset and slow-onset asthma with fatal outcome. *Virchows Archiv,* Vol.441, No.5, (November 2002), pp. 494-499, ISSN 0945-6317

Vonk, J.M., Jongepier, H., Panhuysen, C.I., Schouten, J.P., Bleecker, E.R., & Postma, D.S. (2003). Risk factors associated with the presence of irreversible airflow limitation and reduced transfer coefficient in patients with asthma after 26 years of follow up. *Thorax,* Vol.58, No.4, (April 2003), pp. 322-327, ISSN 0040-6376

Wark, P.A., Johnston, S.L., Moric, I., Simpson, J.L., Hensley, M.J., & Gibson, P.G. (2002). Neutrophil degranulation and cell lysis is associated with clinical severity in virus-induced asthma. *European Respiratory Journal,* Vol.19, No.1, (January 2002), pp. 68-75, ISSN 0903-1936

Wenzel, S., Wilbraham, D., Fuller, R., Getz, E.B., & Longphre, M. (2007). Effect of an interleukin-4 variant on late phase asthmatic response to allergen challenge in asthmatic patients: results of two phase 2a studies. *Lancet,* Vol.370, No.9596, (October 2007), pp. 1422–1431, ISSN 0140-6736

Wenzel, S.E., Balzar, S., Cundall, M., & Chu, H.W. (2003). Subepithelial basement membrane immunoreactivity for matrix metalloproteinase 9: association with asthma severity, neutrophilic inflammation, and wound repair. *Journal of Allergy and Clinical Immunology,* Vol.111, No.6, (June 2003), pp. 1345–1352, ISSN 0091-6749

Wong, C.K., Ho, C.Y., Ko, F.W., Chan, C.H., Ho, A.S., Hui, D.S., & Lam, C.W. (2001). Proinflammatory cytokines (IL-17, IL-6, IL-18 and IL-12) and Th cytokines (IFN-γ, IL-4, IL-10 and IL-13) in patients with allergic asthma. *Clinical & Experimantal Immunology,* Vol.125, No.2, (August 2001), pp. 177-183, ISSN 0009-9104

Wright, J.L., Lawson, L.M., Pare, P.D., Wiggs, B.J., Kennedy, S., & Hogg, J.C. (1983). Morphology of peripheral airways in current smokers and ex-smokers. *American Review of Respiratory Disease,* Vol.127, No.4, (April 1983), pp. 474-477, ISSN 0003-0805

Xystrakis, E., Kusumakar, S., Boswell, S., Peek, E., Urry, Z., Richards, D.F., Adikibi, T., Pridgeon, C., Dallman, M., Loke, T.K., Robinson, D.S., Barrat, F.J., O'Garra, A., Lavender, P., Lee, T.H., Corrigan, C., & Hawrylowicz, C.M. (2006). Reversing the defective induction of IL-10-secreting regulatory T cells in glucocorticoid-resistant asthma patients. *Journal of Clinical Investigation,* Vol.116, No.1, (January 2006), pp. 146–155, ISSN 0021-9738

Zheng, T., Zhu, Z., Wang, Z., Homer, R.J., Ma, B., Riese, R.J. Jr., Chapman, H.A. Jr., Shapiro, S.D., & Elias, J.A. (2000). Inducible targeting of IL-13 to the adult lung causes matrix metalloproteinase- and cathepsin-dependent emphysema. *Journal of Clinical Investigation,* Vol.106, No.9, (November 2000), pp. 1081-1093, ISSN 0021-9738

Zhou, Y., Schneider, D.J, Blackburn, M.R. (2009). Adenosine signaling and the regulation of chronic lung disease. *Pharmacology & Therapeutics*, Vol.123, No.1, (July 2009), pp. 105-116, ISSN 0163-7258

Zhu, J., Qiu, Y.S., Majumdar, S., Gamble, E., Matin, D., Turato, G., Fabbri, L.M., Barnes, N., Saetta, M., & Jeffery, P.K. (2001). Exacerbations of bronchitis: bronchial eosinophilia and gene expression for interleukin-4, interleukin-5, and eosinophil chemoattractants. *American Journal of Respiratory and Critical Care Medicine*, Vol.164, No.1, (July 2001), pp. 109-116, ISSN 1073-449X

Part 4

Smoking Hazards and Cessation Protocols

5

Motivational Intervention and Nicotine Replacement Therapies for Smokers: Results of a Randomized Clinical Trial

Jennifer Lira-Mandujano[1] and Sara Eugenia Cruz-Morales[2]
[1]*Facultad de Psicología, Universidad Michoacana de San Nicolás de Hidalgo*
[2]*Psicofarmacología, UNAM, FES-Iztacala*
México

1. Introduction

The World Health Organization (WHO, 2003, 2011) estimated that at international level approximately 1.3 million people currently smoke cigarettes or other products. Almost one billion men and 250 million women, and about 6 million people die each year from diseases related to smoking. Related diseases comprise different types of cancer (lung, larynx, oral cavity), cardiovascular (atherosclerosis, stroke), respiratory diseases (acute and chronic), alterations in the reproductive system, dental problems (leukoplakia, gingivitis, among others), peptic ulcer and some diseases of eye, diabetes.

In the last two decades different interventions have been developed for smoking cessation, resulting from the World Health Organization Framework Convention on Tobacco Control (abbreviated WHO FCTC), in which emphasize among other actions, the importance of scientific research to develop programs for smoking cessation and for the treatment of nicotine addiction (WHO, 2003). Such interventions include non-pharmacological (psychological) and pharmacological approaches (nicotinic and non-nicotine treatments). Some authors point out that the combination of a psychological intervention with any pharmacological intervention significantly increases the likelihood of success for quitting, however, the results are not conclusive (Ingersoll & Cohen 2005; Prochazca, 2000). In this sense, there have been different clinical trials with the purpose of evaluate systematically and empirically the effectiveness of the combination of these interventions.

2. Psychological interventions for smoking cessation

Different studies showed that psychological treatments, specifically those that employ behavioral and cognitive-behavioral techniques are effective for smoking cessation (Lancaster & Stead, 2011). These techniques include control of stimuli, cue exposure, the handling of contingencies, smoking fast, gradual reduction of ingestion of nicotine and tar (GRINT) technique, nicotine fading, self- control techniques and coping skills (prevention of relapses, skills training), solution of problems and social support (Dodgen, 2005; Fiore, et al., 2000; Foxx & Brown, 1979). Behavioral cognitive interventions focus on cognitive and emotional processes associated to the consumption of tobacco. Recognizes the existence risk situations in which it is likely the person smokes, and identify them. These risk situations could include cognitive aspects, and/or emotional expectations, as well as places, friends or holidays. The identification of situations of risk provides training in coping skills, which can also be cognitive and emotional (cognitive dissonance, restructuring of thought, relaxation), and/or behavioral (avoidance of the situation, social skills, etc.).

3. Nicotine Replacement Therapies (NRT)

Nicotinic replacement therapies seek to reduce smoking and the withdrawal symptoms, consequently increase the probability of remaining abstinent. Reviews of various clinical trials indicate that all types of nicotine replacement therapy (nicotine gum, transdermal nicotine patch, nasal spray, inhaler, and sublingual tablets / pills) can help the people who try to quit smoking to increase the likelihood of maintaining abstinence and all are superior to placebo (Einsenberg, Filion & Yavin (2008)). Also remarks that the effectiveness of nicotine replacement therapy does not increase with the inclusion of some support program as a psychological intervention (Stead, et al., 2011). Some clinical trials in this regard, incorporate in experimental conditions the combination of a psychological intervention with some nicotine replacement therapy mainly with nicotine patch and gum with nicotine.

Richmond, Kehoe and Almeida (1997) analyzed different clinical trials showing that the combination of nicotine replacement therapy and cognitive behavior intervention is more effective. The purpose of the study was to determine the effectiveness of transdermal nicotine patch in combination with a cognitive-behavioral program. Participants (305) were randomly assigned to two groups: the active nicotine patch or the placebo patch group. The subjects of the active group received weekly patches until completing 10 weeks, 21 mg of nicotine / day for 6 weeks, followed by a dose of 14 mg/day for two weeks, and 7 mg of nicotine / day in the past two weeks. All subjects attended to a multicomponent cognitive behavioral program designed to promote the attitude and behavioral change in smokers, consisting in-group sessions of 2 hours/ week for five consecutive weeks. All measures (point prevalence, continuous and prolonged abstinence), abstinence rates at 12 months were consistently twice higher for those who wore nicotine patch compared with placebo.

Another clinical trial shows that telephone counselling in addition to NRT also increases abstinence rates. In this clinical trial 854 smokers were assigned to NRT (nicotine transdermal patches 21 mg, 14 and 7 mg for 10 weeks) alone or NRT and telephone counselling (5 sessions spaced according to a relapse-sensitive call schedule). Abstinence rates were significantly higher in participants receiving telephone counselling than among those not receiving telephone counselling at both 3 and 6 months. In addition, abstinence rates at 6 months were significantly higher for participants receiving counseling. The combination of telephone counselling and NRT was superior compared with NRT alone (in 28 continuous day abstinence at 3 months, 1.6% vs. 25.1%, and at 6 months 30.1% vs. 22.4%) and for 90 continuous day abstinence at 6 months 26.7% vs. 18.6 % (Macleod, Arnaldi & Adams, 2003).

Alterman, Gariti and Mulvaney (2001) evaluated the efficacy and cost of three levels of medical-behavioral treatment intensity in combination with NRT. A low-intensity group received eight weeks of NRT and one advice and education session, a moderate-intensity group received NRT and four advice and education sessions, and a high-intensity group received the combination of NRT, four advice and education sessions, and 12 weeks of individualized cognitive-behavioral therapy. Abstinence rates confirmed biochemically at week 9, 26 and 52 after the beginning of the treatment, were higher for the treatment of high-intensity (45 %, 37 % and 35 %, respectively), followed by low-intensity (35 %, 30 % and 27 %, respectively) and moderate intensity (27 %, 12 %, 12 %, respectively). The cost calculated for the treatment of low-intensity was $308, for the moderate intensity $338 and for the high-intensity $582. The results showed that better abstinence rates confirmed biochemically after a year occurred in the groups that received the high and low intensity interventions. Similar results were obtained for African American smokers (Webb, et al., 2010). In such study, 154 smokers using transdermal nicotine patches for eight weeks (four weeks with 21 mg, two weeks with 14 mg, and 2 mg for seven weeks), were randomly assigned to one of two groups, either cognitive–behavioral therapy or general health education. Results showed that 7-day point prevalence abstinence was higher for cognitive behavioral therapy than for general health education, after the intervention (51% vs. 27%), at three (34% vs. 20%) and 6 months (31% vs. 14%).

However, different clinical trials have found negative results. In one study, the effectiveness of NRT alone and in combination with behavioral interventions was evaluated on a population of smokers from a New England Veterans Affairs Medical Center. Participants (2,054 smokers) were assigned to one of four conditions: stage-matched manuals (the manuals were consistent with their stage of readiness to change; NRT (16 hrs / 15 mg for 6 weeks) and manuals; expert system, NRT and manuals; and automated counselling, NRT, manuals, and expert system. The effectiveness at 30 months of stage-matched manuals was of 20.3%. Intervention did not increase with the addition of NRT (19.3%), nor expert system interventions (17.6%), or automated telephone counselling (19.9%) (Velicer et al., 2006), it is interesting to note that in this study the participants were ready to quit.

The effectiveness of cue exposure treatment in smoking relapse prevention in addition to other NRT, nicorette gum 2mg, and cognitive behavioral intervention was at evaluated 1, 3, 6 and 12 months. A sample of motivated smokers received a counselling session and was randomly assigned to one of the four treatments for the prevention of relapses: a) brief intervention; b) cognitive behavioral intervention and gum nicotine; c) cognitive behavioral intervention and cue exposure; and d) cognitive behavioral intervention, cue exposure and nicotine gum. The addition of NRT to the standard treatments did not increase abstinence rates; no differences were observed for the cue exposure conditions, however the same authors questioned the imaginal cue exposure paradigm used (Niaura et al., 1999).

4. Non nicotinic pharmacological therapies

Non nicotinic pharmacological treatments are one option for people who want to quit smoking and need medical prescription. One of the options for this type of treatment is the use of antidepressants, like bupropion, doxepin, fluoxetine, imipramine, moclobemide, nortriptyline, paroxetine, selegiline, sertraline, tryptophan and velanfaxine. Hughes, Stead and Lancaster (2011a) reviewed the results on the effectiveness to quit smoking with the administration of antidepressants finding that bupropion and nortriptyline have long-term positive effects similar to nicotine replacement therapy, while fluoxetine, a selective serotonin reuptake inhibitor, had minor effects.

Different reviews coincide with the efficacy of the different non-nicotinic pharmacological treatments, being varenicline and bupropion the most effective to increase abstinence rates (Hughes, Stead & Lancaster, 2011a), and varenicline with higher effectiveness (Einsenberg, Filion & Yavin (2008)). Cytisine is an agonist of nicotinic receptors that has been used to treat tobacco dependence for 40 years in Eastern Europe (Etter, 2005) and varenicline is an analog of cytisine (Coe et al., 2005).

Varenicline (Chantix or Champix) is a partial nicotinic receptor agonist that also inhibits dopamine, and it was suggested for smoking cessation (Coe et al., 2005). Reviews of its effectiveness conclude that increases the chances of quitting successfully in the long term between two and three times in comparison with the attempts to quit smoking without pharmacological aid. In addition, varenicline seems to be more effective than bupropion, but the effectiveness compared with nicotine replacement therapy has not fully studied (Cahill, Stead & Lancaster, 2011). Bupropion (Zyban Wellbutrin, Zyban, Voxra, Budeprion) is a non-tricyclic antidepressant that inhibits norepinephrine and dopamine reuptake, and acts as a nicotinic acetylcholine receptor antagonist (Dwoskin et al., 2006; Richmond & Zwar, 2003). Clinical studies showed that bupropion was as effective as the standard antidepressants used at that time in the treatment of major depression, and it was helpful in patients resistant to typical antidepressants (James & Lippmann, 1991). Some reports demonstrated its efficacy in the treatment of smokers (Ferry & Burchette, 1994; Ferry et al., 1992). Bupropion has also been evaluated in combination with psychological interventions under the assumption that in combination with cognitive behavioral therapy abstinence rates are increased. Tonnesen et al. (2003) conducted a randomized, double blind, placebo-controlled study with 707 smokers, 527 smokers received bupropion 300 mg daily for 7 weeks and attended to a behavioral cognitive intervention, and 180 received placebo and a behavioral cognitive intervention. The results showed that abstinence rates were significantly higher for bupropion compared with placebo group. At 12 months continuous abstinence rates were 21% for bupropion and 11% for the placebo group. The authors conclude that bupropion in combination with counselling increases abstinence rates compared to placebo. In addition, McCarthy et al. (2008) conducted a clinical trial with 463 smokers who were randomly assigned to one of four groups: 1) placebo 2) placebo and counselling, 3) bupropion and 4) bupropion with counselling. Counselling sessions were focused in: a) preparation for quitting, b) cope abilities and problems solution (identification of triggers for relapse, analysis of past relapses and relapses in current attempts to quit smoking, and providing psycho education in relation to the distraction and coping), c) relapse prevention (planning long-term relapse) d) social support (empathy, support), e) keep the motivation to quit smoking by encouraging the participants to identify and record the reasons for quit smoking and developing strategies to remind themselves these reasons after they quit smoking. Prolonged abstinence rates obtained at the end of the treatment, at 6 and 12 months were for placebo group 25.1%, 16.8%, 14.2%; for bupropion (50%, 25% and 18.1%), and for bupropion and counselling (50%, 25% and 18.1%). The authors concluded that the group that received bupropion was more effective than the groups receiving placebo, and the inclusion of counselling plus bupropion did not increased abstinence rates significantly.

The combinations of bupropion with cognitive behavioral interventions of different intensity have been evaluated. In a randomized clinical trial, 1524 smokers were randomly assigned to one of four groups: 1) bupropion (150 mg) and moderate behavioral counselling (telephone program based on cessation strategies), 2) bupropion (150 mg) and minimal counselling (self-help mailed materials), 3) bupropion (300 mg) and moderate behavioral counselling, or 4) bupropion (300 mg) and minimal behavioral counselling. Three month follow up shows that groups of bupropion with doses of 300 mg and minimal and moderate behavioral counselling had higher abstinence rates (35% and 26.7% respectively) than the groups that received bupropion (150 mg) and minimal and moderate behavioral (24.4% y 24.2% respectively). At 12 months the abstinence rates changed mainly in the groups of moderate behavioral intervention; groups that used bupropion 150 and 300 mg with a moderate behavioral program had higher abstinence rates (31.4 % and 33.2 %, respectively) than with the bupropion 150 mg and 300 mg groups with a minimal behavioral program (23.4% and 25.7%, respectively) (Swan et al., 2003). The results show that there is an advantage associated with high doses of bupropion for smoking cessation in a three months period but not in 12 months, similarly to other clinical trials. In a similar study with 1524 participants using the same doses of bupropion in combination with behavioral interventions of minimal intensity (tailored mailings) or moderate intensity (proactive telephone calls), it was found that 150 mg of bupropion combined with either behavioral intervention was the most cost effective (Javitz et al., 2004).

Venlafaxine, a reuptake inhibitor of serotonin and norepinephrine (Redrobe, Bourin, Colombel & Baker (1998)) is another antidepressant used to quit smoking. In a study 147 participants were assigned to one of two groups, velanfaxine or placebo in combination with cognitive behavioral intervention (nine weekly sessions: six personally, three by phone) and nicotine patches (22 mg/day). The results showed that the inclusion of venlafaxine in a treatment program including behavioral intervention and nicotine replacement therapy does not improve rates of abstinence. Venlafaxine improves the abstinence of smokers who consume less than a packet, and has positive benefits on negative affect for all smokers 6 weeks after cessation, time in which there is a greater chance of having a relapse (Cinciripini et al., 2005).

Under the same logic, the search conducted identified two studies, which assessed the effectiveness of the combination with the antidepressant nortriptyline and behavioral intervention. Nortriptyline (Sensoval, Aventyl, Pamelor, Norpress, Allegron, Noritren and Nortrilen) is a second-generation tricyclic antidepressant that inhibits the reuptake of norepinephrine and serotonin with small effects on dopamine reuptake (Fuxe et al., 1977; Robinson et al., 2000).

In the first study, nortriptyline (12 weeks) was more effective than placebo increasing abstinence rates independently of depression history and alleviated a negative affect after smoking cessation; while cognitive behavioral therapy was more helpful in participants with a depression history. Participants were 199 smokers, stratified according depression history and number of cigarettes; participants were randomly assigned to cognitive behavioral treatment or health education program and one of two treatments, nortriptyline or placebo. Nortriptyline produced higher abstinence rates than placebo, independent of depression history. Cognitive behavioral therapy was more effective for participants with a history of depression. Nortriptyline alleviated the negative affect occurring after smoking cessation (Hall et al., 1998). In the second study, the effect of long-term nortriptyline treatment (52 weeks) in combination with a psychological intervention was evaluated. One hundred sixty smokers were randomly assigned to four different conditions, brief nortriptyline (12 weeks) or extended treatment with their respective placebo groups; all participants received nicotine patches (4 weeks, 21 mg; 2 weeks 14 mg, 2 weeks, 7 mg) and five counselling sessions. Participants in extended treatment continued with drug or placebo until week 52 and 9 monthly additional counselling sessions. The abstinence rates were superior for extended treatment, and superior to placebo; the authors conclude that extended period in combination with psychological interventions induce high abstinence rates (Hall et al., 2004).

Other clinical trials assessed two types of antidepressants with behavioral interventions. The abstinence rates with 12 weeks of treatment with nortriptyline versus bupropion versus placebo, and the addition of behavior therapy intervention versus medical management involving (brief advice and counselling) was evaluated by Hall et al. (2002). In the study, 220 smokers were randomly assigned to one experimental condition: 1) placebo and medical management, 2) placebo and a psychological intervention, 3) nortriptyline and medical management, 4) nortriptyline and psychological intervention, 5) bupropion and medical management and 6) bupropion and psychological intervention. Bupropion and the nortriptyline were more effective than placebo after one year follow up; the effectiveness of bupropion and nortriptyline was similar (bupropion, nortriptyline and placebo with medical advice 29%, 23% and 13% respectively and bupropion, nortriptyline and psychological intervention 29%, 23% and 21%). The authors conclude that the inclusion of a psychological intervention or the increase of contact does not increase abstinence. Another study carried out with 220 cigarette smokers, comparing bupropion vs. nortriptyline vs. placebo in addition with two behavioral interventions; calculate the cost-effectiveness at 52 weeks. Nortriptyline costs was lower than bupropion, psychological intervention cost less than the two drug treatments; however in both cases the differences were not significant (Hall et al., 2005).

Fluoxetine (Prozac) is a specific serotonin reuptake inhibitor (SSRI) antidepressant also used in smoking cessation interventions (Cornelius et al., 1999). Niaura et al. (2002) explored the dose-effect of fluoxetine in smoking cessation. In a blind study, 989 smokers received nine sessions of a cognitive behavioral therapy and were assigned to one of three treatments: 1) fluoxetine 30 mg, 2) fluoxetine 60 mg, 3) placebo. Follow ups at four, 8, 16 and 26 weeks were conducted to identify abstinent participants. The rates of abstinence reached were of 13% for placebo, 12% for fluoxetine 30 mg, and 14 % for fluoxetine 60 mg, at the end of the treatment no significant differences were detected among groups, the authors suggest that there is not enough support to consider fluoxetine as either a first- or even a second-line treatment for smoking cessation.

In another clinical trial using fluoxetine, Saules et al. (2004) evaluated the combination of fluoxetine, the cognitive behavioral therapy and NRT to quit smoking in 150 people aged between 21 and 65 years. It was a double-blind, placebo controlled study, with three groups, a group receiving treatment with fluoxetine 20 mg, a second group 40 mg and a third group received placebo; all participants received 10 weeks of nicotine patch (20 or 40 mg/day) and six weeks of cognitive behavioral therapy. At the end of treatment abstinence rates obtained were of 35.4 % in the placebo group, 43.1% for the fluoxetine 20 mg group and 43.1 % for the group fluoxetine 40 mg. The results suggest that fluoxetine can moderate withdrawal symptoms, but not improved abstinence rates. Thus, the results obtained by different studies show that behavioral interventions in combination with bupropion, nortriptyline and fluoxetine increase the probability of quitting, although the effectiveness of the first two compounds compared with placebo is substantially higher than fluoxetine.

Naltrexone (Narpan, Revia, Antaxona, Depade) and naloxone (Narcan), opioid receptor antagonists, employed mainly for of alcohol and opioid dependence are other compounds used for the treatment for smoking cessation. There are few studies with naloxone, with contradictory findings. For example, naloxone seems to increase craving (Krishnan-Sarin, Rosen & O´Malley, 1999), and no significant effects on nicotine withdrawal are described (Gorelick, Rose & Jarvik 1988; Wewers, Dhatt & Tejwani, 1998). Regarding the number of cigarettes smoked, a decline was observed with naloxone compared with placebo group (Gorelick et al., 1988; Karras & Kane, 1980), while also negative results are reported (Nemeth-Coslett & Griffiths, 1986). The results obtained with naltrexone are also ambiguous. Covey, Glassman & Stetner (1999), described significant abstinence rates at 3 and at 6 months (26.7% for naltrexone; 15.2% for placebo). The administration of naltrexone with NRT do not induce significant effects on smoking abstinence; 100 participants were given 12 weeks treatments: either placebo, naltrexone (50 mg daily), placebo with nicotine patches (21 mg/24-hour during first 8weeks, 14 mg/24-hour the last 4weeks), or naltrexone with nicotine patches (Wong et al., 1999). The use of naltrexone and nicotine patches in combination with cognitive behavioral treatment based on the community reinforcement approach (CRA) was evaluated in 25 abstinent smokers (smoking 15 cigarettes daily for at least 5 years, with 3 attempts to quit smoking in the last 5 years). The treatment lasted 8 weeks; the first week naltrexone from 5 mg to 25 mg was given orally, all participants received nicotine patches (21 mg/ 24 hrs to 7 mg /24hrs). On week 2, naltrexone doses were administered to four groups: 1) 25 mg of naltrexone, 2) 25 mg of naltrexone and CRA 3) naltrexone 50 mg, and 4) 50 mg of naltrexone and CRA. The craving decreases in each measurement and abstinence to the 3-month follow up rates were higher for groups who received the CRA and naltrexone compared with those that only received naltrexone (46 % and 25 %). In the 18-month follow up the abstinence rates were higher (17 % and 31 %) in the groups receiving the combination of treatments than that using only naltrexone (Roozen et al., 2006). The meaning of this study is questionable since the follow up was done just at 3 months, it is not a blind study and a placebo group was not included. However, since there are few studies of its effectiveness David et al. (2011) indicate that it cannot confirm or refute whether naltrexone helps people to quit smoking. In addition, the anxiolytics drugs do not have empirical evidence indicating that they are effective for smoking cessation (Hughes, Stead & Lancaster , 2011b).

5. Justification

The results of the literature support and justify the importance of conducting clinical randomized controlled trials, given that the results of this kind of studies derive from practice based-evidence, in other words, results show information about treatment options which allows clinical practice supported by scientific evidence (Nathan et al., 2000).

Specifically in México, in the national survey of addiction conducted in 2008, in the population among 12-65 years, 14 millions (18.5%) were active smokers, the 17.1%

ex-smokers and the 64.4% were not smokers (Secretaría de Salud [SS], 2008). The total number of annual deaths attributable to smoking by associated diseases is more than 60 thousand (daily killed 165 people). Specifically, 38% of these deaths (22 778 deaths) were from ischemic heart disease, 29% (17 390 deaths) due to emphysema, chronic bronchitis, and chronic obstructive pulmonary disease (COPD), 23 % (13, 751 deaths) from stroke and 10% by cancer of lung, bronchus and trachea (6,168 deaths) (Kuri-Morales et al., 2006).

The National Council Against Addictions (Consejo Nacional Contra las Adicciones [CONADIC], Spanish abbreviation), pointed out that in public health institutions the programs developed and currently in use are characterized by using different theoretical and methodological assumptions; the range include from rational emotive therapy, hypnosis, systemic therapy, therapy, cognitive behavioral interventions to NRT (SS, 2002).

So we propose that is necessary to consider aspects related to the effectiveness of treatments, such as: a) the systematic evaluation of interventions to stop smoking in order to know the real impact on the consumption pattern; b) the assessment of psychological interventions when combined with pharmacological treatments; c) the theoretical-methodological congruence of psychological treatments; d) evaluation of abstinence rates at the end of the treatment and follow up (for at least six months), that is, evaluate whether abstinence rates are maintained in the long term. Therefore, the hypothesis underlying this work is that the combination of a brief behavioral intervention with the NRT will induce abstinence rates higher at the end of treatment and follow up (6 months) than each one of the treatments.

5.1 Objective

Then the objective of present study was to assess the effectiveness of brief motivational intervention for smoking cessation applied alone and combined with nicotine replacement therapies.

5.2 Method

Participants: 71 smokers (38 man and 33 women), recruited via advertising and fliers which attended to the Communitarian Center and wanted to participate in the study.

Inclusion criteria: Being between 19 and 60 years; signed informed consent.

Exclusion criteria: Present specific medical condition (hypertension, ulcers, diabetes, some types of cancer, chest pain in the last month), pregnant women, and people who were taking any medication for the diagnosis of major depression, severe anxiety or any other psychiatric disorder.

Setting: Communitarian Center "Acasulco", Psychology Faculty, UNAM.

Instruments and assessment tools:

- Pre-selection questionnaire: consists of ten questions related to the criteria of inclusion and exclusion.
- Initial interview: To obtain socio demographic data, family and social history, work history and place of residence, history of alcohol and drugs (Ayala et al., 1998).

- Fagerström Test for Nicotine Dependence (FTND) (Heatherton, Kozlowski, Frecker & Fagerström, 1991).
- Brief Questionnaire for Situational Confidence (BQSC) (Sobell et al., 1996; adapted by Ayala, et al., 1998).
- Beck Depression Inventory (BDI) (Beck et al., 1988; adapted by Jurado et al., 1998).
- Composite International Diagnostic Interview (CIDI), in this study only the B section that refers to "Disorders due to tobacco" was used (WHO, CIDI, 1990).
- Beck Anxiety Inventory (BAI) (Beck et al., 1988; adapted by Robles et al., 2001)
- The timeline follow-back (TLFB) (Sobell, Brown, Leo & Sobell, 1996; adapted by Lira, 2002).
- Stages of Change Readiness and Treatment Eagerness Scale (SOCRATES8D), (Miller, 1999; adapted by Cuevas et al., 2005).

Material used in the brief motivational intervention for smoking (BMIS)

- Brochure No. 1 "Deciding to quit"
- Brochure No. 2 "Identifying my situations related to smoking"
- Brochure No. 3 "Plans of action to stop smoking"
- Registration form of cigarettes consumption.

Procedure:

Smokers attending to the Community Center had an admission session. In this in which several instruments were applied to select participants according to inclusion and exclusion criteria: pre-selection questionnaire, informed consent, initial interview, FTND, and CIDI.

Following the identification of the participants according to inclusion and exclusion criteria, all participants undergoing an initial assessment from the application of the following instruments: BQSC, BDI, BAI, TLFB, SOCRATES 8D.

Subsequent to the initial assessment participants were randomly assigned to one of five experimental conditions: 1) BMIS, 2) nicotine inhaler, 3) gum nicotine, 4) BMIS combined with nicotine inhaler, 5) BMIS combined with nicotine gum. At the end of the treatment and at 6 month follow up the initial assessment instruments were applied (see Figure 1).

Brief Motivational Intervention for smokers (BMIS)

The intervention is individual and consists of an admission session, an evaluation session, four sessions of treatment and six months follow up. In the program, the participants receive three booklets of work and self - reports of consumption (Lira-Mandujano et al., 2009). The BMIS is based in the social cognitive theory (Bandura, 1986), uses as main strategy the motivational interview (Miller, 1999; Miller & Rollnick, 1991), the relapse prevention approach (Carroll, 1999; Marlatt, Parks & Witkiewitz, 2002; Piasecki, 2006) and self-control techniques (Cooper, Heron & Heward, 2007; Muñoz, Labrador & Crusader, 2008).

Nicotine Inhalator (10 mg)

This kind of dose NRT was used by the people according to the level of dependency following the doses indicated by the manufacturer (Table 1). All participants were cited once a week to register the consumption pattern and know if they were having severe withdrawal symptoms and giving them, if necessary, more cartridges for the next week.

Dependence Level	Duration	Nicotine gum 2 mg	Inhalator 10 mg
Severe	3 weeks	2mg / 1 -2 hr *	1 cartridge / 1 -2 hr **
	3 weeks	2mg / 2- 4 hr	1 cartridge / 2- 4 hr
	2 weeks	2mg / 4 - 8 hr	1 cartridge / 4 - 8 hr
Low	3 weeks	2mg / 2 - 4 hrs	1 cartridge / 2 - 4 hrs
	3 weeks	2mg / 4 - 8 hr	1 cartridge / 4 - 8 hr
	2 weeks	2mg / 4 - 8 hr	1 cartridge / 4- 8 hr

* No more than 10 gums /day
** No more than 12 cartridges/day

Table 1. Doses for nicotine gum and inhalator

Nicotine Gum (2 mg)

The dose regimen of nicotine gum was according to the dependence level indicated by the manufacturer (Table 1). All participants were cited once a week to register the consumption pattern and know if you were having severe withdrawal symptoms and giving them, if necessary, more gum for the next week.

5.3 Results

The results showed in Figure 1, include all 71 participants (mean age = 43.5) assigned to one of each experimental conditions and with the initial evaluation; only 47 participants with 6 month follow up finished the treatment.

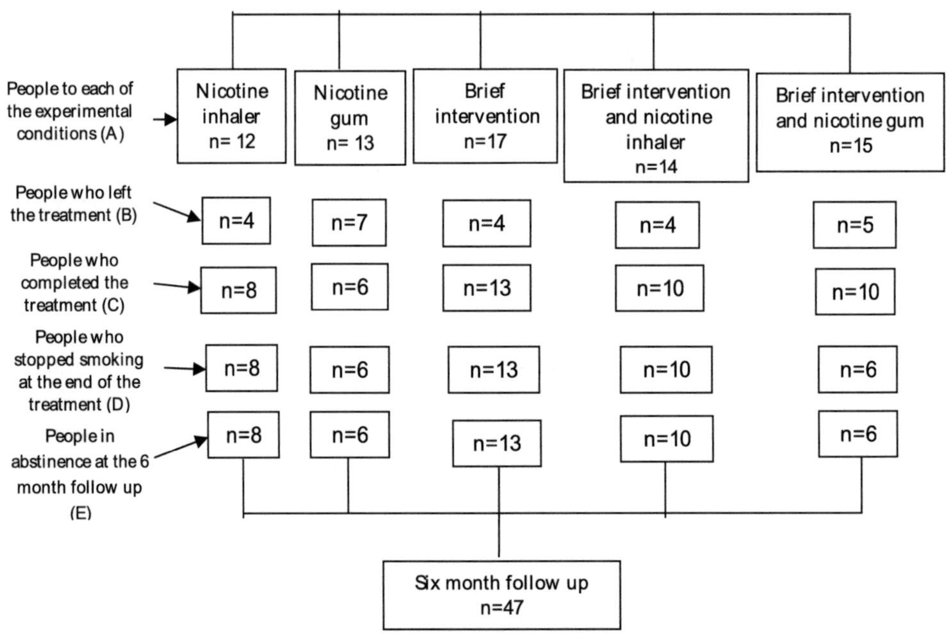

Fig. 1. Number of people in each experimental condition (A); number of persons who left the treatment (B); people who completed the treatment (C); people who stopped smoking at the end of the treatment (D) and people at six-month follow up (E).

In concordance analysis of results of smokers that finish the treatment, comprise:

Initial evaluation

Only the data of participants that finish the treatment and the 6 month follow up were included. Descriptive analysis of demographic variables contained in the initial interview and the corresponding tests were conducted to find out if the variables were homogeneous among groups.

Independent ANOVAS were carried for each variable, age, onset of consumption, number of years of regular smoking, as well as previous attempts to quit smoking. Significant statistically differences were detected for age variable ($F_{4, 62}$=2.55, p=0.048); post hoc test did not detect significant differences; a Kruskal Wallis detected significant differences for the academic level (H (4) = 3. 806, p < 0.001) in the inhaler group compared with the other groups.

Consumption Pattern

A second data obtained were abstinence rates (percentage of smokers that completed a specific treatment and self-declared smoking cessation) obtained at the end of each treatment and at six month follow up. Figure 2 shows that at the end of the treatment, the abstinence rates were higher for the BMIS plus the nicotine inhaler (30%, 40%). At the 6 month follow up a similar picture occurred, followed by BMIS (23% and 38.4 %), nicotine gum group (16.6% and 16.6%), BMIS plus nicotine gum (10% and 20%) and nicotine inhaler (0% and 25%).

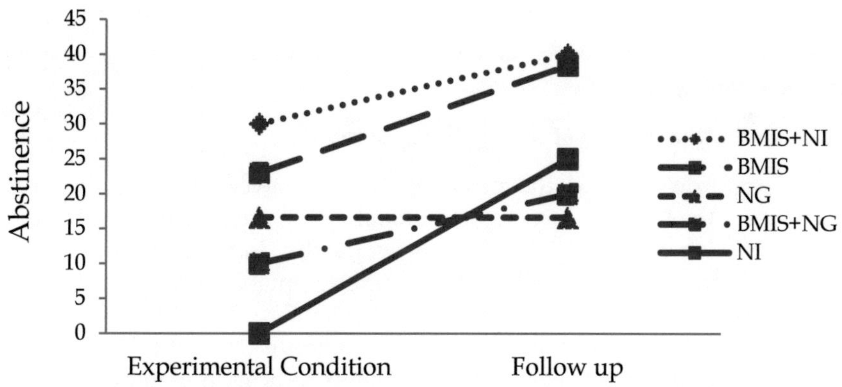

Fig. 2. Abstinence rates obtained in each of the experimental condition at the end of the treatment and 6-month follow up.

A repeated ANOVA (5 x 3; experimental condition x phase of treatment) detected significant differences (F [2.68] = 47. 429, p < 0.001) in consumption pattern for phase of treatment (Figure 3); however, no difference were found for the experimental condition (F [4.34] = 58. 78, p > 0.05). No differences were observed for the interaction experimental condition x phase of treatment (F [6.003, 51.024] = 2. 105, p > 0.05); for this parameter degrees of freedom correction was applied because the data violated the sphericity assumptions. Significant differences on consumption pattern were detected in between baseline, and treatment (p < 0.001) and with regard to the follow up (p < 0.001), but no significant differences between treatment and follow up (p > 0.05).

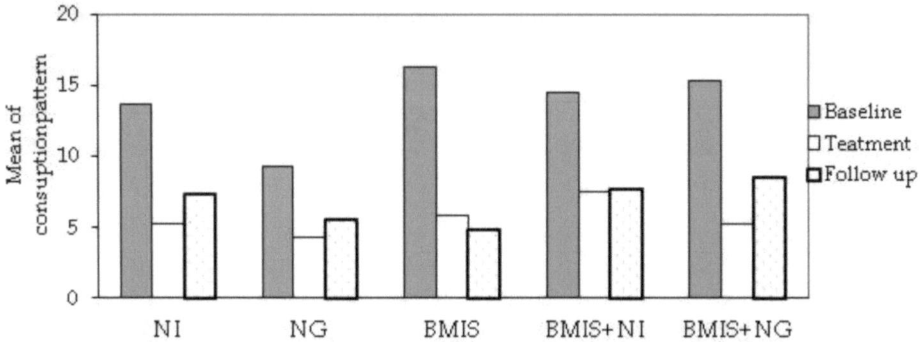

Fig. 3. Shows the mean of consumption pattern of each of the experimental groups (NI = nicotine inhaler, NG = nicotine gum; BMIS = brief intervention, BMIS + NI= brief intervention plus inhaler, and BMIS + NG = brief intervention and nicotine gum) in baseline, treatment and 6 month follow up (n = 47).

Relationship between the observed variables, and the change in consumption pattern

To assess whether there was any relationship between the changes in consumption pattern, a regression analysis was conducted to see if there was a linear relationship between the change in consumption pattern during the treatment and follow up with regard to the variables. The variables proposed as predictors of change are demographic variables (e.g. sex, age, marital status, etc.), variables related to the initial pattern of consumption, level dependence and group to which he belonged during the study; psychological state related variables as depression and anxiety, and variables of readiness to change in recognition, ambivalence and taking steps.

Change in consumption pattern of during the treatment

This variable was calculated as the mean difference between the initial consumption pattern and during the treatment, regression model points out that the involved variables explain a 59.7% (R^2 corrected =. 597, Se = 5.14) variability in the pattern of consumption during the treatment, which is not a broad but quite acceptable percentage. In Table 2 the standardized partial regression coefficients, the probability that these coefficients were observed in the population and the coefficients confidence interval (95%) are presented. As we know, the standardized regression coefficients indicate the amount of change, in typical scores that will occur in the dependent variable for each change unit in the corresponding independent variable (keeping constant the rest of independent variables). Variables with more weight are more important as predictors of consumption pattern change. In order of importance the variables are: 1) initial consumption pattern (β =. 908), that is, when people had a high initial consumption, declined more his pattern of consumption; 2) level of depression (β =-.884), the sign of the coefficient indicates that when the level of depression was higher in initial evaluation, the change in the pattern of consumption was lower; (3) with respect to the level of readiness to change in recognition (β = 0. 542) when the initial evaluation was high, people decreased more their consumption pattern. The level of anxiety (β = 0. 276), the level of readiness to change in ambivalence (β = 0. 184), and the level of dependency (β = 0. 131) are similar but in much smaller proportion. It is important to mention that belonging to the experimental condition variable was not significant to predict the improvement in consumption pattern, nor readiness to change in taking before treatment.

Model	No standardized Coefficients		Standardized Coefficients	t	Sig.	95% Confidence interval for B	
	B	Std. Error.	Beta			B	Std. Error
(Constant)	-17.381	5.620		-3.093	0.004	-28.874	-5.887
Experimental condition	0.325	0.654	**0.053**	0.497	0.062	-1.012	1.661
Dependence level	1.219	1.309	0.131	0.931	0.004	-1.459	3.896
Initial consumption pattern	0.817	0.127	0.908	6.428	0.000	0.557	1.077
Initial Anxiety	0.186	0.083	0.276	0.223	0.001	-0.152	0.189
Initial Depression	-0.656	0.098	-0.884	-0.670	0.005	-0.266	0.135
Readiness to change in initial recognition	0.545	1.134	0.542	0.480	0.006	-1.775	2.865
Readiness to change in initial ambivalence	1.885	1.126	0.184	1.674	0.001	-0.418	4.189
Readiness to change in initial taking steps	0.687	1.094	**0.697**	0.628	0.535	-1.549	2.924

Table 2. Regression coefficients (no standardized and standardized, significance levels, and confidence intervals), dependent variable is change of consumption during treatment.

Change of consumption pattern in follow up

This variable was calculated as the difference between the means of initial consumption pattern and the consumption in the follow up, regression model points out that the involved variables explain a 39.9% (R ^ 2 corrected =. 399, = 5.66) of the variability in consumption pattern during the treatment. This means, a missing of prediction with proposed variables between the treatments and the follow up, although the proportion explained by proposed variables is still appropriate, additionally the weight of independent variables differed from the previous analysis. Table 3 shows the standardized and no standardized regression and error estimation, the confidence interval and significance levels. The significant coefficients with more weight are: 1) initial consumption pattern (β = 0. 769), 2) level of readiness to change in taking steps before treatment (β=0,290), 3) level of readiness to change in ambivalence before treatment (β = 0, 229), 4) initial level of depression (β = 0, 220), 5) level of dependence (β = 0, 052), and 6) level of readiness to change in recognition before to treatment (β = 0, 038), the coefficients in this analysis are much smaller than previously. Both analyses met the assumptions of regression, both in independence as in the non-collinearity among the variables involved in the analysis.

Changes in anxiety, depression, and readiness to change by experimental condition

- **Anxiety scores**

The analysis of anxiety was carried out with global scores; however, the descriptive statistics was done account for each assessment period. Analysis of variance shows that there are

Coefficients(a)

	No Standardized Coefficients		Standardized Coefficients	t	Sig.	95% Confidence interval for B	
	B	Std. Error	Beta			B	Std. Error
(Constant)	-12,191	6,184		-1,97	0,058	-24,838	0,457
Initial consumption pattern	0,624	0,140	0,769	4,457	0,000	0,337	0,910
Readiness to change in initial taking steps	2,398	1,159	0,290	2,069	0,048	0,028	4,768
Readiness to change in initial ambivalence	2,112	1,240	0,229	1,704	0,010	-0,423	4,647
Initial depression	-0,147	0,108	-0,220	-1,36	0,018	-0,368	0,073
Group	0,402	0,719	**0,073**	0,559	0,058	-1,069	1,873
Dependence level	0,435	1,441	0,052	0,302	0,008	-2,511	3,382
Readiness to change in initial recognition	0,342	1,248	0,038	0,274	0,008	-2,211	2,895
Readiness to change in initial taking steps	0,263	1,203	**0,030**	0,219	0,828	-2,198	2,724
Initial Anxiety	0,007	0,092	**0,012**	0,078	0,094	-0,181	0,195

Table 3. Regression coefficients (no standardized and standardized, significance levels, and confidence intervals), dependent variable is change of consumption during follow up.

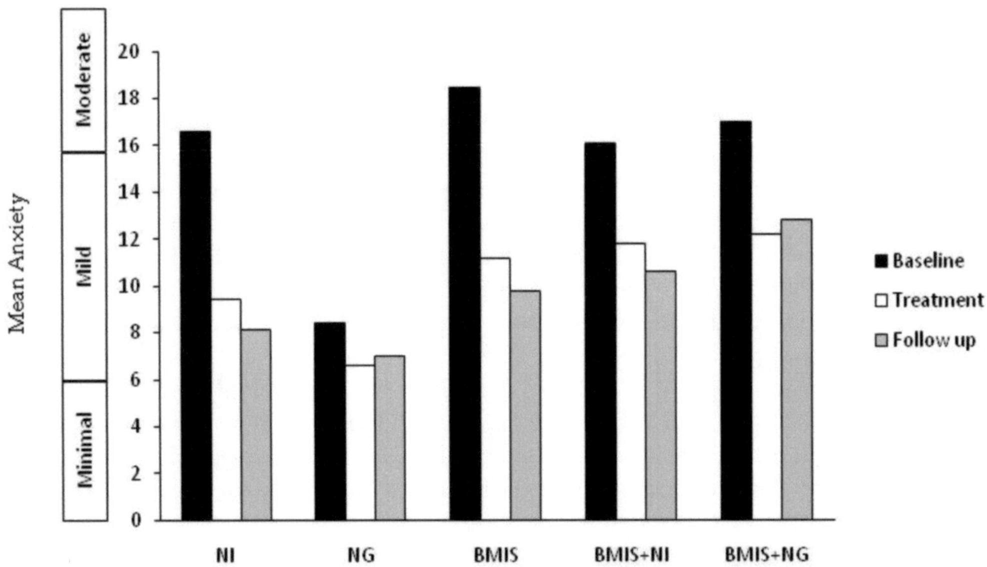

Fig. 4. Shows the mean of anxiety scores for each experimental condition (NI = nicotine inhaler, NG = nicotine gum; BMIS = brief intervention, BMIS + NI= brief intervention plus inhaler, and BMIS + NG = brief intervention and nicotine gum) in baseline, treatment and 6 month follow up.

differences dependent on the assessed period (F [2.68] = 13. 54, p < 0.001), the Bonferroni test post hoc demonstrated that there are differences in the baseline with respect to the phase of treatment (p < 0.001) and on follow up (p < 0.001). No differences for experimental condition (F [4.34] = 0. 748, p > 0.05) or for the interaction between experimental condition and the phase of treatment (baseline, treatment and follow up) ([5.37, 45.66] F = 24. 85, p > 0.05) were detected (Figure 5).

- **Depression scores**

With the use of an ANOVA again significant differences were found for phase of assessment (F [2.68] = 12.59, p < 0.001), significant differences were detected in initial depression scores and phase of treatment (p < 0.05) and in the follow up (p < 0.05); but not between the phase of treatment with regard to the follow up. No difference for experimental conditions (F [4.34] = 0. 74, p > 0.05), and for the interaction of both factors ([6.06, 51.54] F = 0. 888, p > 0.05) (Figure 5).

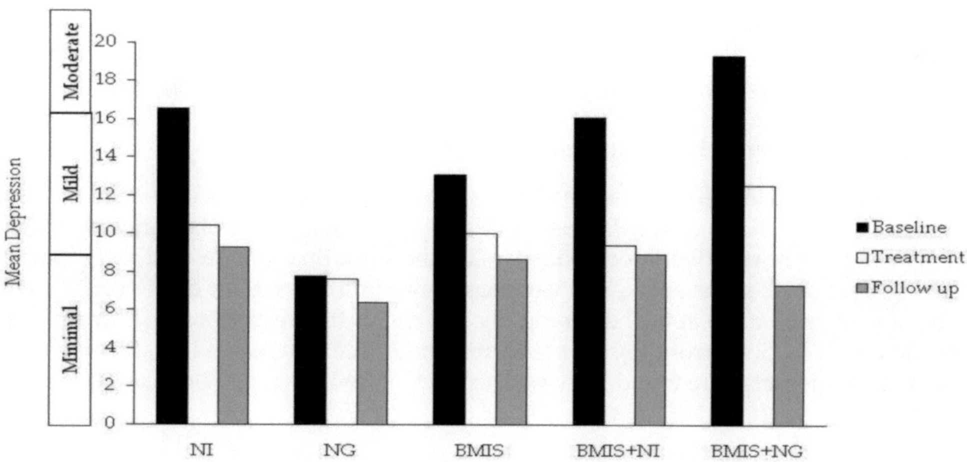

Fig. 5. Shows the mean of anxiety scores for each experimental condition (NI = nicotine inhaler, NG = nicotine gum; BMIS = brief intervention, BMIS + NI= brief intervention plus inhaler, and BMIS + NG = brief intervention and nicotine gum) in baseline, treatment and 6 month follow up.

Stages of Change Readiness and Treatment Eagerness Scale (SOCRATES 8D)

a. Readiness to change in recognition

According to Prochaska and DiCemente (1983) readiness to change in recognition refers to people who directly acknowledge that have problems related to the consumption of cigarettes, these people have a tendency to express a desire for change and perceive that the damage will continue if they do not do any changes. Analysis of variance did not detect significant differences for experimental condition (F [4.34] = 2.19, p > 0.05), changes in the level of readiness to change depending dependent on phase of evaluation ([1.68, 7.29] F = 1,196, p > 0.05), or for the interaction between the two factors.

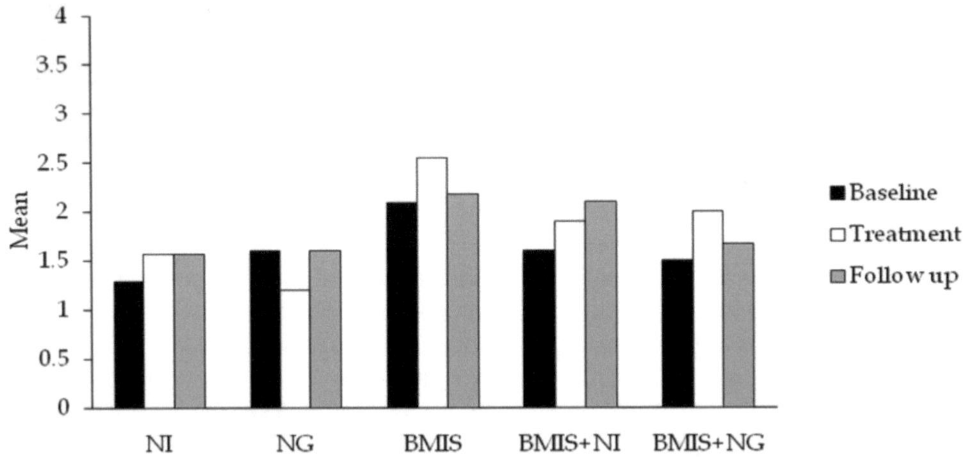

Fig. 6. Shows the mean of stages of change readiness and treatment eagerness scale scores for recognition in each experimental condition (NI = nicotine inhaler, NG = nicotine gum; BMIS = brief intervention, BMIS + NI= brief intervention plus inhaler, and BMIS + NG = brief intervention and nicotine gum) in baseline, treatment and 6 month follow up.

b. Readiness to change in ambivalence

The ambivalence factor of readiness to change, according to the stages of change proposed by Prochaska and DiClemente (1983) refers to the person that is at a point in which knows that smoking can bring adverse consequences on their health, economy and social but find advantages for smoke. The analysis of variance showed differences for ambivalence relying on the time of evaluation, at the beginning, the the end of the treatment or follow up ([2.68] $F = 6.36$ $p < 0.05$); Bonferroni test was used to identify the differences in pairs of variables (Figure 7), differences were found between the baseline and the treatment ($p < 0.05$) as well

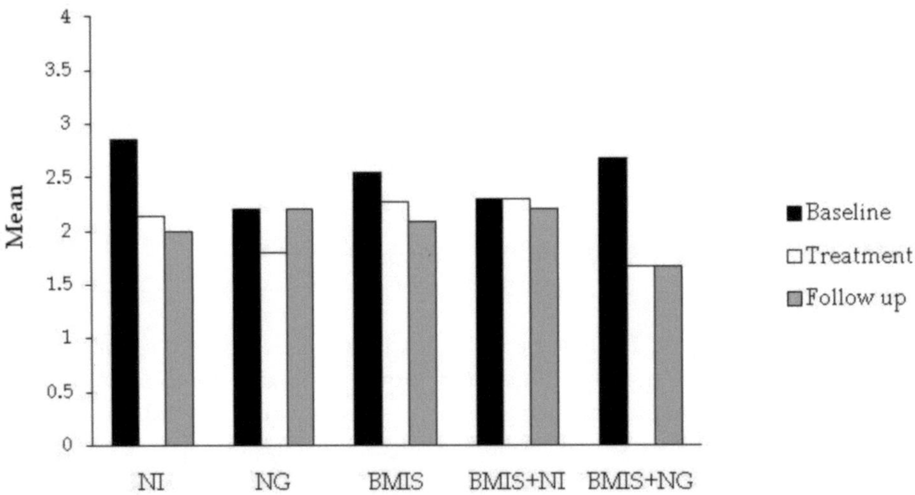

Fig. 7. Shows the mean of stages of change readiness scores for ambivalence factor in each experimental condition (NI = nicotine inhaler, NG = nicotine gum; BMIS = brief

intervention, BMIS + NI= brief intervention plus inhaler, and BMIS + NG = brief intervention and nicotine gum) in baseline, treatment and 6 month follow up.

as between the baseline and the follow up ($p < 0.05$), but there no differences between treatment and follow up; no differences were obtained for experimental condition (F [4.34] =. 37.5, $p > 0.05$), or fo the interaction between variables (F [5.66,48.13] = 1.07, $p > 0.05$).

c. Readiness to change in taking steps

Analysis of variance for the level of readiness to change in action showed that there are significant differences for the moment in which the instrument was applied (F [2.68] = 8.36, $p < 0.001$), Bonferroni test detected differences between the baseline with regard to treatment ($p < 0.05$) and six months follow up ($p < 0.05$), but not between the treatment and the the follow (Figure 8). No differences were found for groups (F [4,348] = 0.765, $p > 0.05$), or due to the interaction between variables (F [5.95,50.59] = 0.23, $p > 0.05$).

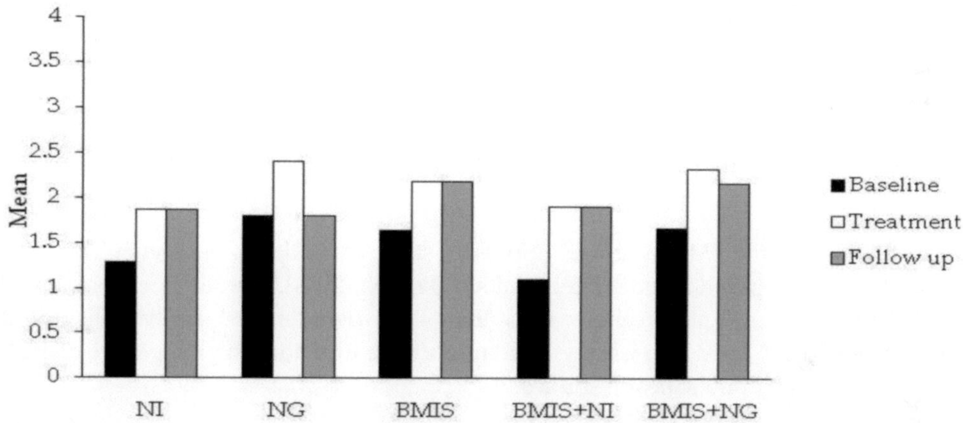

Fig. 8. Shows the mean of stages of change readiness scores for action factor in each experimental condition (NI = nicotine inhaler, NG = nicotine gum; BMIS = brief intervention, BMIS + NI= brief intervention plus inhaler, and BMIS + NG = brief intervention and nicotine gum) in baseline, treatment and 6 month follow up.

One of the specific purposes of the present investigation was to know if there was any relationship between the changes in the pattern of consumption during the treatment and follow up with regard to the observed variables (demographic, initial pattern of consumption, level dependence, group to which it belonged, depression, anxiety and willingness to change in recognition, ambivalence and action). The results obtained from regression analysis showed that no sociodemographic variable (age, sex, marital status) was predictive for reducing tobacco use. However, from a regression analysis, it was noted that the pattern of initial consumption, depression and anxiety as well as the readiness to change in recognition were good predictors to modify the consumption pattern but not to maintain it in the follow up, since their predictive power was lost. Variable with greater weight to change consumption from the baseline to treatment was the initial consumption pattern, i.e. when people had an initial high consumption, after treatment more decreased their consumption pattern.

5.4 Conclusions

Present study assessed the effectiveness of BMIS alone or combined with NRT in the consumption patterns of people who want to quit smoking. The results showed that abstinence rates (Hughes et al., 2003) for inhaler experimental condition combined with BMIS, was much higher at the end of the treatment and at 6 month follow up, followed by the BMIS experimental condition. This is consistent with a previous finding where BMIS has proven to be effective because the people learn a set of skills that allows addressing the specific factors that trigger the consumption of cigarettes (Lira-Mandujano et al., 2009). In the case of the inhaler, different studies have shown its effectiveness to relieve withdrawal symptoms because the absorption of nicotine depends on the administration route (Schneider et al., 2001). In other words, considering only abstinence rates, the hypothesis that increase abstinence rates when combined therapies (NRT and BMIS) are employed, can be accepted.

Clinical trials of last ten years combining NRT with a psychological intervention, show that nicotine patches in combination with a psychological intervention induce higher abstinence rates than the nicotine patch alone (Macleod et al., 2003) and when compared with a placebo group (Richmond et al., 1997). In present study significant differences were not observed between nicotine gum and inhalator in present study, results consistent with last Cochrane review that concludes that all NRT are equally effective and are better than no treatment (Stead et al., 2011).

The effectiveness of the BMIS observed in present study is similar to the reviews indicating the effectiveness of psychological interventions (Becoña, 2004). For all these reasons, the BMIS showed that is equally effective as the NRT. Then present study validates the technique previously used empirically and support the idea that the integrative model is useful for clinical and public health studies.

The brief motivational intervention for smokers initiate by obtaining baseline data related to the history of consumption, factors associated with the consumption of tobacco (depression, anxiety, and willingness to change consumption patterns). Subsequently, the results of such data are provided in order to give a personalized feedback that allows undertaking a decisional balance and thus choosing the technique that the user wants for abstinence. From the delivery of results and choice of technique to achieve abstinence, the user must register their daily consumption and withdrawal symptoms. Then, in the four treatment sessions, where the therapist applies motivational interviewing strategies (express empathy, show reflective listening, support and promote a sense of self-efficacy, develops discrepancy, avoid discussions and arguing) will work the following aspects:

1. Identify the three main triggers of the consumption of cigarettes (situations, states of mood, places, and people), the positive and negative consequences of the consumption of the user from a functional analysis of behavior.
2. With the three main triggers of the consumption, the user set up three strategies to implement them and to reach the abstinence. With the support of the therapist a viable and feasible strategy is selected to cope with the triggers.
3. The user develops an action plan that includes a specific description of how the strategy chosen is going to be applied prior to the trigger.

4. Later, the user must apply the action plan to evaluate the proposed strategies and in this form to apply them to other triggers or to change them to identify the strategies that turn out to be effective to stop smoking.

In the last session of treatment, information related to the consumption of tobacco is obtained to compare with the data obtained initially and a graph is presented where the daily consumption pattern from the baseline and during the treatment sessions to evaluate the advances reached at the end of the intervention and a follow up session is settled. In the session of follow up new information is obtained again with respect the application of strategies to new triggers, to the development of new strategies and for the identification of strategies that already were ineffective, and for the maintenance of the abstinence, for the lapses and relapses.

The analysis of present results suggests that is necessary to include new instruments in the BMIS. The factors inducing the smokers to quit the treatments, like the side effects (e. g. headache, dizziness, nervous, etc.) and the presence of withdrawal symptoms like irritability, anxiety, depression, etc. (Kenford et al., 2002) to different populations, need to be assessed. The literature only identifies seven scales in which the person registers the withdrawal symptoms: 1) *Cigarette Withdrawal Scale* (Etter, 2005), 2) *Mood & Physical Symptoms Scale* (West & Hajek, 2004), 3) *Profile of Mood States Manual* (McNair, Lorr & Droppelman, 1992), 4) *Shiffman Jarvik Withdrawal Scale* (Shiffman & Jarvik, 1976), 5) *Smoker Complaints Scale* (Schneider & Jarvik, 1984), 6) *Wisconsin Smoking Withdrawal Scale* (Welsch, Smith, Wetter, Jorenby, Fiore & Baker, 1999) and 7) *Scale to use on a hand-held computer* (Shiffman, Paty, Gnys, Kassel & Hickcox, 1996).

It is important to develop and instrument equivalent to the Drug Taking Confidence Questionnaire (DTCQ; Annis, Sklar & Turner, 1997) focused on the consumption of tobacco in the Mexican population. One of the components in the relapse prevention model is to identify risk situations and according to this to implement a personalized intervention to prevent relapse that allow maintaining long-term abstinence. That is, this kind of instrument may be included in the package of instruments of the initial component of the BMIS.

Another aspect to assess is the cost effectiveness of the BMIS and the NRT. It has been reported that psychological interventions are more expensive for the training cost and requires much time (Hall et al., 2005). Hall et al. (2005) showed that the psychological intervention was more cost-effective than the nortriptyline, bupropion, but the differences were not statistically significant. However in the case of BMIS, capacitating the personnel is inexpensive and the number of sessions require just 8 sessions. Therefore is important to perform a cost effectiveness analysis of BMIS in order to know which has better cost effectiveness between BMIS and pharmacological treatments. In a preliminary analysis considering only the cost of NRT for 8 weeks, and the material used, the BMIS showed a better cost-effectiveness ratio. It will be important to evaluate the cost effectiveness for new compounds like varenicline (Jorenby et al., 2006; Tonstad et al., 2006), in combination with behavioral interventions.

And finally, an aspect not analyzed but that would be necessary to include are the measurement of biological markers (carbon monoxide in expired air, cotinine concentration in urine or plasma). This will increase the motivation respect of initial consumption, during and after the intervention and also will help to verify the pattern of consumption reported by the users (Benowitz et al., 2002).

A limitation of present study is the difference in the number of participants in each group at the end of the study, because two factors were not considered. The first factor was the use of a simple random assignment for allocate the participants. The second one was the number of people that abandoned the study. Based on the results obtained in present study, in future clinical trials it would be essential to pay attention in the method of randomization and as a consequence in the number of people assigned to each condition for of a clinical trial.

Lazcano Ponce et al. (2004) proposed the method of randomization of balanced blocks. In his method a series of blocks are assembled, consisting of a certain number of cells, which include the different types of treatment. The number of blocks is determined by the number of participants to be included in the study and the number of cells decided to be included in each block. "Each block will contain in each cell of treatment alternatives and within each block must be a balanced number of possible treatments" (p.569).

In present study data obtained in the initial assessment were used to match groups with regard to the level of dependency to nicotine, age, sex, previous attempts to quit smoking, the use of any NRT, so the groups were homogeneous in regard of these variables. An alternative is identified through the systematic or narrative literature review, in consultation with experts or of the same experience, those factors or variables that at any given time could modify the impact of the treatment on the outcome variable; depending on the feasibility of the size of the sample decide how many layers set up as a priori the allocation of the maneuver (Lazcano-Ponce et al., 2004) and to use the method of stratified randomization, which guarantees treatment balance on these known predictive variables, allowing easy interpretation of outcomes without adjustment.

Finally, an essential methodological aspect regarding the measure of abstinence is to explain the results in terms of: 1) prolonged abstinence (continuous abstinence after an initial grace period or the period of continuous abstinence in two follow ups) as a main measure; (2) the use of the term continuous abstinence only to refer to the prolonged abstinence without grace period; (3) not to use the term of sustained abstinence; (4) include the use of tobacco products other than cigarettes in the definition of failure; (5) do not include the use of nicotine (e.g. the use of NRT) in the definitions of failure and 6) present the results of the analysis of the history of survival (Hughes et al., 2003).

The variable group or experimental condition in relation to the treatment used to quit smoking, was not a good predictor, perhaps by the sample size or because it is interacting with all the other variables and this interaction interacting blur its action. The group CONSORT (Consolidated standards of reporting trials) indicates that would be important to address in the clinical trial the size of the sample, randomization, statistical methods, instrumentation, flow of participants, recruiting and reporting of results (Moher, Schulz & Altman, 2001).

Depression was found to be a predictive variable of change in consumption pattern during treatment, when the level of depression was higher in the initial assessment, the change in the pattern of consumption was lower. In other words, there is a relationship between the presence of increased symptoms of depression and more difficult to reduce consumption or smoking cessation (Brody, Hamer & Haaga, 2005; Paperwalla, Levin, Weiner & Saravay, 2004; Vázquez, Becoña & Míguez, 2002). Vázquez and Becoña (1999) previously reported that subjects who continued smoking in 12 month follow up presented depressive symptoms in the initial assessment with the Beck Depression Inventory. In addition, Kinnunen et al. (1996) conducted a research with the idea of examine if smokers with high symptoms of depression were less likely to succeed in the treatment to quit smoking than smokers with minor symptoms of depression. The results showed that depressive symptoms were an obstacle to the success of abstinence from smoking.

Theoretically, this is in agreement with the assumption that smoking cessation induces depressive symptoms, since smoking modulates negative affection. People with depressive symptoms are more likely to smoke (this happens more often in women) and when smokers with depressive symptoms are trying to quit smoking have higher probability of not maintaining abstinence (Moreno-Coutiño & Medina- Mora, 2008). For this reason in present study, people with medical diagnosis of major depression where not included, however, some participants showed severe depression according to the BDI. Nevertheless in some cases they stopped smoking or decreased their consumption, therefore in forthcoming studies would be necessary to measure the depression during treatment and obtain abstinence data for more than six months.

A second particular aim of this study was to compare the level of anxiety, depression, and the readiness to change in the application of NRT and the brief intervention alone and combined. The results showed that there were no significant differences among treatments in these variables; only significant differences were detected for phases (baseline, treatment and follow up). Specifically in depression and anxiety significant differences were found between baseline and treatment and between baseline and follow up; in readiness for change in ambivalence existed changes from baseline to treatment and baseline and follow up, and readiness for taking steps action between baseline and treatment. Not any treatment resulted in a significant reduction in depression and anxiety. These results confirm that NRT do not lessen the symptoms of depression and anxiety by which have been used antidepressants and anxiolytics for smoking cessation (Hughes, Stead & Lancaster, 2005a; Hughes, Lancaster & Stead, 2005b; Hughes, Stead, Lancaster, 2008a; Hughes, Stead, Lancaster, 2008b).

Different reports show that there is a strong association between a history of depression and anxiety, and difficulty to smoke cessation (Becoña, 2003; Scheitrum & Akillas, 2002). Goldstein (2003) explains that for people with depression and anxiety antecedents that want to quit smoking and decide to use some NRT, it would be important to use an antidepressant or anxiolytic during the attempt to quit smoking, and for those who despite this combination fail in their attempt to quit would be advisable to combine bupropion with NRT or bupropion with other antidepressant; however, should be assessed its effectiveness (Hughes et al., 2005b; Hughes et al., 2008b).

In present study, the BAI was used to assess anxiety, however, would be important to use the instrument "Anxiety, trait and State" (Spielberger et al., 1998 in, Becoña, 2003) to know if the people who want to quit smoking and present anxiety trait or state have higher rates of abstinence when they employ a NRT, when they attend to any psychological therapy or when treatments are combined. In addition it is important to investigate whether the anxiety trait or state is a predictor of treatment abandonment or relapse in the follow up. People who stopped using nicotine gum reported that the taste was unpleasant, that they did not feel better and that they continued with craving so they were not interested in continue using it; a possible explanation could be that 2 mg nicotine gum did not decrease withdrawal symptoms, perhaps with the use of nicotine gum of 4 mg effectiveness could increase.

Taken together, the results of this clinical trial including the BMIS and NRT show that the effectiveness for this program did not differ of the effectiveness of NRT, implying that it is just as effective to stop smoking with nicotine gum and nicotine inhaler. Present study is one of the first trials evaluating the effectiveness of the combination inhaler with a psychological intervention.

6. Acknowledgment

Correspondence should be addressed to: Dra. Sara E. Cruz Morales, Div. de Investigación y Posgrado, UIICSE, FES-Iztacala, UNAM.Av. Barrios, No. 1, Los Reyes Iztacala, Tlalnepantla, Edo. México, 54090, México. saracruz@unam.mx

7. References

Annis, H.M., Sklar, S.M. & Turner, N.E. (1997). *The Drug-Taking Confidence Questionnaire (DTCQ): User's Guide.* Toronto, Canada: Addiction Research Foundation, Centre for Addiction and Mental Health.

Alterman, A.I., Gariti, P. & Mulvaney, F. (2001). Short- and Long-Term Smoking Cessation for Three Levels of Intensity of Behavioral Treatment. *Psychology of Addictive Behaviors,* Vol.15, No.3, (September 2001) pp. 261-264, ISSN 0893-164X.

Ayala, V.H., Cárdenas, L. G., Echeverría, L., y Gutiérrez, L. M. (1998). *Manual de auto ayuda para personas con problemas en su forma de beber.* Porrúa. UNAM. ISBN 968-842-850-7, México.

Bandura, A. (1986). *Social foundations of thought and action. A social cognitive theory.* Prentice Hall, ISBN 013815614X, New Jersey.

Beck, A. T., Epstein, N., Brown, G. & Steer, R. A. (1988). An inventory for measuring clinical anxiety: Psychometric properties. *Journal of Consulting and Clinical Psychology,* Vol. 56, No.6, (December 1988) pp. 893–897, ISSN 0022-006X.

Beck, A. T., Steer, A. R. & Garbin, G. M. (1988). Psychometric properties of the Beck Depression Inventory: twenty-five years of evaluation. *Clinical Psychology Rewiew,* Vol. 8, No. 1, pp. 77-100, ISSN 0272-7358.

Becoña, I. E. (2003). Tabaco, ansiedad y estrés. *Salud y Drogas,* Vol.3, No. 1, pp.71-92, ISSN 1578-5319.

Becoña, I. E. (2004). Eficacia del Tratamiento Psicológico en el Tabaquismo. *Revista Thomson Psicología,* Vol. 1, No. 1, pp. 19- 34, ISBN: 0-01-665636-9.

Benowitz, N. L., Jacob, P., Ahijevych, K., Jarvis, M. J., Hall, S., LeHouezec, J., et al. (2002). Biochemical verification of tobacco use and cessation. SRNT Subcommittee on Biochemical Verification. *Nicotine and Tobacco Research, Vol. 4,* No.2, pp. 149-159, ISSN 1462-2203.

Brody, C. L., Hamer, D. H. & Haaga, D. A. (2005). Depression vulnerability, cigarette smoking, and the serotonin transporter gene. *Addictive Behaviors*, Vol. 30, No. 3, (March 2005) pp.557- 566, ISSN 0306-4603.

Cahill, K. Stead, L. & Lancaster, T. (2011). Nicotine receptor partial agonists for smoking cessation. Cochrane database of systematic reviews. In: *The Cochrane Library*, Issue 06, 30.07.2011, Available from http://cochrane.bvsalud.org/cochrane/main.php?lib=COC&searchExp=smoking &lang=pt

Carroll, M. K. (1999). Behavioral and Cognitive Behavioral Treatments. In: McCrady, S. B., Epstein, E. E. (Eds.). *Addictions. A Comprehensive Guidebook.* New York: Oxford University Press.

Cinciripini, P. M., Tsoh, J. Y., Wetter, D. W., Lam, C., de Moor, C., Cinciripini, L., Baile, W., Anderson, C. & Minna, J. D. (2005). Combined Effects of Venlafaxine, Nicotine Replacement, and Brief Counseling on Smoking Cessation. *Experimental and Clinical Psychopharmacology*, Vol.13, No. 4, (November 2005) pp. 282-292, ISSN 1064-1297.

Coe, J. W., Brooks, P. R., Vetelino, M. G., Wirtz, M. C., Arnold, E. P., Huang, J., Sands, S. B., Davis, T. I., Lebel, L. A., Fox, C. B., Shrikhande, A., Heym, J. H., Schaeffer, E., Rollema, H., Lu, Y., Mansbach, R. S., Chambers, L. K., Rovetti, C. C., Schulz, D. W., Tingley, F. D. & O'Neill, B. T. (2005). Varenicline: an alpha4beta2 nicotinic receptor partial agonist for smoking cessation. *Journal of Medicinal Chemistry*. 19, Vol.48, No.10,(April 2005), pp.3474-3477, ISSN 0022-2623.

Cooper, J. O., Heron, T. E., & Heward, W. L. (2007). *Applied Behavior Analysis* (2^a ed.). Pearson, ISBN 131421131, New Jersey.

Covey, L. S., Glassman, A. H. & Stetner, F. (1999). Naltrexone effects on short-term and long-term smoking cessation. *Journal of Addictive Diseases*, Vol. 17, No.1, (March 1999), pp.31-40, ISSN 1055-0887.

Cornelius, J. R., Perkins, K. A., Salloum, I. M., Thase, M. E. & Moss, H. B. (1999). Fluoxetine versus placebo to decrease the smoking of depressed alcoholic patients [letter]. *Journal of Clinical Psychopharmacology*, Vol. 19, No.2, (April 1999), pp.183–184, ISSN 0271-0749.

Cuevas, E. Luna, G. Vital, G. & Lira, J. (2005, septiembre). *Validez Interna de la Escala de las Etapas de Disposición al Cambio y Anhelo de tratamiento (SOCRATES 8D)*. Proceedings of XVII Congreso Mexicano de Análisis de la Conducta. San Luis Potosí, September, México.

David, S., Lancaster, T., Stead, L. F., Evins, A. E. & Cahill, K. (2011). Opioid antagonists for smoking cessation. Cochrane database of systematic reviews. In: *The Cochrane Library*, Issue 06, 30.07.2011, Available from http://cochrane.bvsalud.org/cochrane/main.php?lib=COC&searchExp=smoking&lang=pt

Dodgen, E. C. (2005). *Nicotine dependence. Understanding and applying the most effective treatment interventions*. American Psychological Association, ISBN 978-1591472339, Washington, D.C.

Dwoskin, L. P., Rauhut, A. S., King-Pospisil, K. A., & Bardo, M. T. (2006). Review of the pharmacology and clinical profile of bupropion, an antidepressant and tobacco use cessation agent. *CNS Drug Reviews*, Vol. 12, No.3-4, (Fall/Winter 2006), pp.178-207, ISSN 1527-3458.

Eisenberg, M. J., Filion, K. B., & Yavin, D. (2008). Pharmacotherapies for smoking cessation: A meta-analysis of randomized controlled trials. *Canadian Medical Association Journal*, Vol. 179, (July 2008), pp.135-144, ISSN 1488-2329.

Etter, J. F. (2005). A self-administered questionnaire to measure cigarette withdrawal symptoms: The Cigarette Withdrawal Scale. *Nicotine and Tobacco Research*, Vol.7, No.1, (February 2005), pp.47-57, ISSN 1462-2203.

Ferry, L. H. &, Burchette, R. J. (1994). Efficacy of bupropion for smoking cessation in non-depressed smokers [abstract]. *Journal of Addictive Diseases*. Vol.13, p.249, ISSN 1055-0887.

Ferry, L. H., Robbins, A. S., Scariati, P. D., Masterson, A., Abbey, D.E. & Burchette, R. J. (1992). Enhancement of smoking cessation using the antidepressant bupropion hydrochloride [abstract]. *Circulation*. Vol.86, p. 671, ISSN 0009-7322.

Fiore, M. C., Bailey, W. C., Cohen, S. J. et al. (2000). Treating tobacco use and dependence. Clinical practice guideline. Rockville: U.S. Deparment of Health and Human Services, Public Health Service.

Foxx, R.M. & Brown, R.A. (1979). Nicotine fading, self-monitoring for cigarette abstinence or controlled smoking. *Journal of Applied Behavior Analysis*, Vol. 12, pp.115-125.

Fuxe, K., Ogren, S. O., Agnati, L., Gustafsson, J. A. & Jonsson, G. (1977). On the mechanism of action of the antidepressant drugs amitriptyline and nortriptyline. Evidence for 5-hydroxytryptamine receptor blocking activity. *Neuroscience Letters*, Vol. 6, No. 4, (December 1977), pp. 339-343, ISSN 0304-3940.

Goldstein, M. G. (2003). Pharmacotherapy for smoking cessation. In Abrams, D. B., Niaura, R., Brown, R., Emmons, K., Goldstein, M. & Monti, P. (Eds.), *The Tobacco Dependence Treatment Handbook. A Guide to Best Practices*. The Guilford Press. ISBN 1-57230-849-4, New York.

Gorelick, D. A., Rose, J. E. & Jarvik, M. E. (1988). Effect of naloxone on cigarette smoking. *Journal of Substance Abuse*, Vol. 1, No. 2, pp.153-159, ISSN 0899-3289.

Hall, S., Humfleet, G., Reus, V., Muñoz, R. & Cullen, J. (2004). Extended Nortriptyline and Psychological Treatment for Cigarette Smoking. *American Journal of Psychiatry*, Vol.161, (November 2004), pp. 2100–2107, ISSN 0002-953X.

Hall, S., Humfleet, G., Reus, V., Muñoz, R., Hartz, D., & Maude-Griffin, R. (2002). Psychological Intervention and Antidepressant Treatment in Smoking Cessation. *Archives of General Psychiatry*, Vol. 59, (October 2002), pp. 930 – 936, ISSN 003-990X.

Hall, S., Lightwood, J., Humfleet, G. L., Bostrom, A., Reus, V. & Muñoz, R. (2005). Cost-Efectiveness of Bupropion, Nortriptyline, and Psychological Intervention in Smoking Cessation. *The Journal of Behavioral Health Services & Research*. Vol. 32, No. 4, (October/December 2005), pp. 381- 393, ISSN 1094-3412.

Hall, S. M., Reus, V. I., Muñoz, F. R., Sees, L. K., Humfleet, G., Hartz, T. D., Frederick, S. & Triffleman, E. (1998). Nortriptyline and Cognitive-Behavioral Therapy in the Treatment of Cigarette Smoking. *Archives of General Psychiatry*, Vol.55, (August 1988), pp. 683-690, ISSN 003-990X.

Heatherton, T., Kozlowski, L., Frecker, R. & Fagerström, K. (1991). The Fagerström Test for Nicotine Dependence: A Revision of the Fagerström Tolerance Questionnaire. *British Journal of Addiction*, Vol. 86, pp. 1119-1127, INSS 0952-0481.

Hughes, J. R., Keely, J. P., Niaura, R. S., Ossip-Klein, D. J., Richmond, R. L. & Swan, G. E. (2003). Measures of abstinence in clinical trials: issues and recommendations. *Nicotine & Tobacco Research*, Vol.5, No.1, pp. 13–25, ISSN 1462-2203.

Hughes, J. R., Stead, L. F. & Lancaster, T. (2005a). Ansiolíticos para dejar de fumar. *La Biblioteca Cochrane Plus*. 3. Available from www.cochrane.es

Hughes, J. R., Stead, L. F. & Lancaster, T. (2005b). Antidepresivos para el abandono del hábito de fumar. *La Biblioteca Cochrane Plus*. 3. Recuperado el Febrero 10, 2006 en www.cochrane.es

Hughes, J. R., Stead, L. F. & Lancaster, T. (2008a). Ansiolíticos para dejar de fumar. *La Biblioteca Cochrane Plus*. 2. Recuperado el 7 de Julio 2008 en www.cochrane.es

Hughes, J.R., Stead L. F. & Lancaster, T. (2008b). Antidepresivos para el abandono del hábito de fumar. *La Biblioteca Cochrane Plus*. 2. Recuperado el 7 de Julio 2008 en www.cochrane.es

Hughes, J. R., Stead, L. F. & Lancaster, T. (2011a). Antidepressants for smoking cessation. Cochrane database of systematic reviews. In: *The Cochrane Library*, Issue 06, 30.07.2011, Available from http://cochrane.bvsalud.org/cochrane/main.php?lib=COC&searchExp=smoking&lang=pt

Hughes, J., Stead, L. & Lancaster, T. (2011b). Anxiolytics for smoking cessation. Cochrane database of systematic reviews. In: *The Cochrane Library*, Issue 06, 30. 07. 2011, Available from http://cochrane.bvsalud.org/cochrane/main.php?lib=COC&searchExp=smoking&lang=pt

Ingersoll, K. S. & Cohen, J. (2005). Combination Treatment for Nicotine Dependence: State of the Science. *Substance Use & Misuse*, Vol. 40, NO. 13-14, (January 2005), pp.1923–1943, ISSN 1082-6084.

James, W. A. & Lippmann S. (1991). Bupropion: overview and prescribing guidelines in depression. *South Medical Journal*, Vol. 84, No. 2, (February 1991), pp. 222-224, ISNN 0038-4348.

Javitz, H., Swan, G., Zbikowski, S., Curry, S., McAfee, T., Decker, D., et al. (2004). Cost-Effectiveness of Different Combinations of Bupropion SR Dose and Behavioral Treatment for Smoking Cessation: A Societal Perspective. *The American Journal of Managed Care*, Vol.10, pp. 217–226, ISSN 1088-0224.

Jorenby, D. E., Hays, T. Rigotti, N. A., Azoulay, S. Watsky, E., Williams, K., Billing, C. B. Gong, J. & Reeves, K. (2006). Efficacy of Varenicline, an α4β2 nicotinic acetylcholine receptor partial agonist vs placebo or sustained- release Bupropion for smoking cessation. *Journal of the American Medical Association*. Vol. 296, No.1, (July 2006), pp.56-63, ISSN 0098-7484.

Jurado, S., Villegas, M. E., Méndez, L., Rodríguez, F., Loperena, V. & Varela, R. (1998). La Estandarización del Inventario de Depresión de Beck para los Residentes de la Ciudad de México, *Salud Mental*, Vol. 21, No.3, (Junio 1998), pp.26-31, ISSN 0185-3325.

Kenford, S., Smith, S., Wetter, D., Jorenby, D., Fiore, M. & Baker, T. (2002). Predicting Relapse Back to Smoking: Contrasting Affective and Physical Models of Dependence. *Journal of Consulting and Clinical Psychology*, Vol. 70, No. 1, (February 2002) pp.216-227, ISSN 0022-006X.

Karras, A. & Kane, J. M. (1980). Naloxone reduces cigarette smoking. *Life Sciences*, Vol. 27, No. 17, (October 1980) pp. 1541–1545, ISSN 0024-3205.

Kinnunen, T., Doherty, K., Militello, F. S., & Garvey, A. J. (1996). Depression and smoking cessation: Characteristics of depressed smokers and effects of nicotine replacement. *Journal of Consulting and Clinical Psychology, Vol. 64*, No. 4, (August 1996) pp.791-798, ISSN 0022-006X.

Krishnan-Sarin, S., Rosen, M. I. & O'Malley, S. S. (1999). Naloxone challenge in smokers. Preliminary evidence of an opioid component in nicotine dependence. *Archives of General Psychiatry*, Vol.56, (July 1999), pp.663-668, ISSN 0003-990X.

Kuri-Morales, P. A., González-Roldan, J. F., Hoy, M. M. & Cortés-Ramírez, M. (2006). Epidemiología del Tabaquismo en México. *Salud Pública de México*, Vol.48 (Suppl. 1), pp. s91- s98, ISSN 0036-3634.

Lancaster, T. & Stead, L. F. (2011). Individual behavioural counselling for smoking cessation. Cochrane database of systematic reviews. In: *The Cochrane Library*, Issue 06, 30.07.2011, Available from http://cochrane.bvsalud.org/cochrane/main.php?lib=COC&searchExp=smoking&lang=pt

Lazcano-Ponce, E., Salazar-Martínez, E., Gutiérrez-Castrellón, P., Angeles-Llerenas, A., Hernández-Garduño, A. & Viramontes, J.L. (2004). Ensayos clínicos aleatorizados: variantes, métodos de aleatorización, análisis, consideraciones éticas y regulación. *Salud Pública de México*, Vol.46, No. 6, pp.559-584, ISSN 0036-3634.

Lira, M. J. (2002). Desarrollo y evaluación de un programa de tratamiento de la dependencia a la nicotina. Tesis de Maestría. FES- Iztacala. UNAM.

Lira-Mandujano, J., González-Betanzos, F., Carrascoza, V. C., Ayala, V. H. & Cruz-Morales, S. E. (2009). Evaluación de un programa de intervención breve motivacional para fumadores: resultados de un estudio piloto. *Salud Mental*. Vol 32, No.1, (Enero-Febrero 2009), pp.35-41, ISSN 0185-3325.

Macleod, Z., C., M. Arnaldi, V. & Adams, I. (2003). Telephone Counselling as an Adjunct to Nicotine Patches in Smoking Cessation: A Randomised Controlled Trial. *Medical Journal of Australia*, Vol.179, No. 7, pp.349- 352, ISSN 0025-729X.

Marlatt, G. A, Parks, A. G. & Witkiewitz, K. (2002). *Clinical Guidelines for Implementing Relapse Prevention Therapy*. Seattle: University of Washington.

McCarthy, D. E, Piasecki, T. M., Lawrence, D. L., Jorenby, D. E., Shiffman, S., Fiore, M. C. & Baker T. B. (2008). A randomized controlled clinical trial of bupropion SR and individual smoking cessation counseling. *Nicotine & Tobacco Research*. Vol.10, No. 8, pp.717–729, ISSN 1462-2203.

McNair, D. M., Lorr, J. & Droppelman, L. F. (1992). *Profile of Mood States Manual*. North Tonawanda, NY: Multi-Health Systems.

Miller, W. (1999). *Enhancing Motivation for Change in Substance Abuse Treatment*. Rockville: U. S. Department of Health and Human Services.

Miller, R. W. & Rollnick, S. (1991). *Motivational Interviewing*. Guilford Press. ISBN 1-57230-563-0,New York.

Moher, D., Schulz, K. F., & Altman, D. G. (2001). The CONSORT statement: Revised recommendations for improving the quality of reports of parallel group randomized trials. *BMC Medical Research Methodology, 1*, 2. Retrieved from www.scopus.com

Moreno-Coutiño, A. & Medina-Mora, I.M. E. (2008). Tabaquismo y Depresión. *Salud Mental*, 31, 409-415.

Muñoz, L. M., Labrador E. F. & Cruzado, R., J. (2008). *Manual de técnicas de modificación y terapia de conducta*. Ediciones Pirámide, ISBN 9788436813746, España.

Nathan, P., Stuart, S. & Dolan, S. (2000). Research a Psychotherapy Efficacy and Effectiveness: Between Scylla and Charibdis?. In: Kazdin (Eds.). *Methodological Issues y Strategies in Clinical Research*. APA. ISBN 978-1-55798-958-1, Washington, DC.

Nemeth-Coslett, R., & Griffiths, R. R. (1986). Naloxone does not affect cigarette smoking. *Psychopharmacology Berl., Vol.* 89,No. 3, pp. 261-2644, ISSN 0033-3158.

Niaura, R., Abrams, D. B., Shadel. W. G., Rohsenow, D. J., Monti, P. M. & Sirota, A. D. (1999). Cue exposure treatment for smoking relapse prevention: a controlled clinical trial. *Addiction*, Vol.94, No.5 (May 1999), pp. 685-95, ISSN 1360-0443.

Niaura, R., Borrelli, B., Goldstein, M. G., Depue, J., Chiles, A. J., Spring, B., et al. (2002). Multicenter Trial of Fluxetine as an Adjunct to Behavioral Smoking Cessation Treatment. *Journal of Consulting and Clinical Psychology*, Vol.70, No. 4, (August 2002) pp.887-896, ISSN 0022-006X.

Paperwalla, N. K., Levin, T. T., Weiner, J. & Saravay, S. M. (2004). Smoking and depression. *The Medical Clinics of North America*. Vol.88, pp.1483- 1494, ISSN 00257-125

Piasecki, T. (2006). Relapse to Smoking. *Clinical Psychology Review*. Vol.26, No. 2, (March 2006) pp.196-215, ISSN 0272-7358.

Prochaska, J. O. & DiClemente, C. (1983). Stages and Processes of Self-Change of Smoking: Toward an Integrative Model of Change. *Journal of Consulting and Clinical Psychology*, Vol. 51, No. 3, (June, 1983) pp. 390-395, ISSN 0022-006X .

Prochazca, V. A. (2000). New Developments in Smoking Cessation. *Chest*. 117, 169s-175s.

Redrobe, J. P., Bourin, M., Colombel, M.C. &, Baker, G. B. (1998). Dose-dependent noradrenergic and serotonergic properties of venlafaxine in animal models indicative of antidepressant activity. *Psychopharmacology (Berl)*, Vol. 138, pp.1-8, ISSN 0033-3158.

Richmond, R., Kehoe, L., & Almeida, N. (1997). Effectiveness of a 24-hour Transdermal Nicotine Patch in Conjunction with a Cognitive Behavioural Programme: One Year Outcome. *Addiction*, Vol.92, No. 1 (January 1997),pp. 27- 31, ISSN 1360-0443.

Richmond, R. & Zwar, N. (2003). Review of bupropion for smoking cessation. *Drug and Alcohol Review*. Vol. 22, No.2 (June 2003) 203-220, ISSN 1465-3362.

Robles, R., Varela, R., Jurado, S. & Páez, F. (2001). Versión Mexicana del Inventario de Ansiedad de Beck: Propiedades Psicométricas. *Revista Mexicana de Psicología*, Vol.2, pp.211-218, ISSN 0185-6073.

Robinson, R. G., Schultz, S. K., Castillo, C., Kopel, T., Kosier, T, J., Newman, M., Curdue, K., Petracca, G. & Starkstein, S. E. (2000). Nortriptyline Versus Fluoxetine in the Treatment of Depression and in Short-Term Recovery After Stroke: A Placebo-Controlled, Double-Blind Study. *The American Journal of Psychiatry*. Vol.157, (March 2000), pp.351-359, ISSN 0002-953X.

Roozen, H. G., Vann Beers, S., Weevers, H., Breteler, M., Willemsen, M., Postmus, P. & Kerkhof, J. (2006). Effects on Smoking Cessation: Naltrexone Combined with a Cognitive Behavioral Treatment Based on the Community Reinforcement Approach. *Substance Use & Misuse*, Vol.41, no. 1, (January 2006), pp.45- 60, ISSN 1082-6084.

Saules, K. K., Schuh, L. M., Arfken, C. L. Reed, K., Kilbey, M. M. & Schuster, C. R. (2004). Double- Blind Placebo- Controlled Trial of Flouxetine in Smoking Cessation Treatment Including Nicotine Patch and Cognitive - Behavioral Group Therapy. *The American Journal on Addictions*, Vol.13, No.5 (October- December 2004), pp.438-446, ISSN 1521-0391.

Scheitrum, R. R. & Akillas, E. (2002). Effects of Personality Style, Anxiety, and Depression on Reported Reasons for Smoking. *Journal of Applied Biobehavioral Research*. Vol. 7, No.1, (January 2002), pp.57-64, ISSN 1071-2089.

Schneider, N. G. & Jarvik, M. E. (1984). Time course of smoking withdrawal symptoms as a function of nicotine replacement. *Psychopharmacology*, Vol.82, No. 1-2, pp. 143-144, ISSN 0033-3158.

Schneider, N. G., Olmstead, R., Franzon, M. & Lunell, E. (2001). The Nicotine Inhaler. Clinical Pharmacokinetics and Comparison with Other Nicotine Treatments. *Clinical Pharmacokinetics*, Vol. 40, No. 9, pp.661-684, ISSN 1179-1926.

Secretaría de Salud (2002). Benchmarking: *Mejores Prácticas en la Prestación de Servicios para Dejar de Fumar*. CONADIC, ISBN 970-721-150-4, México.

Secretaría de Salud (2008). Encuesta nacional de adicciones. México: CONADIC, INP, INSP, Fundación Rio Arronte.

Shiffman, S. & Jarvik, M. E. (1976). Smoking withdrawal symptoms in two weeks of abstinence. *Psychopharmacology*, Vol. 50, No. 1, pp.35-39, ISSN 0033-3158.

Shiffman, S., Paty, J. A., Gnys, M., Kassel, J. A. & Hickcox, M. (1996). First lapses to smoking: Within-subjects analysis of real-time reports. *Journal of Consulting and Clinical Psychology*, Vol.64, No.2, (April 1996) pp. 366-379, ISSN 0022-006X.

Sobell, L., Brown, J., Leo, G. I., & Sobell, M. B. (1996). Reliability of the alcohol Timeline Followback when Administered by telephone and by computer. *Drug and Alcohol Dependence*, Vol.42, No.2, (September 1996), pp 49-54, ISSN 0376-8716

Stead, L. F., Perera, R., Bullen, C., Mant, D. & Lancaster, T. (2011). Nicotine Replacement Therapy for Smoking cessation. Cochrane database of systematic reviews. In: *The Cochrane Library*, Issue 06, 30.07.2011, Available from http://cochrane.bvsalud.org/cochrane/main.php?lib=COC&searchExp=smoking&lang=pt

Swan, G., McAfee, Curry, S. Jack, L., Javitz, H., Dacey, S. & Bergman, K. (2003). Effectiveness of Bupropion Sustained Release for Smoking Cessation in a Health Care Setting. *Archives of Internal Medicine*, Vol. 27, No. 163, (October 2003), pp. 2337-2344, ISSSN 1538-3679.

Tonnesen, P., Tonstad, S., Hjalmarson, A., Lebargy, F., Van Spiegel, P., Hider, A., Sweet, R. & Townsend, J. (2003). A multicentre, randomized, double-blind, placebo-controlled, 1-year study of bupropion SR for smoking cessation. *Journal of Internal Medicine*, Vol. 254, No. 2, (August 2003,) pp. 184–192, ISSSN 1365 2796.

Tonstad, S., Tonnesen, P., Hajek, P., Williams, K., Billing, C. & Reeves, K. (2006). Effect of Maintenance Therapy with Varenicline on Smoking Cessation. *Journal of the American Medical Association*. Vol. 296, No. 1, (July 2006), pp.64- 71, ISSN 0098-7484.

Vázquez, G. F., Becoña, I. E., & Míguez, C. (2002). Fumar y depresión: Situación actual en España. *Salud y Drogas*, Vol. 2, No. (1), pp. 17-28, ISSSN 1988 205X.

Vázquez, G. F. & Becoña, I. E. (1999). Depression and Smoking in a Cessation Programme. *Journal of Affective Disorders*, 55, Vol. 55, No. 2-3, (October 1999), pp. 125-132, ISSSN 1573 2517.

Velicer, W. F., Friedman, R. H., Fava, J. L., Gulliver, S. B., Keller, S., Sun, X., Ramelson, H. & Prochaska, J. O. (2006). Evaluating Nicotine Replacement Therapy and Stage-Based Therapies in a Population-Based Effectiveness Trial. *Journal of Consulting and Clinical Psychology*, Vol.74, No. 6, (December 2006) pp.1162–1172, ISSN 0022-006X.

Webb, M. S., Rodríguez, D., Baker, E., Reis, I. M.& Carey, M. P. (2010). Cognitive–Behavioral Therapy to Promote Smoking Cessation Among African American Smokers: A Randomized Clinical Trial. *Journal of Consulting and Clinical Psychology*. Vol 78, No. 1, (February 2002) pp.24–33, ISSN 0022-006X.

Welsch, S. K., Smith, S. S., Wetter, D. W., Jorenby, D. E., Fiore, M. C. & Baker, T. B. (1999). Development and validation of the Wisconsin Smoking Withdrawal Scale. *Experimental and Clinical Psychopharmacology*, Vol. 7, No.4, (November 1999), pp. 354-361, ISSN 1064-1297.

West, R. & Hajek, P. (2004). Evaluation of the mood and physical symptoms scale (MPSS) to assess cigarette withdrawal. *Psychopharmacology*, Vol. 177, No. 1-2, (June 2004), pp. 195-199, ISSSN 1432 2072.

Wewers, M. E., Dhatt, R. & Tejwani, G. A. (1998). Naltrexone administration affects ad libitum smoking behavior. *Psychopharmacology Berl.*, Vol. 140, No. 2, (November 1998), pp. 185-190, ISSSN 1432 2072

WHO (1990). Composite International Diagnostic Interview (CIDI), Version 1.0. Geneva, World Health Organization. 05.06.2008, Available from http://www.hcp.med.harvard.edu/wmhcidi/about.php

WHO (2003). *Framework Convention for Tobacco Control, ISBN 9789241501316, 09.08.2011,* Available from www.scopus.com

WHO (2011). *MPOWER a Package to Reverse the Tobacco Epidemic.* World Health Organization. ISBN 978 92 4 068781 3, Geneva.

Wong, G. Y., Wolter, T. D., Croghan, G. A., Croghan, I. T., Offord, K. P. & Hurt, R. D. (1999) A randomized trial of naltrexone for smoking cessation. *Addiction*, Vol. 94, No. 8, (August 1999), pp. 1227-37, ISSSN1360-0443.

Part 6

Interstitial Lung Diseases

6

Respiratory Diseases Among Dust Exposed Workers

Weihong Chen, Yuewei Liu, Xiji Huang and Yi Rong
Department of Occupational and Environmental Health, School of Public Health, Tongji Medical College in Huazhong University of Science & Technology
China

1. Introduction

Airborne contaminants occur in the gaseous form (gases and vapours) or as aerosols. Aerosols may exist in the form of airborne dusts, sprays, mists, smokes and fumes. In the occupational setting, all these forms may be important because they relate to a wide range of occupational diseases. Airborne dusts are of particular concern because they are well known to be associated with classical widespread occupational lung diseases such as the pneumoconiosis, chronic obstructive pulmonary disease, occupational asthma, etc. Occupational exposure to dust particles occurs everywhere but is especially prevalent in low- and middle-income countries. Table 1 shows some examples of the types of dust found in the work environment.

TYPE OF DUST	EXAMPLES
mineral dusts	free crystalline silica, coal and cement dusts
metallic dusts	lead, cadmium, nickel, and beryllium dusts
other chemical dusts	many bulk chemicals and pesticides
organic and vegetable dusts	flour, wood, cotton and tea dusts, pollen
biohazards	viable particles, moulds and spores

Table 1. Common types of dust in the work envrionment

2. Commonest type of occupation dust particles

2.1 Silica

Silica, also known as silicon dioxide (SiO_2), is formed from silicon and oxygen atoms. It has a melting point of 1,600°C and is a colorless, odorless, and noncombustible solid. Since oxygen and silicon make up about 75% of the Earth, the compound silica is quite common in surrounding environment[1]. Silicates comprise about 25% of known minerals, nearly 40% of the common minerals, and well over 90% of the earth's crust[1]. It is found in many rocks, such as marble, sandstone, flint and slate, and in some metallic ores. Silica can also be in soil, mortar, plaster, and shingles.

Silica occurs in three forms: crystalline, microcrystalline (or cryptocrystalline) and amorphous (non-crystalline). "Free" silica is composed of pure silicon dioxide, not combined with other elements, whereas silicates (e.g. talc, asbestos, and mica) are SiO_2 combined with an appreciable portion of cations. Crystalline silica exists in seven different forms (polymorphs), depending upon the temperature of formation. The main 3 polymorphs are quartz, cristobalite, and tridymite. Quartz is subdivided into alpha and beta forms. In nature, most quartz is alpha-quartz and alpha-quartz comprises the bulk of crystalline silica. Quartz is the second most common mineral in the world. Amorphous forms of silica, such as opal, diatomaceous earth, silica-rich fiberglass, fume silica, mineral wool, and silica glass (vitreous silica), are generally considered as less harmful[2].

Occupational exposure to crystalline silica can occur in any workplace situation where airborne dust, containing a proportion of crystalline silica, is generated. Industries where crystalline silica is present include quarrying, mining, mineral processing (eg drying, grinding, bagging and handling), slate working, stone crushing and dressing, foundry work, brick and tile making, some refractory processes, construction work, including work with stone, concrete, brick and some insulation boards, tunnelling, building restoration and in the pottery and ceramic industries. Figure 1 shows some of the job processes that generate and disperse large quantities of respirable silica dusts into the air. Silica dust is an inhalation hazard. Workers may be at risk of silicosis from exposure to silica dust when high-velocity impact shatters the sand into smaller, respirable (< 0.5 to 5.0 μm in diameter) dust particles. From recent reports, more than 23 million workers are exposed to crystalline silica in China

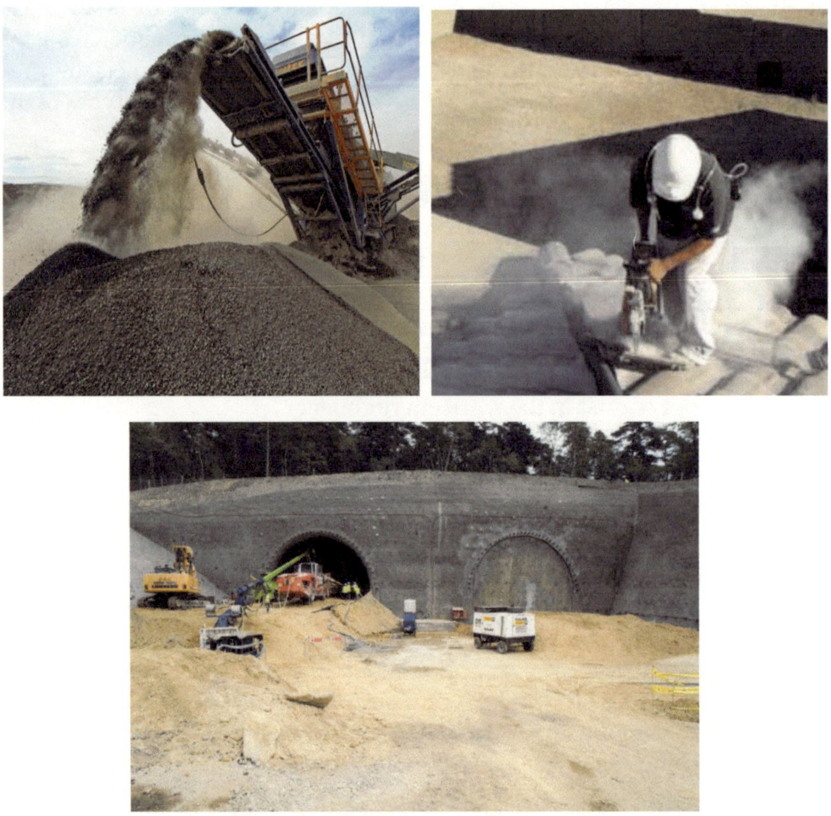

Fig. 1. Job processes that generate and disperse respirable silica dusts into the air

and more than 10 million in India, as well as over 3 million workers in Europe and at 1.7 million in the United States[3].

2.2 Asbestos

Asbestos is a set of six naturally occurring silicate minerals exploited commercially which possess high tensile strength, flexibility, resistance to chemical and thermal degradation, and electrical resistance. Six minerals are defined by the United States Environmental Protection Agency as "asbestos" including those belonging to the serpentine class chrysotile and those belonging to the amphibole class amosite, crocidolite, tremolite, anthophyllite and actinolite[4]. They have different physical and chemical properties but share a fibrous form. Mineralogists have taken a particle with a length-to-breadth ratio (aspect ratio) of 10:1 or more to be a fibre. In milled asbestos most of the particles have aspect ratios that range from 5:1 to 20:1 or more and, in the case of chrysotile , mostly greater than 50:1. In medical and environmental literature a regulated fibre has been defined as a mineral particle with a length which is at least three times greater than its diameter, of length greater than 5 micrometers and diameters less than 3 micrometres. There are essentially two major varieties of asbestos viz. serpentine and amphibole. Table 2 shows the species and varieties[5].

SPECIES	VARIETY
Chrysotile	Serpentine
Anthophyllite	Amphibole
Amosite	Amphibole
Actinolite	Amphibole
Tremolite	Amphibole
Crocidolite	Amphibole

Table 2. Asbestos

Asbestos is used for insulation in buildings and as ingredient in a number of products, such as roofing shingles, water supply lines, fire blankets, plastic fillers, and medical packing, as well as clutches and brake linings, gaskets and pads for automobiles. Table 3 illustrates certain kinds of work involve high exposure to asbestos. All forms of asbestos are

work involve high exposure to asbestos	
asbestos mining and milling	manufacture of asbestos tiles
building demolition	manufacture of asbestos fabrics
manufacture of brake linings	drywall installation
shipbuilding trades	drywall removal
insulation work in construction	other asbestos removal
plasterers	firefighting
pipe fitters	asbestos tile setters
railroad workers	aluminum plant workers

Table 3. Certain kinds of work involve high exposure to asbestos

carcinogenic to humans, and may cause mesothelioma and cancer of the lung, larynx and ovary. Asbestos exposure is also responsible for other diseases, such as asbestosis (fibrosis of the lungs), pleural plaques, thickening and effusions.

Currently, about 125 million people in the world are exposed to asbestos at the workplace. According to the most recent WHO estimates, more than 107 000 people die each year from asbestos-related lung cancer, mesothelioma and asbestosis resulting from exposure at work. One in every three deaths from occupational cancer is estimated to be caused by asbestos. In addition, it is estimated that several thousand deaths annually can be attributed to exposure to asbestos in the home[6].

2.3 Coal mine dust

Coal is a valuable and plentiful natural global resource. It is found throughout the world. Coal is classified into four main types or ranks (anthracite, bituminous, subbituminous, and lignite), depending on the amounts and types of carbon it contains and on the amount of heat energy it can produce. Coal is mined by two methods: surface mining and underground mining. The choice of mining method is largely determined by the geology of the coal deposit. Underground mining currently accounts for a bigger share of world coal production than opencast. Coal mine dust is a mixture that contains more than 50 substances. The mineral content depends on the particle size of the dust and the coal seam. The most commonly found minerals in coal mine dust include kaolinite, illite, calcite, pyrite and quartz (silica). Dust from high rank coals usually contains more silica particles than dust of lower rank coals. Most workplace exposure to coal dust occurs during mining; however exposure can also occur during handling of the mined product during cleaning and blending processes or bulk handling at large coal fired facilities[7].

3. Main respiratory diseases related to occupational dust particles

3.1 Pneumoconiosis

Pneumoconiosis is an occupational lung disease and a restrictive lung disease caused by the inhalation of dust. A longer, factitious term is pneumonoultramicroscopicsilicovolcanoconiosis. Depending upon the type of dust, the disease is given different names:

1. Coal worker' pneumoconiosis(CWP): caused by inhaling coal dust;
2. Asbestosis: caused by inhaling asbestos;
3. Berylliosis: caused by inhaling beryllium;
4. Kaolin pneumoconiosis: caused by inhaling china clay;
5. Siderosis: caused by inhaling iron oxide;
6. Silicosis: caused by inhaling silica dust;
7. Metallic pneumoconiosis: caused by inhaling barium, cobalt, tin, tungsten dust;
8. Talc pneumoconiosis: caused by inhaling talc dust;
9. Popcorn pneumoconiosis: caused by inhaling fumes produced when manufacturing microwave popcorn

Some more types of pneumoconiosis include graphite pneumoconiosis, carbon black pneumoconiosis, talc pneumoconiosis, cement pneumoconiosis, mica pneumoconiosis, aluminosis, electric welder pneumoconiosis, foundry worker's pneumoconiosis.

3.2 Silicosis

Silicosis is a form of pneumoconiosis caused by inhalation of crystalline silica dust, and is marked by inflammation and scarring in forms of nodular lesions in the upper lobes of the lungs[6] (Figure 2).

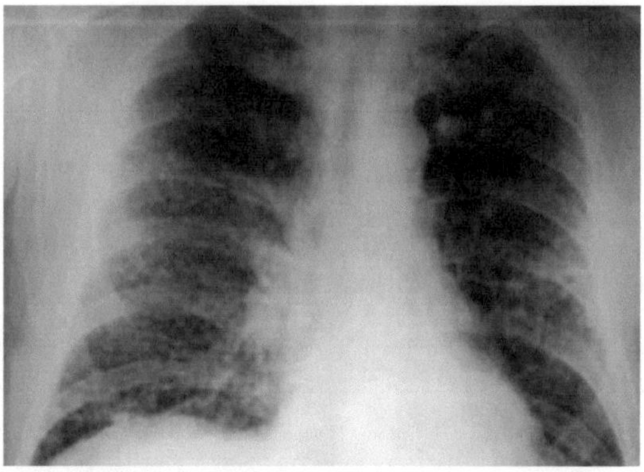

Fig. 2. Silicosis showing as nodular mass on a chest x-ray

Silicosis is the commonest occupational lung disease worldwide. It occurs everywhere but is especially prevalent in low- and middle-income countries. China is the country with the largest number of silicosis patients, with more than 500,000 cases in records from 1949 to 2010. During 1991 to 2010, more than 6,000 new cases and more than 24,000 deaths occurred annually. The problem is particularly acute in small-scale mines in China[3]. High risk of silicosis also reported in other countries. The proportions of gold miners with silicosis increased from 0.03 to 0.32 for black miners and from 0.18 to 0.22 for white miners in a 33-year period in South Africa. Among ornamental stone carvers in Brazil, the prevalence of disease remains over 50 percent. Although U.S. silicosis mortality declined between 1968 and 2002, silicosis deaths and new cases continue to occur, even in young workers[6].

The most common form of silicosis (chronic) will often develop between 15 to 45 years after first exposure, but certain rare forms of the disease can occur after a single heavy dose or heavy exposures to a very high concentration of silica in a short period of time. Workers with Silicosis may have following symptoms: Shortness of breath following physical exertion, severe and chronic cough, fatigue, loss of appetite, chest pains and fevers.

Silicosis is generally divided into three types as below:

1. Acute Silicosis: Occurs after heavy exposure to high concentrations of silica. The symptoms can develop within a few weeks or as long as 5 years after the exposure.
2. Chronic Silicosis: Occurs after long term exposure (over 10 years) of low concentrations of silica dust. This is most common form of the disease, and is often undetected for many years because a chest X-Ray often will not reveal the disease for as long as 20 years after exposure. This type of the disease severely hinders the ability of the body to fight infections because of the damage to the lungs, making the person more susceptible to other lung illnesses, including tuberculosis.
3. Accelerated Silicosis: Occurs after exposure to high concentrations of silica. The disease develops within 5 to 10 years after exposure.

The development of silicosis is associated with content of free silica in the dust, type of silica, concentration of dust, dispersion, years of exposure, prevention and individual factors. The cumulative dose of silica (respirable dust concentration x crystalline silica content x exposure duration) is probably the most important factor for the development of silicosis[8].

Pathology

Pathological varieties of silicosis include simple (nodular) silicosis, progressive massive fibrosis, silicoproteinosis (acute silicosis) and diffuse interstitial fibrosis.

Alveolar macrophages engulf inhaled free silica particles and enter lymphatics and interstitial tissue. The macrophages cause release of cytokines (tumor necrosis factor-α, IL-1), growth factors (tumor growth factor-β), and oxidants, stimulating parenchymal inflammation, collagen synthesis, and, ultimately, fibrosis.

When the macrophages die, they release the silica into interstitial tissue around the small bronchioles, causing formation of the pathognomonic silicotic nodule. These nodules initially contain macrophages, lymphocytes, mast cells, fibroblasts with disorganized patches of collagen, and scattered birefringent particles that are best seen by polarized light microscopy. As they mature, the centers of the nodules become dense balls of fibrotic scar with a classic onion-skin appearance and are surrounded by an outer layer of inflammatory cells. In low-intensity or short-term exposures, these nodules remain discrete and do not compromise lung function (simple chronic silicosis). But with higher-intensity or more prolonged exposures (complicated chronic silicosis), these nodules coalesce and cause progressive fibrosis and reduction of lung volumes (total lung capacity, ventilatory capacity) on pulmonary function tests, or they coalesce, sometimes forming large conglomerate masses (called progressive massive fibrosis).

Silica quartz crystals in lung tissue can be observed under polarised light microscopy. Figure 3 illustrates a slide under polarised light microscopy of lung tissue containing crystalline silica quartz. The white spots represent silica crystals in the specimen of lung tissue. The silica crystals present in the lung tissue are of different size and represent

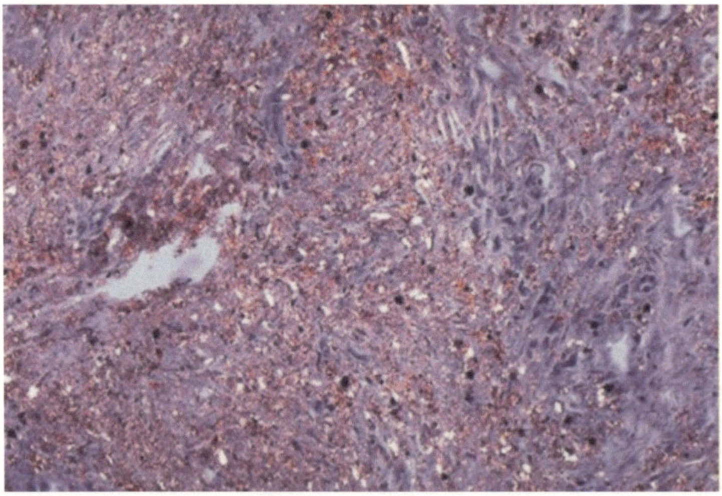

Fig. 3. Lung tissue observed under polarized light microscopy containing crystalline silica

therefore a typical picture of silica crystal distribution in lung tissue of a worker exposed to crystalline silica.

The primary feature that develops in lungs of silica quartz exposed workers is nodule formation in the upper zones of the lung[9]. Nodule formation is usually the result of many years of exposure to relatively low levels of dust that contain silica quartz[10]. Figure 4 represents a photo of silicotic nodule. The classical silicotic nodule is usually located in the area of the respiratory bronchiole.The nodule is composed of reticulin fibres in the periphery and collagen fibresin the center. Fibroblastic activity is usually evident around the periphery of the concentric lesion[11].

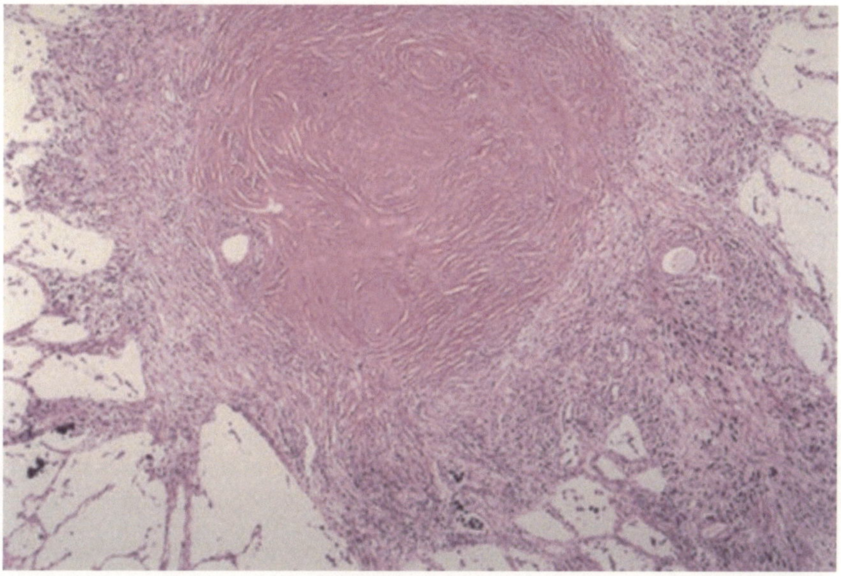

Fig. 4. A microscopic photo of a typical silicotic nodule containing collage fibres in a whorled pattern

The airway and blood vessels are frequently destroyed by being entrapped in the fibrotic nodule. Silica particles are difficult to identify in tissue section by polarized light microscopy. Therefore, special techniques involving high resoluton microscopy are required. It appears that the extent of lesion bears little association with amount of silica present[11].

Diagnosis

The diagnosis of silicosis generally rests upon history of substantial exposure to silica dusts and compatible radiological features, together with the exclusion of other competing diagnoses, like miliary tuberculosis, fungal infections, sarcoidosis, idiopathic pulmonary fibrosis, other interstitial lung diseases, or carcinomotosis.

History: The individual may report a history of exposure to silica dust. Although initially there may be no symptoms, symptoms may eventually include difficulty breathing, shortness of breath, a cough (either dry or productive), and/or chest tightness.

Physical exam: Auscultation (listening to breath sounds through a stethoscope) may reveal changes in breath sounds that may indicate obstruction in the upper lobes of the lung. Wheezing only occurs when other conditions such as bronchitis or asthma are present. In chronic complicated silicosis or subacute silicosis, right-sided heart failure (cor pulmonale) may be noted. Rales are often heard.

Tests: Lung tissue changes in progressive silicosis are often detected by chest x-ray before they cause any symptoms. Pulmonary function tests will be used to evaluate lung function and confirm the presence of lung disorders. These may include spirometry and lung volume measurement to detect any restriction of normal lung expansion or obstruction of air flow, peak flow measurement to detect narrowing of the airways, and diffusing capacity to assess the efficiency of gas absorption into the blood. Arterial blood gases (ABGs) are performed to assess the efficiency of gas exchange in the lungs by measuring oxygen and carbon dioxide (CO2) in arterial blood. CT scanning may also be useful for identifying lung nodules. It's generally accepted that the advent of high-resolution computed tomography (HRCT) has been the major diagnostic technique which is more sensitive than conventional radiography in detecting nodular lung parenchymal changes, progressive massive fibrosis, bulla, emphysema, pleural and hilar changes in silicosis. Qualitative and quantitative parameters on HRCT may also be used as indirect measures of functional impairment in silicosis. Therefore, HRCT has been widespread used. Sputum (phlegm) may be cultured to identify any causative organisms and to rule out tuberculosis.

Treatment

Damage to the lungs from silicosis is irreversible; there is no standard treatment other than reducing symptoms and treating complications. Lung tissue changes due to silicosis are often detected by a chest x-ray before they cause any symptoms. If dust exposure is stopped at this point, further progression of the disease can sometimes be prevented.

The disease is otherwise treated symptomatically. Appropriate drug therapy may be given to control symptoms; these may include drugs to reduce inflammation (anti-inflammatory), antibiotics to treat or prevent infections, and drugs to widen the airways in the lungs (bronchodilators). Sleeping in a semi-upright position may help reduce shortness of breath. Because smoking can aggravate the symptoms of silicosis and increase the risk of lung cancer, people with the condition who smoke cigarettes are urged to quit. In severe or advanced cases, a lung transplant may be required[12].

Prevention

Silicosis are preventable. In 1995, the ILO/WHO Global Program for the Elimination of Silicosis (GPES) was established by a joint ILO/WHO committee. GPES is encouraging and supporting countries with silica hazard to establish their national action programs to control silicosis.

It is recommended to assess the potential of silica exposure before a job begins, especially in the industries where silicosis cases were reported before[13]. Periodic respirable silica monitoring should be performed in all industries involving silica exposure. Currently enforced or suggested permissible exposure limits (PEL) for respirable silica are between 0.025 mg/m^3 and 0.35 mg/m^3 in different countries [14-16]. The current standards have not been confirmed by epidemiology studies to be fully protective. For example, the quantitative risk assessments by NIOSH predicted excess lifetime risks of 19/1000 for lung cancer mortality, 54/1000 for lung disease other than cancer and 75/1000 for radiographic silicosis with exposure at the current US Occupational Safety and Health Authority standard for respirable cristobalite dust (about 0.05 mg/m3) over 45-year working lifetime[17].

For workers in workplaces with high dust levels, administrative measures can also be used to reduce exposure to silica dust e.g., by cutting short their working hours or job rotation. Exposure control at the worker level includes training and education on work practices, and personal protection. Personal protection equipment such as respirators is a good solution for short duration tasks. Respirators can be used in combination with engineering controls. However, they should only be considered as the last resort for routine full shift protection. They cannot be heavily relied upon because they may not be fully effective in workplaces with high dust concentrations. NIOSH recommends the use of half-facepiece particulate respirators with N95 or better filters for exposure to crystalline silica at concentrations less than or equal to 0.5mg/m^3 [18].

Regular medical evaluation may detect adverse health effects among exposed workers before disease reaches advance stages[13].Medical evaluation commonly includes respiratory questionnaires, physical examination, chest radiography and spirometry. There is no universal standard as to how frequent such evaluation should be performed, because the decision may be influenced by past and current respirable silica concentration, dust particulate characteristics and economic conditions. The WHO recommends routine evaluation every 2-5 years, ideally 'life-long' for workers exposed to silica dust[19]. American College of Occupational and Environmental Medicine (ACOEM) recommended evaluation at baseline and after 1 year, then 3-yearly for the first 10 years and 2-yearly thereafter when silicosis is the major concern and respirable silica levels are below 0.05 mg/m^3[20]. Biomarkers of early disease could potentially benefit prevention efforts and clinical diagnosis. While a number of biomarkers have shown some promising results, none of them have been validated fully for clinical use so far[21]. The occurrence of a new case of silicosis is a sentinel health event to prompt a thorough evaluation of silica exposure levels and control measures in workplace[22]. In addition to reporting new cases, occupational health doctors or hygienists should periodically analyze health records from all workers in an industry or plant and assess the effects of prevention activities.

3.3 Chronic obstructive pulmonary diseases

In the past few years a new definition has been presented by Global Initiative on Obstructive Lung Disease (GOLD) and by a Task Force of the American Thoracic Society (ATS) and the European Respiratory Society (ERS). Both GOLD and ATS/ERS state that "COPD is a disease state characterized by airflow limitation that is not fully reversible. The airflow obstruction is usually both progressive and associated with an abnormal inflammatory response of the lungs to noxious particles and gas." The ATS/ERS definition also state that COPD is both preventable and treatable and that COPD is systemic disease[23].

Epidemiology

According to WHO estimates, 80 million people have moderate to severe chronic obstructive pulmonary disease (COPD). More than 3 million people died of COPD in 2005, which corresponds to 5% of all deaths globally. In 2002 COPD was the fifth leading cause of death, and expected to become the third leading cause of death globally by 2030, trailing only ischemic heart disease and cerebrovascular disease[24].

During 2000--2005, COPD was the underlying cause of death for 718,077 persons overall aged >25 years in the United States. In 2005, approximately one in 20 deaths in the United States had COPD as the underlying cause[25]. COPD has a prevalence of 4 to 10 percent in adults in populations in whom lung function has been measured. The National Health Interview Survey, an annual survey of approximately 40,000 United States households, has yielded an estimate of 10 million adults in the United States with a physician-based diagnosis of COPD. Other estimates, such as that from the Third National Health and Nutrition Examination Survey (NHANES III), that included spirometry along with questionnaires and a physical examination, done between 1988 and 1994, have yielded even more impressive prevalence figures. According to NHANES III, COPD affects 23.6 million adults in the United States, of whom 2.4 million have severe disease. Thus, approximately 10 percent of the United States adult population might be classified as having COPD, and of this group about 10 percent have advanced disease[23].

According to data published by the Chinese Ministry of Health, COPD ranks as the fourth leading cause of death in urban areas and third leading in rural areas [16]. The overall prevalence of COPD in China was 8.2% (95% CI, 7.9–8.6) according to GOLD diagnostic criteria. The crude prevalence of COPD was the highest in Chongqing and lowest in Shanghai among urban areas and was highest in Guangdong and lowest in Liaoning and Shangxi among rural areas. The COPD prevalence was significantly higher in rural areas compared with urban areas[26]. Both crude and age-adjusted COPD mortality rates have fluctuated but have displayed a decreasing trend from 1990 which is probably because of improved management of COPD, upgraded technologies, and awareness of the disease[24].

Risk factors

There are two types of risk factors for COPD: host factor and exposures (table 4).

ENVIRONMENT EXPOSURES	HOST FACTORS
Smoking	Genetic mutations
Occupational exposures	Airway hyperresponsiveness
Air pollution	Reduced lung growth
Childhood respiratory infections	
Low socioeconomic status	

Table 4. Common risk factors for COPD

Cigarette smoking is the major risk factor for COPD. However, relevant information from the literature published within the last years, either on general population samples or on workplaces, indicates that about 15% of all cases of COPD is work-related[27]. A 1989 study of black goldminers showed that the risk of chronic airflow limitation increases with duration of underground exposure and is an effect that is independent of the presence of silicosis. A study of white South African gold miners showed that the forced expiratory volume in one second (FEV1), and the FEV1/FVC ratio, adjusted for age, height, and tobacco smoking, decreased with increasing cumulative respirable dust exposure, in both smokers and non-smokers. The average cumulative dust exposure attributables loss in lung function[28].

Pathology

COPD includes two main diseases: bronchitis - in which inflammation of the bronchi (tubes carrying air to and from the lung) both narrows them and causes chronic bronchial secretions. Chronic bronchitis is defined by the presence of cough and sputum production on most days for three or more months of the year for two or more consecutive years[29]; and emphysema - a permanent destructive enlargement of the airspaces within the lung without any accompanying fibrosis of the lung tissue. Asthma may also be included within the term COPD if there is some degree of chronic airway obstruction.

In COPD, inflammation causes direct destruction of lung tissues and also impairs defense mechanisms used to repair damaged tissues. This results in not only destruction of the lung parenchyma, but also mucus hypersecretion, and airway narrowing and fibrosis.

A wide range of inflammatory cells and mediators are involved in the pathogenesis of COPD, namely neutrophils, macrophages, and CD8+ T cells in different areas of the lung.

Overall, COPD pathogenesis can be summarized as resulting from a combination of genetic susceptibility combined with environmental exposures which lead to inflammatory processes that disrupt the balance of proteases and antiprotease. These abnormal inflammatory mechanisms result in tissue destruction, airway inflammation and remodeling, and ultimately airway limitation. These imbalances and the presence of inflammation may result in a "positive feedback loop," in which inflammation induces these imbalances, and the imbalances promote more inflammation. Once the inflammatory responses are set in motion, three types of damages to the lung occur: disruption of the alveolar walls, mucus hypersecretion contributing to airway obstruction, and fibrosis of the bronchioles.To support the inflammation mechanism further, a study shows there is a stepwise increase in alveolar inflammation has been found in surgical specimens from patients without COPD versus patients with mild or severe emphysema. As part of the peripheral airway system, the bronchioles are the major site of airway obstruction in COPD[30].

Diagnosis

The diagnosis of COPD, classification of its severity, and progression of the disease can be monitored with spirometry. A test that measures the forced expiratory volume in one second (FEV1), which is the greatest volume of air that can be breathed out in the first second of a large breath. Spirometry also measures the forced vital capacity (FVC), which is the greatest volume of air that can be breathed out in a whole large breath. Normally, at least 70% of the FVC comes out in the first second (i.e. the FEV1/FVC ratio is >70%). A ratio less than normal defines the patient as having COPD. More specifically, the diagnosis of COPD is made when the FEV1/FVC ratio is <70%. The GOLD criteria also require that values are after bronchodilator medication has been given to make the diagnosis, and the NICE criteria also require FEV1%. According to the ERS criteria, it is FEV1% predicted that defines when a patient has COPD, that is, when FEV1% predicted is < 88% for men, or < 89% for women[31]. Once airflow obstruction is established, the severity of the disease is classified by the reduction of FEV 1 compared with a healthy reference population. Table 5 shows the widely used GOLD classification of COPD severity based on the FEV1.

STAGE	CHARACTERISTICS
I Mild COPD	FEV_1 80% predicted
II Moderate COPD	FEV_1 50% - 79% predicted
III Severe COPD	FEV_1 30% - 49% predicted
IV Very Severe COPD	FEV_1 < 30% predicted or < 50% predicted with room air Pao_2 < 60 mmHg (8.0KPa)

Table 5. Classification of COPD severity

On chest x-ray, the classic signs of COPD are overexpanded lung, a flattened diaphragm, increased retrosternal airspace, and bullae[32]. A high-resolution computed tomography scan of the chest may show the distribution of emphysema throughout the lungs and can also be useful to exclude other lung diseases.

Treatment

Directions about the management and prevention of work-related diseases [33-35], can be applied to COPD as well. Physicians should attempt to understand the patient's occupational exposure and whether he/she has been adequately trained in the dangers of these exposures and how to manage them. Removal of the respiratory irritants and substitution of non-toxic agents are the best approach because they eliminate the work-related COPD hazard. If substitution is not possible, ongoing maintenance of engineering controls, such as enclosure of the industrial process and improving work area ventilation, are useful. Administrative controls (e.g., transfer to another job or change in work practices), and personal protective equipment (e.g., masks or respirators) should be mentioned, although less effective in decreasing exposures to respiratory tract irritants.

3.4 Asthma

Occupational asthma is a lung disorder in which substances found in the workplace cause the airways of the lungs to swell and narrow, leading to attacks of wheezing, shortness of breath, chest tightness, and coughing.

Causes and prevalence

Though the actual rate of occurrence of occupational asthma is unknown, it is suspected to cause 2 - 20% of all asthma cases in industrialized nations. In the USA, OA is considered the most common occupational lung disease[33]. At present, over 400 workplace substances have been identified as having asthmagenic or allergenic properties. Their existence and magnitude vary from region to region and the type of industry and can be as varied as wood dust (cedar, ebony, etc.), persulfates (Hairsprays), zinc or even seafood like prawns. In south-eastern Nigeria, a study was done to determine the magnitude of the problem among woodworkers exposed to high level of wood dust. Five hundred and ninety one woodworkers were selected using a stratified random sampling. The prevalence of occupational rhinitis was 78%, while that of asthma was 6.5%. As period of woodwork increased the prevalence of rhinitis and asthma increased (rhinitis: chi2 trend = 53.015, df = 1, P = 0.000; asthma, chi2 trend = 19.721, df = 1, P = 0.000). It demonstrates that the prevalence of rhinitis and asthma in woodworkers was high and significantly increased with years of working as a woodworker[34].

Occupations at risk

The riskiest occupations for asthma are: adhesive handlers (e.g. acrylate), animal handlers and veterinarians (animal proteins), bakers and millers (cereal grains), carpet makers (gums), electronics workers (soldering resin), forest workers, carpenters and cabinetmakers (wood dust), hairdressers (e.g. persulfate), health care workers (latex and chemicals such as glutaraldehyde), janitors and cleaning staff (e.g. chloramine-T), pharmaceutical workers (drugs, enzymes), seafood processors, shellac handlers (e.g. amines), solderers and refiners (metals), spray painters, insulation installers, plastics and foam industry workers (e.g. diisocyanates), textile workers (dyes) and users of plastics and epoxy resins (e.g. anhydrides)[35].

Mechanism

Even if the precise causative mechanism of occupational asthma is unknown, several mechanisms have been proposed, i.e. immunological, pharmacological and genetic mechanisms, and airway and neurogenic inflammation. More than one mechanism may be operative in occupational asthma. Whether various mechanisms are involved in occupational asthma induced by different agents is also unknown. An agent which causes asthma may be considered as "inducer" (i.e. causing reversible airway bronchoconstriction associated with long-lasting airway hyperresponsiveness to nonspecific and/or specific agents) or as "inciter" (i.e. triggering asthma attacks)[36]. Among the mechanisms proposed in the pathogenesis of occupational asthma, the immunological one plays a key role[35].

Diagnosis

Diagnosis of OA is a process and has to be done over a period of time. First, the patient's occupational and clinical history is taken and his symptoms are charted (Charting is usually done at the end of a typical work week and within 24 hours of the occurrence of symptoms in order to get objective information). Once this has been established, the following diagnostic methods are used:

1. Blood tests to look for antibodies to the substance;
2. Bronchial provocation test (test measuring reaction to the suspected allergen);
3. Chest x-ray;
4. Complete blood count;

5. Peak expiratory flow rate;
6. Pulmonary function tests.

Treatment

According to the Canadian Centre for Occupational Health and Safety (CCOHS), better education of workers, management, unions and medical professionals is the key to the prevention of OA. This will enable them to identify the risk factors and put in place preventive measures like masks or exposure limits, etc.

Avoiding exposure to the substance which causes you asthma is the best treatment. The best option is to change your jobs, or using a respiratory device to protect yourselves is an alternative option.

Anyone diagnosed with Asthma will have to undergo medical treatment. This is complementary to either removing or reducing the patient's exposure to the causal agents.

3.5 Pulmonary tuberculosis

Pulmonary tuberculosis, or TB, is a communicative disease caused by the bacterium *Mycobacterium tuberculosis* and, less frequently, *M.bovis*. Lesions most often occur in the lungs.

Species of *Mycobacterium* are characterized by unusual "acid fast" staining properties, slow growth, relative resistance to chemical disinfectants, and ability to survive for decades with cells in the infected animal. The few studies of TB as an occupational hazard suggest that physicians, nurses, medical laboratory workers, and miners are at increased risk of TB.

The symptoms of active TB of the lung are coughing, sometimes with sputum or blood, chest pains, weakness, weight loss, fever and night sweats. Tuberculosis is treatable with a six-month course of antibiotics.

Epidemiology

Roughly a third of the world's population has been infected with M. tuberculosis, and new infections occur at a rate of one per second. In 2007, an estimated 13.7 million people had active TB disease, with 9.3 million new cases and 1.8 million deaths; the annual incidence rate varied from 363 per 100,000 in Africa to 32 per 100,000 in the Americas[37]. In 2007, the country with the highest estimated incidence rate of TB was Swaziland, with 1200 cases per 100,000 people. India had the largest total incidence, with an estimated 2.0 million new cases[37]. According to the statistic data released by the Chinese Ministry of Health in July 2011, the recorded cases of pulmonary tuberculosis is 112647 which is the second in the recorded cases of notifiable disease, and 170 deaths.

However, few studies of TB incidence among various occupational have been reported. Therefore, only general and somewhat unsatisfactory comments can be made about TB as an occupational hazard.

Miners and others who work in poorly ventilated areas are more likely to be infected by a fellow worker who has TB than a person who works in a well-ventilated areas[38].

Silicotuberculosis

Both silica dust exposure and silicosis are risk factors for TB. Tuberculosis in a person with established silicosis is termed silicotuberculosis. The risk of developing TB increases with duration of exposure to silica dust even in the absence of silicosis. The presence of silicosis increases the risk of pulmonary TB approximately four fold, with the risk rising as radiological become more severe. This increased risk of TB associated with silicosis is lifelong, continuing after silica exposure ceases.

The presence of silicosis in the lungs can be modify the natural history of TB and may alter its radiological appearance. The interaction of TB and silicosis is very damaging to the lung, unless the TB is diagnosed and treated early.

Pathology

Infection with *Mycobacterium tuberculosis* results most commonly from infected aerosol exposure through the lungs or mucous membranes. In immunocompetent individuals, this usually produces a latent/dormant infection, only about 5% of these individuals later show evidence of clinical disease.

TB infection begins when the mycobacteria reach the pulmonary alveoli, where they invade and replicate within the endosomes of alveolar macrophages[39]. The primary site of infection in the lungs is generally located in either the upper part of the lower lobe, or the lower part of the upper lobe[39]. Bacteria are picked up by dendritic cells, which do not allow replication, although these cells can transport the bacilli to local (mediastinal) lymph nodes. Further spread is through the bloodstream to other tissues and organs where secondary TB lesions can develop in other parts of the lung (particularly the apex of the upper lobes), peripheral lymph nodes, kidneys, brain, and bone[40].

Workers exposed to silica are more likely to have TB because silica interferes with the function of the pulmonary macrophages[38].

Diagnosis and Treatment

The diagnosis of tuberculosis is confirmed by the growth of *Mycobacterium tuberculosis* from culture of sputum, CSF, urine, lymph nodes, or other infected tissue. If necessary, the patient should have a positive tuberculin shin test.

The goal of treatment is to cure the infection with drugs that fight the TB bacteria. Treatment of active pulmonary TB will always involve a combination of many drugs (usually four drugs). All of the drugs are continued until lab tests show which medicines work best. The most commonly used drugs include: Isoniazid, Rifampin, Pyrazinamide and Ethambutol.

Prevention

Transmission of TB can be prevented by the rapid identification and treatment of persons with disease and by the identification and treatment of those persons infected but not yet diseased.

As indicated above, chronic inhalation of dust particles has been linked for decades with lung diseases such as silicosis and silicotuberculosis. Also studies have suggested that dust particles may increase risk of lung cancer as well as some other diseases.

4. References

[1] James A . Merchant, M.D., Dr. P.H., *Silicate pneumoconisis.* Occupational respiratory diseases, September 1986: p. 243.

[2] Pannett B, K.T., Toikkanen J et al, *Occupational exposure to carcinogens in Great Britain in 1990–93: preliminary results.* Carex: International Information System on Occupational Exposure to Carcinogens. Helsinki, Finland: Finnish Institute of Occupational Health. , 1998.

[3] *NIOSH Hazard Review.* Health Effects of Occupational Exposure to Respirable Crystalline Silica. DHHS 2002-129: p. 5.

[4] Berman, D.W.C., Kenny S, *Final draft:technical support document for a protocol to assess asbestos-related risk.* . Washington DC: U.S. Environmental Protection Agency., 2003: p. 474.

[5] R. Guild, R.I.E., *Airbone pollutants: asbestos.* Occupational health practice in the South African mining industry. , 2001: p. 88.

[6] Organization, W.H., *Elimination of Silicosis.* The global Occupational Health Network Issue No.12-2007.

[7] *Coal Dust at the Work Site.* CH063 – Chemical Hazards. Government of Alberta, April 2010.

[8] NIOSH., *Health Effects of Occupational Exposure to Respirable Crystalline Silica.* DHHS (NIOSH) Publication No. 2002–129. Cincinnati, OH, USA, 2002.

[9] M., L., *Interspecies comparisons of particle deposition and mucociliary clearance in the tracheobronchial airways.* J Toxicol.Environ.Health., 1984. 13441-69.

[10] MM., F., *Silica, silicosis, and lung cancer: a risk assessment.* Am.J Ind.Med, 2000. 38(1):8-18.

[11] James A. Merchant, M.D., Dr. P.H., *Pneumoconiosis: Slicosis.* Occupational respiratory diseases, 1986: p. 230.

[12] *preventing silicosis.* Centers for Disease Control and Prevention. U.S. Department of Health and Human Services., October. 2004.

[13] NIOSH., *A guide to working safety with silica: If it is silica, it is not just dust.* Washington, DC, 1997.

[14] NIOSH., *Health Effects of Occupational Exposure to Respirable Crystalline Silica.* DHHS (NIOSH) Publication No. 2002–129. Cincinnati, OH, USA, 2002. No. 2002–129. Cincinnati, OH, USA.

[15] *American Conference of Governmental Industrial Hygienists.* Cincinnati: ACGIH, 2009.

[16] *Occupational exposure limits for hazardous agents in the workplace part 1: chemical hazardous agents in China.* Beijing: People's Medical Publishing House, 2007.

[17] NIOSH., *High impact: silica, lung cancer, and respiratory disease quantitative risk.* Cincinnati, OH, DHHS (NIOSH) Publication, 2010. No. 2011-120.

[18] NIOSH., *Respiratory Protection Recommendations for Airborne Exposures to Crystalline Silica.* Washington D.C.: DHHS Publication, 2008. No. 2008-140.

[19] Wagner G, W.S., *Screening and surveillance of workers exposed to mineral dust.* Geneva: World Health Organization, 1996.

[20] Raymond, L.W. and S. Wintermeyer, *Medical surveillance of workers exposed to crystalline silica.* J Occup Environ Med, 2006. 48(1): p. 95-101.

[21] Gulumian, M., et al., *Mechanistically identified suitable biomarkers of exposure, effect, and susceptibility for silicosis and coal-worker's pneumoconiosis: a comprehensive review.* J Toxicol Environ Health B Crit Rev, 2006. 9(5): p. 357-95.

[22] Aldrich, T.E. and P.E. Leaverton, *Sentinel event strategies in environmental health.* Annu Rev Public Health, 1993. 14: p. 205-17.

[23] Fishman, A.P., *Chronic Obstructive Pulmonary Disease: Epidemiology, Pathophysiology, and Pathogenesis.* Fishman's Pulmonary Diseases and Disorders: p. 707.

[24] Fang, X., *COPD in China : The Burden and Importance of Proper Management.* Chest., 2011. 10-1393: p. 920-929.

[25] *Deaths from Chronic Obstructive Pulmonary Disease --- United States, 2000--2005.* Centers for Disease Control and Prevention. U.S. , November 2008.

[26] Zhong, N., *Prevalence of Chronic Obstructive Pulmonary Disease in China A Large, Population-based Survey.* AMERICAN JOURNAL OF RESPIRATORY AND CRITICAL CARE MEDICINE, December 2006: p. 753-760.

[27] Boschetto, P., *Chronic obstructive pulmonary disease (COPD) and occupational exposures.* Journal of Occupational Medicine and Toxicology, June 2006. 1:11.

[28] Hnizdo, E., *Chronic obstructive pulmonary disease due to occupational exposure to silica dust: a review of epidemiological and pathological evidence.* Occup Environ Med, August 2002. 60: p. 237-243.

[29] R. Guild, R.I.E., *Ocupational lung diseases.* Occupational health practice in the South African mining industry, 2001: p. 131.

[30] D., P., *The pathogenesis and pathology of COPD: identifying risk factors and improving morbidity and mortality* Advanced Studies in Medicine, November 2004. 4: p. 744-749.

[31] Alleman, J.E., *Asbestos Revisited.* Scientific American November 2010. 54-57.

[32] M., T., *Evaluation of the acutely dyspneic elderly patient.* Clin. Geriatr. Med, May 2007. 307–25.

[33] Bonauto, D., *Diagnosing Work-Related Asthma.* American College of Occupational and Environmental Medicien, 2006.

[34] Aguwa, E.N., T.A. Okeke, and M.C. Asuzu, *The prevalence of occupational asthma and rhinitis among woodworkers in south-eastern Nigeria.* Tanzan Health Res Bull, 2007. 9(1): p. 52-5.

[35] C.E. Mapp, M.S., *Mechanisms and pathology of occupational asthma.* Eur Respir J, July 1993. 7: p. 544-554.

[36] Dolovich, J. and F. Hargreave, *The asthma syndrome: inciters, inducers, and host characteristics.* Thorax, 1981. 36(9): p. 614-44.

[37] *Global tuberculosis control: epidemiology, strategy, financing.* World Health Organization November 2009: p. 6-33.

[38] James A . Merchant, M.D., Dr. P.H., *Tuberculosis as an occupational disease.* Occupational respiratory diseases, 1986: p. 709.

[39] Kumar V, A.A., Fausto N, *Robbins Basic Pathology* Saunders Elsevier: p. 516–522.
[40] Herrmann J, L.P., *Dendritic cells and Mycobacterium tuberculosis: which is the Trojan horse?.* . Pathol Biol 53 (1): p. 35–40.

Part 5

Asthma

7

Oxidative Damage and Bronchial Asthma

Eva Babusikova, Jana Jurecekova, Andrea Evinova,
Milos Jesenak[1] and Dusan Dobrota
Comenius University in Bratislava, Jessenius Faculty of Medicine in Martin,
Department of Medical Biochemistry
[1]Department of Paediatrics
Slovakia

1. Introduction

All organisms live in the environment that contains oxygen which is vital for all aerobic organisms, and **reactive oxygen species** (ROS) which are formed in cells as a consequence of aerobic metabolism. Moreover mitochondrial respiration (a base of energetic production in all eukaryotic organisms) is associated with an inevitable electron leak, resulting in a non-stop production of reactive oxygen species, such as **superoxide anion radical**, **hydrogen peroxide** and **hydrogen radical**. Universal nature of reactive oxygen species is underlined by the presence of one enzyme - **superoxide dismutase**. This enzyme occurs in all aerobic organisms and it is responsible for dismutation of superoxide anions into oxygen and hydrogen peroxide. Genes involved in detoxification of reactive oxygen species are highly conserved among eukaryotes and their deficiency could be limit of several diseases and life span. **Oxidative stress** is a unique pathophysiological condition resulting from the disrupted balance between oxidants and antioxidants. Increased level of reactive oxygen species may cause **oxidative damage** of all biomolecules: nucleic acids, proteins, lipids, saccharides. A progressive grow of oxidative damage is the result of increasing production of reactive oxygen species or an insufficient antioxidant defence system and this damage may contribute to the origin and development of several diseases including bronchial asthma, but on the other hand oxidative damage can be the consequence of them as well (fig. 1).

The lungs have the highest exposure to atmospheric oxygen. This organ is vulnerable to oxidative damage by oxygen and pollutants (tobacco smoke, ozone, silicon, asbestos, oxides of nitrogen and sulphur) because of its location, anatomy and function. The large endothelial surface (100 m^2) makes the lungs a major target site for circulating oxidants and xenobiotics. Bronchial asthma is the most frequent chronic respiratory disease in children. It is characterized by on-going airway inflammation commonly associated with airway remodelling. Oxidative damage is not only result of non-controlled airway inflammation but it can be a significant factor in the provoking of asthma exacerbations and in the maintenance of asthmatic symptoms, and may play one of the essential roles in the development and persistence of bronchial asthma. Oxidative damage may represent a potential target of the treatment of bronchial asthma.

Endogenous production of ROS occurs *in vivo* as by-products of enzymatic redox chemistry and traces of the iron and other metals catalyse oxidative reaction *in vivo*. Production of highly reactive oxygen species causes progressive, causal damage of nuclear DNA, mitochondrial DNA, RNA, enzymes, other proteins as well as unsaturated fatty acids and phospholipids. These kinds of damage may lead to a cell damage, changed cell function, and finally to a cell death.

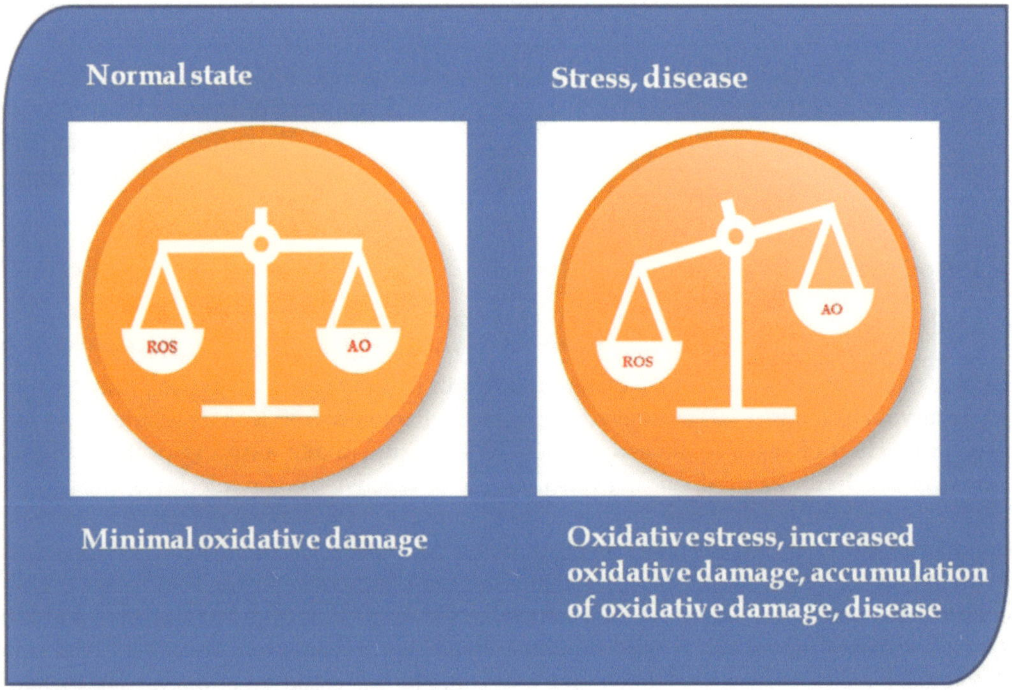

Fig. 1. **Reactive oxygen species in the development of disease.** As a consequence of disturbed equilibrium between reactive oxygen species (ROS) and antioxidants (AO) on the side of ROS, oxidative stress is increased. This causes increased oxidative damage of biomolecules, its accumulation, and the development of several diseases.

2. Origin of reactive oxygen species

Higher eukaryotic organisms cannot exist without oxygen. Molecular **oxygen** is essential for energy production in its diatomic basic state ($^3\sum g\text{-}O_2$ or O_2). During a lot of primary intracellular reactions in which oxygen is necessary, reactive oxygen species are produced. Oxygen and reactive oxygen species have destructive properties that can explain wide palette of medical states which become during origin and duration of many diseases. Single oxygen is not extremely reactive. Oxygen has two unpaired electrons which have parallel spin quantum number and they are localized in different molecular orbital and therefore oxygen molecule is quantified as diradical. If oxygen wants to accept two electrons both of them could have antiparallel spin. This criterion is executed very rarely in a typical electron pair. Therefore oxygen accept electrons for one in time and *in vivo* it is typical two- or four-electron reduction of oxygen using coordinating, serial enzymatic catalysed one-electron reductions (Beckman & Ames, 1998).

Reactive oxygen species are created in the organism under normal physiological conditions after controlled stimulation like by-product of some biological processes. There are several sources of exogenous oxidant production as well (fig. 2). Four from the endogenous sources (mitochondria, phagocytes, peroxisomes, and cytochrome P_{450} enzymes) are responsible for origin of the majority of oxidants produced by cells (Ames et al. 1993).

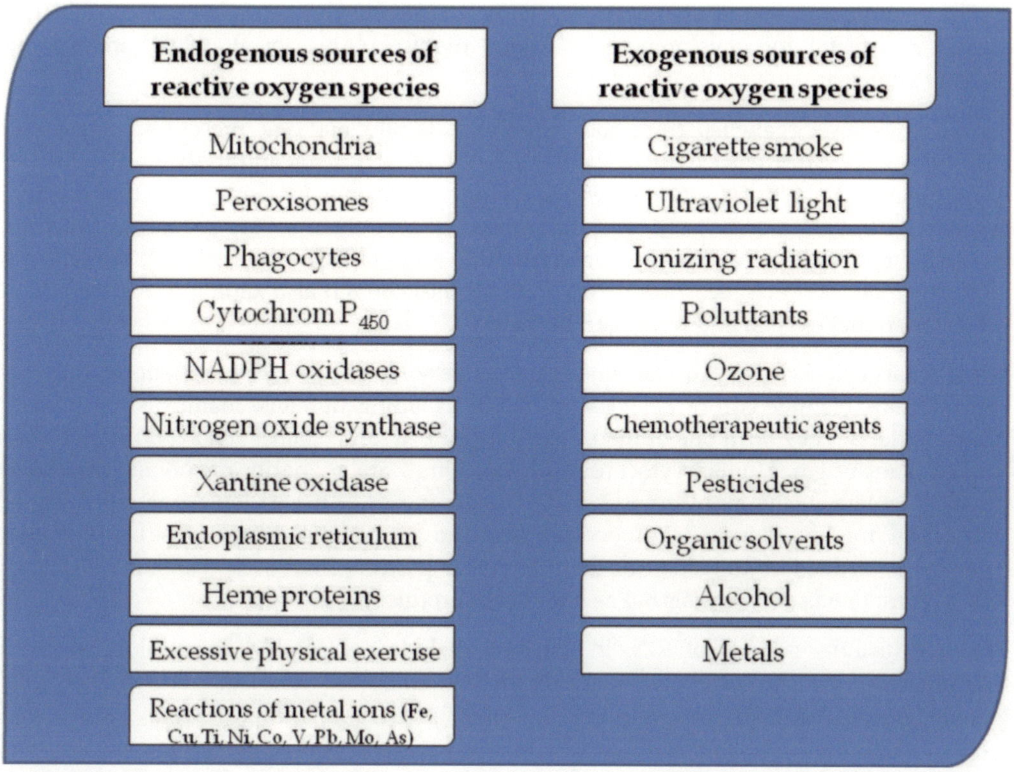

Fig. 2. **Endogenous and exogenous sources of reactive oxygen species.**

The main endogenous source of reactive oxygen species are **mitochondria** which produce reactive oxygen species continuously. The main mitochondrial function is energy production. In normal aerobic respiration mitochondria utilize oxygen that is reduced by serial steps whereby is produced water (H_2O). Mitochondria are the major producer of reactive oxygen species via incomplete reduction of oxygen by electrons leaked out of the respiratory chain in the animal and human cells. It has been demonstrated that NADH-coenzyme Q oxidoreductase (Complex I) and ubiquinol-cytochrome c reductase (Complex III) of the respiratory chain are the major sites that generate reactive oxygen species in animal mitochondria. Mitochondrial oxidative damage can lead to the release of greater amount of reactive oxygen species and cause increased oxidative damage of mitochondrial, cytoplasmic and nuclear components what subsequently may lead to dysfunctional mitochondria. Damage of mitochondrial electron transport may be an important factor in the pathogenesis of many diseases.

Phagocytig cells are another important endogenous source of oxidants. The main function of phagocytosis is the defence of host organisms against pathogens, conditionally pathogenic micro-organisms and foreign as well as body own particles bigger than 0.1 μm. Neutrophils and another phagocytes attack pathogens by mixture of reactive oxygen species: **singlet oxygen** ($O_2^{\bullet -}$), **nitric oxide** ($^{\bullet}NO$), **hydrogen peroxide** (H_2O_2), **hypochlorous acid** (HClO) (Pollack & Leeuwenburgh, 1999). Chronic virus, bacterial or parasite infection results in chronic increased phagocyting activity and finally chronic inflammation, which is a main risk factor for development of several diseases (Ames et al., 1993), and raising oxidative damage.

Peroxisomes are organelles from the microbody family and are present in almost all eukaryotic cells. They participate in the β-oxidation of fatty acids and in the metabolism of many others metabolites. Certain enzymes within peroxisome, by using molecular oxygen, remove hydrogen atoms from specific organic substrates, in an oxidative reaction, producing **hydrogen peroxide**. Hydrogen peroxide is degraded by catalase, another enzyme in peroxisome (Beckman & Ames, 1998). Peroxisomes contain also xanthine oxidase which produces **singlet oxygen** and **hydrogen peroxide**.

Microsomal **cytochrome P_{450} enzymes** are a very large and diverse superfamily of hemoproteins identified from all lineages of life including humans, mammals, birds, fish, plants, bacteria. They form one of the primary defence system against xenobiotic compounds usually plant origin. Human cytochrome P_{450} enzymes are primarily membrane-associated proteins, located in the inner mitochondrial membrane or in the endoplasmic reticulum of cells. They modify thousands of endogenous and exogenous compounds by univalent oxidation or reduction. Induction of these enzymes protects from acute oxidative effects of foreign compounds or chemicals but also results in production of oxidants.

The main cellular sources of ROS in the lung include neutrophils, eosinophils, alveolar macrophages, alveolar epithelial cells, bronchial epithelial cells and endothelial cells (Kinnula et al., 1992, 1995).

2.1 Types of reactive oxygen species

Reactive oxygen species are chemical units which are divided into two groups: **free radicals** and **non-radical compounds** (fig. 3). Free radical or radical is an atom, molecule or compound which has, contrary to non-radical atoms, one or more unpaired electrons.

One of the basic properties of reactive oxygen species is their extreme reactivity. Reactive oxygen species oxidize molecules and therefore they are named **oxidant**. They can also act as a reducing factor, can be electron neutral but also can have positive or negative charge. Radicals are predominantly high reactive and they initiate complex line of consequential reactions by which other new reactive oxygen species are formed. Results of these series reactions are chemical modification of amino acids, peptides, proteins, nucleotides, nucleic acids, fatty acids, lipids and saccharides. Structural changes of biological molecules, which are situated in the proximity of their reactive species cause change of their biological function. Reactive oxygen species participate on regulation of several physiological functions of cells and organisms such as cell signalling, neurotransmission and regulation of neurotransmitters release, gene expression, metabolism, cell proliferation and grow cells, immunity answer, and control of contraction and relaxation of smooth muscles, respiration, cell death (Chan, 2001; Halliwell and Gutteridge, 1999; Hanafy et al., 2001; Kroncke, 2001). Control of signal (Chan, 2001; Kroncke, 2001) and metabolic pathways (Halliwell and Gutteridge, 1999; Hanafy et al., 2001) through reactive oxygen species has meaning not only during physiological state of organism but supposes that during definite conditions deregulation of reactive oxygen species production participate on various kinds of diseases.

OXIDANTS

Radicals		Non-radicals	
$O_2^{\bullet -}$	superoxide anion	H_2O_2	hydrogen peroxide
$^{\bullet}OH$	hydroxyl radical	HClO	hypochlorous acid
$ROO^{\bullet}$	alkyl hydroperoxide radical	$^1O_2$	singlet oxygen
$RO^{\bullet}$	alkoxyl radical	O_3	ozone
$RS^{\bullet}$	thiyl radical	HNO_2	nitrous acid
$^{\bullet}NO$	nitric oxide	N_2O_3	dinitrogen trioxide
$NO_2^{\bullet}$	nitrogen dioxide	NO^-	nitroxyl anion
$ONOO^-$	peroxynitrite	ROONO	alkyl peroxynitrite
$^{\bullet}CCl_3$	trichloromethyl radical		

Fig. 3. **Examples of reactive oxygen species.**

2.2 Antioxidant defense

Reactive oxygen species are necessary for human life. Many vital events are mediated by radical reactions in organism. Reactive oxygen species serve as signal molecules in low concentrations but if they are produced in oversize amount evoke harmful, destructive effects (Dhalla et al., 2000). Toxicity connected with inadequate production of these species is prevented by antioxidant defence systems that provides healthy cell environment. Cells possess **enzymatic** and **non-enzymatic** defence systems (dietary antioxidants, extracellular compounds that have antioxidant activity) (fig. 4) (Bergendi et al., 1999; Pollack & Leeuwenburgh, 1999).

Superoxid dismutase (SOD, EC 1.15.1.1) is universal enzymatic antioxidant. This enzyme is extremely efficient and catalyses the neutralization of superoxide anion to oxygen and hydrogen peroxide. There are three major families of superoxide dismutase, depending on the metal cofactor: Cu/Zn (which binds both copper and zinc), Fe and Mn types (which bind either iron or manganese), and the Ni type (which binds nickel). In humans three form of SOD are present: cytoplasmic Cu/Zn-SOD (SOD1), mitochondrial Mn-SOD (SOD2), and extracellular Cu/Zn-SOD (ECSOD, SOD3).

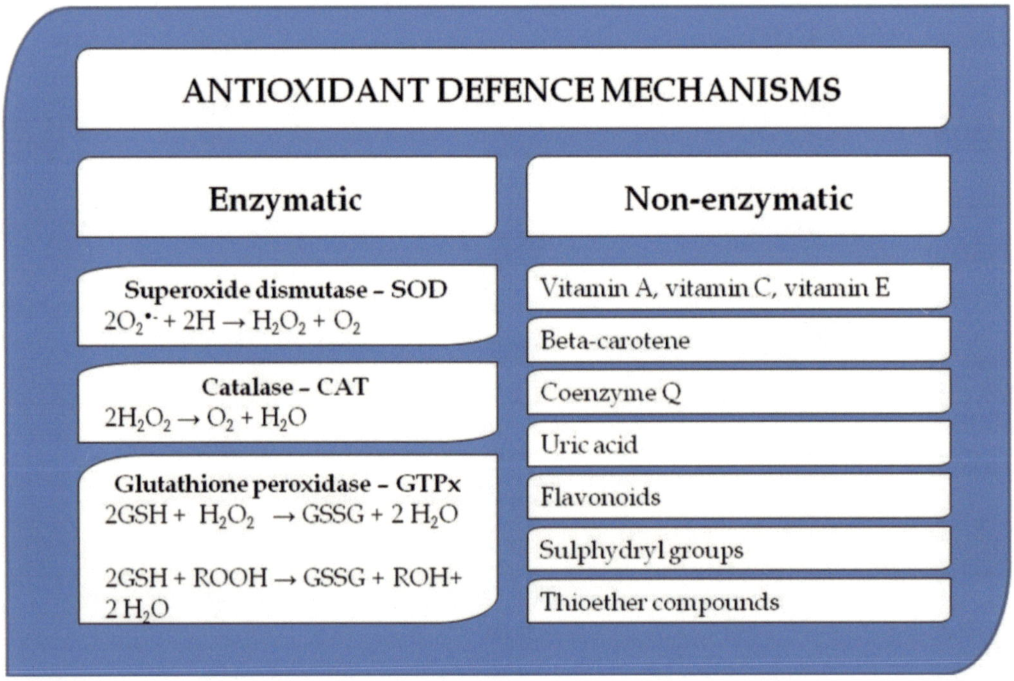

Fig. 4. **Antioxidant defence systems in organism.** $O_2^{\bullet -}$, superoxide anion; GSH, glutathione; GSSG, glutathione disulfide; ROOH, alkyl hydroperoxide.

Catalase (CAT, EC 1.11.1.6) is a common antioxidant enzyme responsible for controlling hydrogen peroxide concentrations in cells. It is ubiquitous to most aerobic cells and is situated in the lungs as well (macrophages, fibroblasts, and pneumocytes) (Kinnula et al., 1995). Catalase as an intracellular antioxidant enzyme catalyzes the decomposition of two molecules of hydrogen peroxide into one molecule of oxygen and two of water and its activity is genetically determined.

Glutathione peroxidases (GPXs, EC 1.11.1.9) are family of enzymes ubiquitously distributed which have peroxidase activity whose a main biological role is to protect the organism from oxidative damage. Glutathione peroxidases reduce hydrogen peroxide to water and reduced glutathione and lipid hydroperoxides to their corresponding alcohols, water and reduced glutathione. Four type of GPXs have been identified: cellular GPX, gastrointestinal GPX, etracellular GPX, and phospholipid hydroperoxide GPX (Tappel, 1984).

Glutathione reductase (GR, EC 1.8.1.7) participates on maintenance of intracellular concentration of glutathione.

Other an essential part of defence mechanism is a super-family of enzymes called **glutathione transferases** (GSTs, EC 2.5.1.18). These enzymes are involved in the cellular detoxification of various electrophilic xenobiotic substances such as chemical carcinogens, environmental pollutants, and antitumor agents. Glutathione transferases inactivate endogenous α,β-unsaturated aldehydes, quinone, epoxides, and hydroperoxides formed as secondary metabolites during oxidative damage. GSTs may reduce reactive oxygen species to less reactive metabolites and protect organism against consequences of lipid peroxidation. Glutathione transferases are of interest to researchers because they provide targets for antiasthmatic and antitumor drug therapies (Ruscoe et al., 2001).

Glutathione (GSH, γ,L-Glutamyl-L-cysteinylglycine) is an important antioxidant which reduces organic hyperoxides and protect organs from lipid peroxidation.

Heme oxygenase (heat shock protein 32, HO; EC 1.14.99.3) plays an important role in organism defence to oxidative stress (Paredi et al., 1999) and inflammation (Otterbien & Choi, 2000). There are known tree isoforms of HO: HO-1, HO-2, and HO-3. HO-1 is activated by a lots of inflammatory mediators, reactive oxygen species and by another stimuli (proinflammatory cytokines: interleukin-1β, interleukin-6, interferon-γ, tumor necrosis factor-α, bacterial toxins; airway viral infection; heme; hemin; reactive oxygen species: superoxide, peroxynitrite, hydrogen peroxide and reactive nitrogen species) (Nath et al., 2001; Sardana et al., 1981). HO-1 is expresses mainly in epithelial cells and endothelial cells of air system (Paredi et al., 1999).

Although cells possess complex net of antioxidant defence, the defence is not completely effective. Small fractions of oxidants escape from elimination and cause molecular damage. Some of these damages are irreversible therefore they are accumulated in time and they make base of functional decline. At specific conditions production of reactive oxygen species is increased and thereby balance between reactive oxygen species and defence systems is disrupted. In consequence, imbalance between oxidants and antioxidants in favour of oxidants and their harmful effects, oxidative damage is increased. Oxidative damage of biomolecules is a major contributor factor to many diseases such as cardiovascular and neurological diseases, lung diseases, ischemia-reperfusion injury, cancer and cataracts (Ames at al., 1993) and to physiological processes such as ageing and protein turnover (Fukagawa, 1999; Stadtman, 1993).

3. Bronchial asthma

Bronchial asthma (BA) is a lung disorder characterized by inflammation and airway hyperresponsiveness. The causes and pathogenic mechanisms of BA are poorly understood, and available treatments do not reverse and stop the disease process. Bronchial asthma has a significant global impact, affecting approximately 300 million individuals worldwide. The prevalence of bronchial asthma increases significantly during past years, especially in children. Asthma has become more common in both children and adults around the world in recent decades. The increase in the prevalence of asthma has been associated with an increase in atopic sensitization, and is paralleled by similar increases in other allergic disorders such as eczema and rhinitis. Asthma is a complex and heterogeneous chronic inflammatory disease of airways that involves the activation of many inflammatory and structural cells, all of which release inflammatory mediators that result in the typical pathophysiological changes in asthma (Barnes at al., 1998). Bronchial asthma is characterized by recurrent episodes of airway obstruction that resolve spontaneously or as a result of treatment, which occurs in individuals who may periodically have normal airway function. The airway mucosal inflammatory response in asthma is characterized by increased vascular permeability with oedema of airway walls, mucus hypersecretion with small airway plugging and infiltration by inflammatory cells, typically eosinophils. Prominent symptoms include wheezing, breathlessness, chest tightness, and cough, particularly at night and/or early in the morning.

Asthma has been recognized as a disease since the earliest times; Hippocrates used the term "αδθμα". The pathogenesis of BA is complicated and at present poorly understood. Asthma is a disorder involving all bronchial structures and depends on a complex interaction between the respiratory tract and inflammatory cells, mediators and adhesion molecules. Release of mediators primes both activation and migration of inflammatory cells that cause various degrees of airway obstruction, alternations in the mucociliary system and hyperreactivity o the bronchial smooth muscles. The cells infiltrating the bronchial mucosa in patients with asthma produce also reactive oxygen species (Andreadis at al., 2003). Oxidative damage plays an important role in the development of bronchial asthma. Increase production of reactive oxygen species leads to mutagenic alternations resulting in many pathological processes and can be implicated in pathogenesis of asthma.

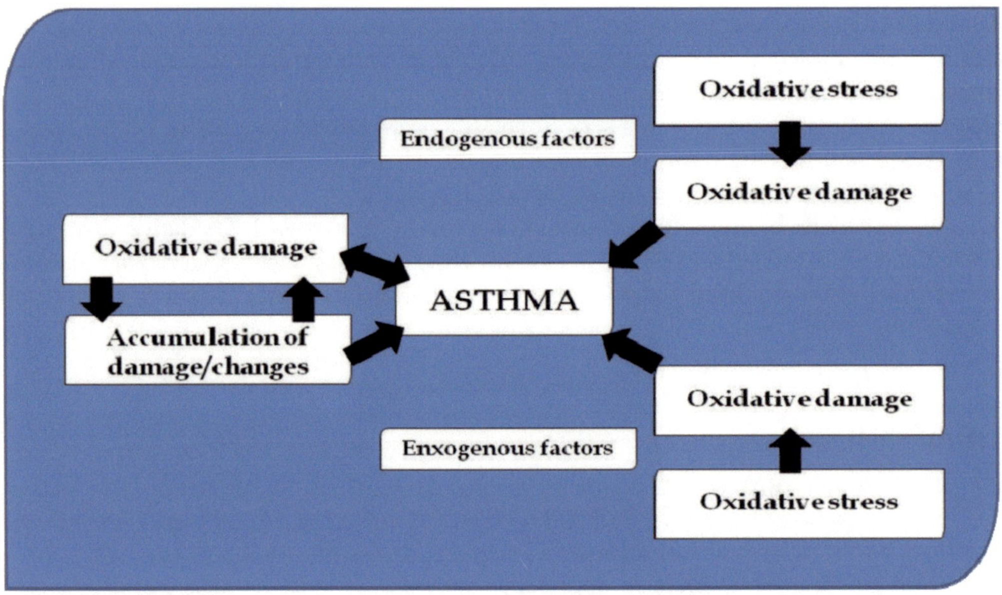

Fig. 5. **Participation of oxidative damage in the bronchial asthma origin.**

Protein oxidation, DNA modification and lipid peroxidation, all of these oxidative changes can be cumulated in airway and may participate to bronchial asthma persistence and lead to further release of mediators from epithelium resulting in further increase of oxidative damage which can again participate in asthma pathogenesis (fig. 5). Oxidative damage represents dynamic balance between a degree of oxidative damage and a degree of repair of this damage. Changes are not happened only in consequence of oxidative damage of biomolecules but also in consequence of damage of repair mechanisms.

Direct evidences of a causal role of reactive oxygen species in asthma are limited. Reactive oxygen species can influence airway cells and initiate lipid peroxidation, protein oxidation, DNA modification, enhancing release of arachidonic acid from cell membranes, contracting airway smooth muscle, increasing vascular permeability, increasing airway reactivity and airway secretion, as well as the synthesis and release of chemoattractants, inducing the release of tachykinins and neurokinins, decreasing cholinesterase and neutral endopeptidase activities, and impairing the responsiveness of β-adrenergic receptors (Barnes, 1994; Barnes et al., 1998; Rahman & MacNee, 2002). Increased oxidative damage can contribute to the origin and development of respiratory disease including bronchial asthma.

3.1 Oxidative damage in bronchial asthma

Oxidative damage has myriad effects and can negatively influence metabolic pathways including amplifying the inflammatory process. Changes in levels of **oxidants**, **antioxidants** and **markers of oxidative damage** can be determined in bronchoalveolar lavage fluid (BAL), plasma, serum, tissue and as well as in exhaled breath condensate. Our measurements are still limited by low concentration of reactive oxygen species, their extreme reactivity and short lifetime and therefore a determination of biomarkers which can reflect existence of reactive oxygen species predominates over direct evidences of increased origin of reactive oxygen species.

The ability to collect and analyse exhaled condensate has allowed the direct assessment of reactive oxygen species in allergic respiratory diseases. Higher concentration of hydrogen peroxide (Emelyanov et al., 2001; Horvath et al., 1998), superoxide anion radical (Jarjour & Calhoun, 1994; Sedgwick et al., 1990; Teramoto et al., 1996), nitric oxide (Ashutosh, 2000; Banovcin et al., 2009) was observed in asthmatic patients. Data about normal physiological value of ROS and oxidative damage biomarkers of DNA, proteins and lipids are missing or very rare in adults or in children population and therefore an implication of relevant conclusion can be uncertain.

3.1.1 Protein oxidative damage

A prominent marker of oxidative damage is **oxidative damage of proteins**. Endogenous proteins are very sensitive to modification by reactive oxygen species. Oxidized proteins can loss their biological function as result of extensive complex protein chemical modifications. These proteins may be changed to proteins which are more sensitive to intracellular proteolysis (Davies, 1987) and are very quickly degraded by endogenous proteases (Stadtman & Bertlet, 1997). Protein oxidation by reactive oxygen species may lead to **oxidation of side chains of amino acids residues** and proteins can contain **new functional groups** (hydroxyl and carbonyl groups) (Fu et al., 1998), to **cleavage of peptide bounds**, to form **new protein-protein cross bounds** (Stadtman & Berlett, 1997). These changes can result in secondary modifications such as protein **fragmentation**, **aggregation**, **unfolding**

(Davies, 1987) whereby these processes are connected with change or loss protein activity and protein function (Stadtman, 1993). Children with bronchial asthma had higher level of **protein carbonyls** compared to the healthy children (Szlagatys-Sidorkiewicz et al., 2005). There was observed a trend for higher concentrations in protein carbonyls in atopic asthmatic children compared with control subjects (Schock et al., 2003). Increased level of protein carbonyls was observed also in BAL of atopic asthmatic children (Foreman et al., 1999). We observed plasma protein modification in our group of asthmatic children (Babusikova et al., 2009). **The total concentration of sulfhydryl groups** was decreased during asthma. The value was lower in asthmatic group of children compared to the healthy subjects. Asthmatic patients with atopy had significantly lower amount of sulfhydryl groups than non-atopic patients. Nadeem et al. (2005) observed significant different in total sulfhydryl groups content between acute and stable asthmatics. Buss et al. (2003) observed **3-chlorotyrosine** in tracheal aspirate in significantly higher amounts in preterm infants with respiratory distress than in control infants. **Nitrotyrosine** was increased in exhaled breath condensate in patients with mild asthma (Hanazawa et al., 2000), in children (Baraldi et al., 2006) and in airway epithelial lining fluid of asthmatic children (Fitzpatrick et al. 2009).

In asthmatic children was observed increased level of eosinophils and mast cells compared to the healthy children (Schock et al., 2003). Several studies observed an increased level of eosinophils in adults with bronchial asthma in peripheral blood, in tissues and in exhaled breath condensate (Venge, 1995; 2010). In asthmatic children, the number of inflammatory cells in BAL fluid correlated significantly with the concentration of protein carbonyls (Schock et al., 2003). Increased respiratory burst can reflect increased oxidative stress, phagocyte auto-oxidation and subsequent intracellular oxidant release leading to additional inflammatory and lung damage in asthmatic children. Tissue damage and phagocyte activation can contribute to increased reactive oxygen species production. Activated phagocyte, neutrophils, eosinophils, monocytes and macrophage generate large amount of superoxide anion radical.

3.1.2 Lipid peroxidation

Lipid peroxidation is example of oxidative damage of biological membranes, lipoproteins and another lipid containing structures. It can be a very destructive process in a living system. Damaged biological membranes have changed biophysical properties. Proteins and lipids have limited mobility in membrane and membrane fluidity is decreased (Kaplan et al., 2003). Peroxidation of membrane lipids leads to the production of **isoprostanes**. Isoprostanes are chemical stable substances and they can contribute to the pathophysiological changes seen in asthma. They are generated *in vivo* and are specific for lipid peroxidation (Praticò et al., 2001). Increased level of 8-isoprostanes was observed in exhaled breath condensate (Baraldi et al., 2003; Caballero Balanza et al., 2010; Montuschi et al., 1999), in plasma (Wood et al., 2000), as well as in urine and BAL (Dworski et al., 1999) of asthmatic patients. **Ethane** can reflect changes that are happened in consequence of lipid peroxidation (Kneepkens et al., 1994). Increased level of ethane which is produced following lipid peroxidation in exhaled breath was observed in adult with bronchial asthma (Paredi et al., 2000). Other markers of lipid peroxidation are **thiobarbituric acid-reactive substances** (TBARS) measuring the concentration of malondialdehyde, an end product of the oxidation of polyunsaturated fatty acids. Oxidative stress can cause accumulation of TBARS. We observed increased levels of hiobarbituric acid-reactive substances in asthmatic children (Babusikova et al., 2009). Concentration of TBARS was significantly higher in exacerbated asthmatic children compared to controlled asthmatics and in atopic children levels of thiobarbituric acid-reactive substances enhanced compared to non-atopic as well. Increased level of TBARS was observed also in exhaled breath of asthmatic patients (Antczak et al., 1997) and in plasma of asthmatic patients (Shanmugasundarasn et al., 2001). Concentration of malondialdehyde was higher in exhaled breath condensate in asthmatic children (Corradi et al., 2003, Kalayci et al., 2000). Increased level of malondialdehyde was observed also in BAL and peripheral blood sample of adult patients (Ozaras R et al., 2000).

3.1.3 Antioxidant changes

Antioxidant deficiencies have been frequently reported in patients with BA. The data are inconsistent, possibly due to variation in disease severity, diet, and ethnic, using techniques and using human fluids for measurement. Activities of enzymatic antioxidants have been reported increased, decreased, and unchanged as well. In children with asthma was observed increased activity of superoxide dismutase in erythrocytes and serum (Liao et al., 2004; Szlagatys-Sidorkiewicz et al., 2005). Decreased and unchanged levels of antioxidant enzymes such as superoxide dismutase, catalase and glutathione peroxidase were observed (Comhair et al., 2000; Novak et al., 1991; Powell et al., 1994; Shanmugasundarasn et al., 2001). Decreased activity of salivary peroxidase was found in children (Bentur et al., 2006). Total antioxidant capacity in serum of asthmatic children was decreased (Liao et al., 2004). Asthmatic patients with severe exacerbation of their disease have decreased serum total antioxidant status (Katsoulis et al., 2003). Concentration of glutathione peroxidase was not changed in asthmatic children (Marcal et al., 2004). Glutathione transferase shared catalytic properties for reaction of glutathione with reactive substrates. GST enzyme family is critical for protecting cells from reactive oxygen species because enzymes can utilize a wide range of products of oxidative damage as substrates. Members of glutathione transferase superfamily play an important role in the lungs during various physiological and pathophysiological conditions (Gilliland et al., 2002a, b, c). Peripheral blood lymphocyte glutathione concentration may potentially serve as a convenient marker of lung inflammation. The increase demand for glutathione production in the face of ongoing inflammation suggests a potential role for supplementation with cysteine donors (Lands et al., 1999). GSTM1 can be an important susceptibility factor for children with bronchial asthma after exposure during the fetal period (Gilliland et al., 2002a). Polymorphism within *GSTP1* does not represent a major genetic factor in the development of bronchial asthma in children (Nickel et al., 2005). Variants of glutathione transferase confer risk to the development of asthma when the children are exposed to smoke (Kabesh et al., 2004). A significant decreased level of α-tocopherol, β-carotene, and ascorbic acid was detected in serum and erythrocytes of asthmatic children (Shanmugasundarasn et al., 2001; Kalayci et al., 2000). Composition of diet can also contribute to the increased development of bronchial asthma. Pulmonary functions are affected by intake of fresh fruit. Low intake of fruit rich in vitamin C is associated with an increased frequency of wheezing symptoms in children. Lung function parameters were lower in children with inadequate antioxidant vitamin intake (Gilliland et al., 2003). Decreased concentration of vitamins can suggest imbalance between antioxidant/oxidant status and it can be related with chronic airflow limitation. Diets and oxidative stress play a role in adults (Ochs-Balcom et al., 2006). Changes in antioxidant-oxidant balance in BAL fluid in children with asthma may be an indicator of ongoing inflammatory event in symptom-free periods. This inflammation is associated with the increased production of reactive oxygen species or oxidative stress in lung.

Individual parameters of oxidative damage influence reciprocally and together participate in the development of bronchial asthma (fig. 6). Estimation of all kind of markers of oxidative damage (proteins, lipids, DNA), together with estimation of antioxidant defence status, production of reactive oxygen species and genotype of relevant genes in the same time in asthmatic patients can be helpful for the selection the best treatment.

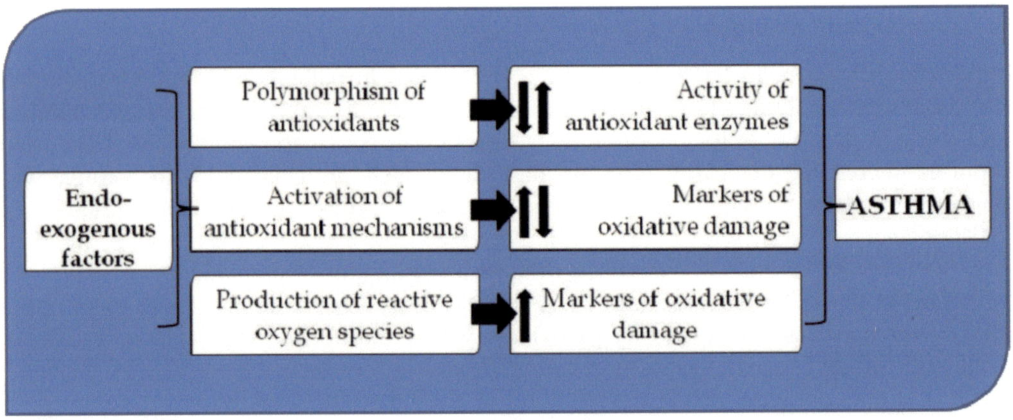

Fig. 6. **Participation of oxidative damage factors in origin of bronchial asthma.** Oxidative damage results from polymorphism of antioxidant genes (influencing enzyme activity), activation of antioxidant pathways, and polymorphism of prooxidant genes and production of reactive oxygen species (influencing increased oxidative damage).

3.1.4 Genetic changes in bronchial asthma related to oxidative damage

Environmental and genetic factors play a role in the development of asthma; however, the exact mechanisms of these factors are not fully determined. A prominent aim of BA research is to understand the genetic and environmental triggers for bronchial asthma. Asthma clusters in families and twin studies suggest a strong genetic component to bronchial asthma. Having a parent with asthma doubles a child's risk of asthma, and having two affected parents increases the risk 4-fold (Gilliland et al., 2001). Many genes as well as gene-gene interactions are associated with asthma (fig. 7).

Superoxide dismutase represents the most important part of an active antioxidant defence. Since superoxide dismutase is decreased in asthma, and its activity is strongly related to BA pathophysiology, it has been hypothesized that genetic variations in superoxide dismutase may play a role in the development of asthma. The genes encoding SOD1, SOD2, SOD3 are located in different chromosomes and in all of them polymorphisms have been described. *SOD1* is encoded on 21q22.1, *SOD2* on 6q25.3, and *SOD3* on 4p16.3-q21. Regulation of *SOD* genes plays a crucial role in balancing the reactive oxygen species concentration. In ***SOD1*** has been observed substitution of A to C at the non-coding position 35. This polymorphism influence SOD1 activity (Flekac et al., 2008). Substitution T to C at position 24, resulting in a valine to alanine substitution at amino acid 16 has been identified in ***SOD2***. Impairment of the mitochondrial superoxide dismutase activity was related to bronchial asthma pathophysiology (Comhair et al., 2005). In ***SOD3*** gene has been identified three single nucleotide polymorphism: alanine to threonine substitution at amino acid 40, phenylalanine to cysteine at amino acid 131, and finally the most studied polymorphism which represents substitution of arginine to glycine at amino acid 213. Studies about superoxide dismutase polymorphisms are very rare in asthmatic population. In Chinese and Finnish asthmatic patients was not found significant differences either in allele or in genotype in *SOD2* (Kinnula et al., 2004; Mak et al., 2006).

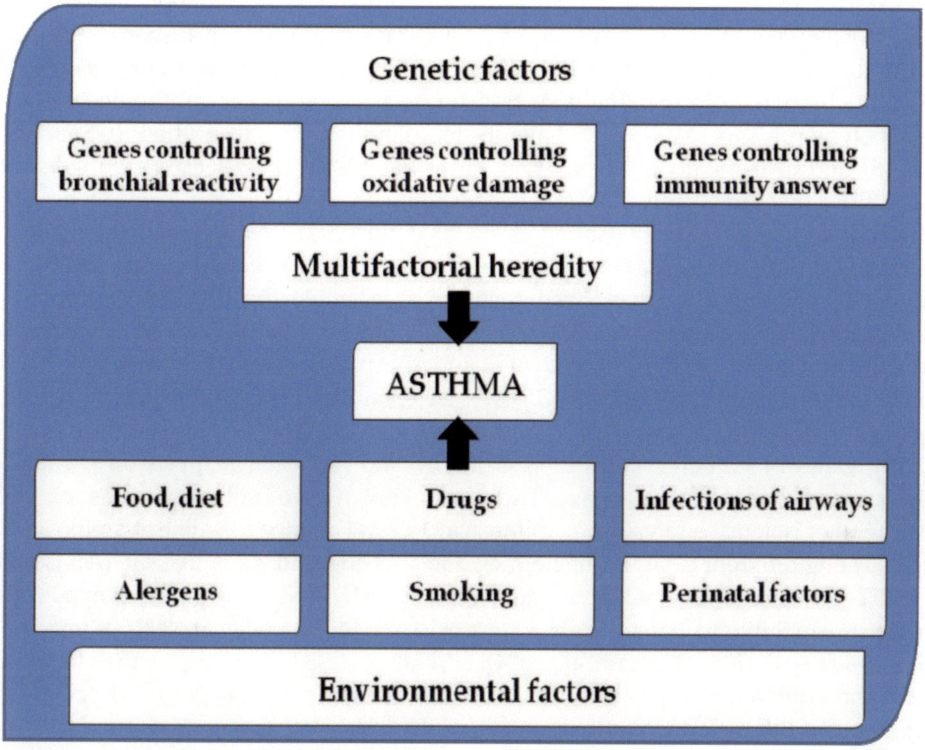

Fig. 7. **Impact of genetic and environmental factors on bronchial asthma development.**

Catalase is a common antioxidant enzyme responsible for controlling hydrogen peroxide concentrations in cells. The catalase gene is located on chromosome 11p13. There are known different polymorphisms of this enzyme in coding regions (Goth, 1998; Kishimoto et al., 1992) and in non-coding regions as well (Casp et al., 2002; Forsberg et al., 2001; Goth et al., 2005; Kishimoto et al., 1992; Ukkola et al., 2001; Zhou et al., 2005; Wen et al., 1990). A common polymorphism in the promoter region of the catalase gene consists of a C to T substitution at position -262 in the 5' region (Forsberg et al., 2001), which is thought to result in reduced activity. *CAT* polymorphism may be associated with increased risk of asthma (Mak et al., 2006; Polonikov et al., 2009). In our study the frequency of TT genotype of catalase -262C→T was 0.226 in asthmatic children and 0.048 in healthy children ($p < 0.001$) and *CAT* polymorphism may be associated with increased oxidative damage in asthmatic subjects (unpublished results).

Glutathione transferase genes have been suggested as candidate genes for BA because they are involved in antioxidant defence pathways and they are expressed in the lungs. Glutathione transferases have historically also been called glutathione-S-transferases, and it is this latter name that gives rise to the widely used abbrevation, GST. Three major families of proteins the cytosolic, mitochondrial and microsomal (membrane-associated proteins in eicosanoids and glutathione metabolism, MAPEG) are known. In some organisms expression of *GSTs* are upregulated by exposure to prooxidants (An & Blackwell, 2003; Desikan et al., 2001; Veal et al., 2002). Seven classes of cytosolic glutathione transferases are recognising in mammals (Alpha, Mu, Pi, Sigma, Theta, Omega, and Zeta) (Hayes & Pulford, 1995). At least 16 cytosolic GST subunits exists in human and display polymorphisms, and this is probably contributing factor to interindividual differences in responses to diseases and xenobiotics. *GSTM1* is one of the genes encoding the Mu class of enzymes. Gene for GSTM1 has been mapped to glutathione transferase mu gene cluster on chromosome 1p13.3. Three polymorphisms of *GSTM1* have been identified: a substitution (*GSTM1A* and *GSTM1B*) and a deletion (Rebbeck, 1997; Xu et al., 1998). The alleles of the substitution variant differ by C to G transition at base position 534, resulting in a lysine to asparagine substitution at amino acid 172 (Cotton et al., 2000; Rebbeck, 1997). There is no evidence to date that *GSTM1A* and *GSTM1B* alleles are functionally different from one another; thus these alleles are typically categorized together as a single functional phenotype. Other polymorphism is a deletion - *GSTM1* null variant that results in a lack of functional gene product. The *GSTT1* gene is located at 22q11.2. Absence of both alleles for this gene represents null variant analogous to *GSTM1*. Deletion of whole gene results in the lack of enzymatic activity (Sprenger et al., 2000). Gene for GSTP1 is one of the most intensive studying genes of glutathione transferase family and has been mapped on chromosome 11q13 and comprising nine exons. There are known two polymorphisms of *GSTP1*: substitution of isoleucine to valine at amino acid 105 and alanine to valine at amino acid 114, demonstrating different catalytic efficiencies due to changes in the active site (Ali-Osman et al., 1997). A number of studies suggest that *GSTM1, GSTT1, GSTM1* polymorphisms increase susceptibility to asthma (Babusikova et al., 2009; Hanene et al., 2007; Kamada et al., 2007; Romieu et al., 2006; Tamer et al., 2004). *GSTM1* and *GSTT1* deficiency may increase the risk for the asthma development of in utero and current smoke exposure (Kabesch et al., 2004). People with a *GSTM1* null variant or *GSTP1* Val/Val genotype show decreased in lung function growth (Gilliland et al., 2002b; Imboden et al., 2007).

Nicotinamide adenine dinucleotide (phosphate) reduced:quinone oxidoreductase (NQO1, EC 1.6.5.2) is phase II enzyme important in response to oxidative stress. NQO1 is highly expressed in the lungs. The gene for this protein is localised on chromosome 16q22.1. NQO1 catalyzes the two-electron reduction of quinones to hydroquinones, thus bypassing the potentially toxic semiquinone radical intermediate (Jaiswal, 2000; Vasiliou et al., 2006) and prevents the generation of reactive oxygen species, and protects cells from oxidative damage. Some evidence suggest that NQO1 may also interact directly with reactive oxygen species (Jia et al., 2008), such as hydroxyl radical and hydrogen peroxide, and may influence the balance between oxidants and antioxidants. This enzyme can act also as an antioxidant enzyme by reducing ubiquinone (coenzyme Q_{10}) and vitamin E quinone to their antioxidant forms (Beyer et al., 1996; Siegel et al., 1997) and bases on its influence on antioxidant mechanisms NQO1 is a candidate gene. Currently, there are 22 reported single-nucleotide polymorphisms in the *NQO1* gene. Only two of these, arginine139tryptophan and proline187serine (Larson et al., 1999; Traver et al., 1992) have been studied extensively. The *NQO1* gene plays an important role in asthma susceptibility (David et al., 2003; Li et al., 2009). Functional polymorphism of *NQO1* gene with conjugation of *GSTM1* null variant can have a protective effect in relation to asthma risk (David et al., 2003). For individuals already exhibiting disease status, a decrease or loss of NQO1 activity due to mutation, can play a role by increasing the risk of severity (Goodrich et al., 2009). Polymorphism in *NQO1* gene may be an important factor determining the intensity of medical therapy in asthmatic children. Asthmatic children with functional polymorphism of *NQO1* may require more intensive pharmaceutical treatment to effectively control their asthma (Goodrich et al., 2009).

Nicotinamide adenine dinucleotide phosphate oxidase (NADPH oxidase, EC 1.6.3.1) is a membrane-associated enzyme that catalyzes the production of superoxide anion. This enzyme is one of the main sources of superoxide anion and is highly expressed in neutrophils and endothelial cells (Azumi et al., 1999). NADPH oxidase is multicomponent enzyme made up from six subunits: Rho guanosine triphosphatase and five subunits of phagocytic oxidases (phox). Gp91phox and gp22phox are transmembrane subunits, and p40phox, p47phox and p67phox are cytosol subunits. The gp22phox is also called cytochrome b α subunit (CYBA) and presence of this protein in the NADPH oxidase determines the enzyme activity and production of superoxide radical (De Keluelanear et al., 1999). There were identified three polymorphisms in gene for gp22phox subunit at position +242 in exon 4, which consists of a C to T substitution resulting in a histidine to tyrosine substitution at amino acid 72; in the 3' untranslated region at position 640 A is substituted by G, and the third polymorphism is located in the promoter region at position -930, which consists of a A to G substitution (Dinauer et al., 1990; Moreno et al., 2003). Polymorphism of *CYBA* can be an important genetic component that determines susceptibility to allergic form of BA (Ivanov et al., 2008).

3.1.5 Antioxidant treatment

Antioxidant therapy may be a useful treatment for bronchial asthma because oxidative damage is increased in asthmatic patients. Epidemiological studies suggest that antioxidant have a significant effect on the incidence and severity of BA (Fogarty & Britton, 2000; Smith et al., 1999). There are several antioxidants, including endogenous metobolites (glutathione, *N*-actylcysteine, heme oxygenase 1, uric acid), natural antioxidants and other nutrients (vitamins C and E, β-carotene, co-enzyme Q10, urate, curcumin, α lipoic acid, fish oil), and herbal molecules and polyphenols (esculitin, sulforaphane, resveratrol, caffeic acid phenethyl ester). Vitamin C and E are powerful antioxidants found in the lungs. Vitamin C is hydrophilic antioxidant and acts to quench radicals within cells and regenerates vitamin E. Vitamin E is a lipophilic chain-breaking antioxidant that acts by stopping the chain reaction involved in lipid peroxidation. Urate is hydrophilic and has chain-breaking properties and stabilizes vitamin C as well. Several authors observed decreased oxidative damage in asthmatic mice treated with antioxidants (Dittrich et al., 2009; Lee et al., 2009; Okamoto et al., 2006). Studies of antioxidant intake have provided conflicting results in asthmatic patients. Epidemiological studies indicate that elevated dietary intake of vitamin C may be associated with a reduced risk of asthma (Hatch, 1995; Soutar et al., 1997). On the other hand, many studies do not indicate any relation between asthma and vitamin C (Fogarty et al., 2003; Troisi et al., 1995). Pearson et al. (2004) observed no benefit of dietary supplementation with vitamin E in adults with mild to moderate asthma. Controlled studies in humans, on both healthy subjects (Chatham et al., 1987; Samet et al., 2001) and individuals with asthma (Trenga et al., 2001), have also suggested that antioxidant supplementation (vitamin C and vitamin E) may protect against the acute effects of ozone on lung functioning. Supplementation with antioxidants might modulate the impact of ozone exposure on the small airways of children with moderate to severe asthma (Romieu et al., 2002). Vitamin A supplementation early in life was not associated with a decreased risk of asthma in an area with chronic vitamin A deficiency (Checkley et al., 2011). Diet supplementation with omega-3 fatty acids, Zn and vitamin C significantly improved asthma control test, pulmonary function tests and pulmonary inflammatory markers in children with moderately persistent bronchial asthma either singly or in combination (Biltagi et al., 2009). Dietary supplementation with vitamins E and C benefits asthmatic adults who are exposed to air pollutants (Trenga et al., 2001).

4. Conclusion

Prevalence of bronchial asthma increases and represents very serious medical problems. Bronchial asthma is a complex multifactorial disease in which environmental factors, oxidative damage and genetic factors are responsible for initiating and modulating the progression of the disease. Several markers of oxidative damage in plasma, serum, exhaled breath, and as well as in bronchoalveolar lavage fluid are rising in patients with asthma. Oxidative damage represents an important factor contributing to the origin and persistence of airway inflammation in asthmatic subjects. The role of mentioned gene polymorphisms and many others gene polymorphisms as risk factors for the occurrence of bronchial asthma is still controversial. We still need new studies for clear determination gene polymorphisms which are related to asthma. Moreover multiple genotype analyses are necessary as well because a single gene polymorphism can be without relationship to increased risk of asthma but the combination of gene polymorphisms may have a significant effect for asthma development. Oxidative damage plays a significant role in the pathology of bronchial asthma therefore this process may represent a potential target of the therapy in asthmatic patients. In summary bronchial asthma is a no single disease; it is an umbrella of diseases associated with increased oxidative stress followed by an accumulation of oxidative damage.

5. Acknowledgment

This work was supported by grants VEGA 1/0071/11 and Ministry of Health 2007/47-UK-12.

6. References

Ali-Osman, F., Akande, O., Antoun, G., Mao, .JX. & Buolamwini, J. (1997). Molecular cloning, characterization, and expression in Escherichia coli of full-length cDNAs of three human glutathione S-transferase Pi gene variants. Evidence for differential catalytic activity of the encoded proteins. *The Journal of Biological Chemistry*, Vol.272, No.15, (April 1998), pp. 10004-10012

Ames, B. N., Shigenaga, M. K. & Hagen, T. M. (1993). Oxidants, antioxidants, and the degenerative diseases of aging. *Proceedings of the National Acadademy of the Sciences of the United States of America*, Vol.90, No.17, (September 1993), pp. 7915-7922

An, J.H. & Blackwell, T.K. (2003). SKN-1 links C. elegans mesendodermal specification to a conserved oxidative stress response. Genes and Development, Vol.17, No.15, (August 2003), pp. 1882-1893

Andreadis, A.A., Hazen, S.L., Comhair, S.A. & Erzurum, S.C. (2003). Oxidative and nitrosative events in asthma. *Free Radical Biology and Medicine*, Vol.35, No.3, (August 2003), pp. 213-225

Antczak, A., Nowak, D., Shariati, B., Król, M., Piasecka, G. & Kurmanowska Z. (1997). Increased hydrogen peroxide and thiobarbituric acid-reactive products in expired breath condensate of asthmatic patients. *The European Respiratory Journal*, Vol.10, No.6, (June 1997), pp. 1235-1241

Ashutosh, K. (2000). Nitric oxide and asthma: a review. *Current Opinion in Pulmonary Medicine*, Vol.6, No.1, (January 2000), pp. 21-25

Azumi, H., Inoue, N., Takeshita, S., Rikitake, Y., Kawashima, S., Hayashi, Y., Itoh, H. & Yokoyama, M. (1999). Expression of NADH/NADPH oxidase p22phox in human coronary arteries. *Circulation*, Vol.100, No.14, (October 1999), pp. 1494-1498

Babusikova, E., Jesenak, M., Kirschnerova, R., Banovcin, P. & Dobrota D. (2009). Association of oxidative stress and GST-T1 gene with childhood bronchial asthma. *Journal of Physiology and Pharmacology*, Vol.60, No.Suppl. 5, (November 2009), pp. 27-30

Banovcin, P., Jesenak, M., Michnova, Z., Babusikova, E., Nosal, S., Mikler, J., Fabry, J. & Barreto M. (2009). Factors attributable to the levels of exhaled nitric oxide in asthmatic children. *European Journal of Medical Research*, Vol.14, Suppl. 4, (December 2009), pp. 9-13

Baraldi, E., Ghiro, L., Piovan, V., Carraro, S., Ciabattoni, G., Barnes, P.J. & Montuschi P. (2003). Increased exhaled 8-isooprostane in childhood asthma. *Chest*, Vol.124, No.1, (July 2003), pp. 25-31

Baraldi, E., Giordano, G., Pasquale, M.F., Carraro, S., Mardegan, A., Bonetto, G., Bastardo, C., Zacchello F. & Zanconato, S. (2006). 3-Nitrotyrosine, a marker of nitrosative stress, is increased in breath condensate of allergic asthmatic children. *Allergy*, Vol.61, No.1, (January 2006), pp. 90-96

Barnes, P.J. (1994). Cytokines as mediators of chronic asthma. *American Journal of Respiratory and Critical Care Medicine*, Vol.150, No.5Pt2, (November 1994), pp. S42-S49

Barnes, P.J., Chung, K.F., & Page C.P. (1998). Inflammatory mediators of asthma: an update. *Pharmacological Reviews*, Vol.50, No.4, (December 1998), pp. 515-596

Beckman, K. B. & Ames, B. N. (1998). The free radical theory of aging matures. *Physiological Review*, Vol.78, No.2, (April 1998), pp. 547-581

Bentur, L., Mansour, Y., Brik, R., Eizenberg, Y. & Nagler R.M. (2006). Salivary oxidative stress in children during acute asthmatic attack and during remission. *Respiratory Medicine*, Vol.100, No.7, (July 2006), pp. 1195-1201

Bergendi, L., Benes, L., Durackova, Z. & Ferencik, M. (1999). Chemistry, physiology and pathology of free radicals. *Life Sciences*, Vol.65, No.18-19, pp. 1865-1874

Beyer, R.E., Segura-Aguilar, J., Di Bernardo, S., Cavazzoni, M., Fato, R., Fiorentini, D., Galli, M.C., Setti, M., Landi, L. & Lenaz, G. (1996). The role of DT-diaphorase in the maintenance of the reduced antioxidant form of coenzyme Q in membrane systems. *Proceedings of the National Acadademy of the Sciences of the United States of America,* Vol.93, No.6, (March 1996), pp. 2528-2532

Biltagi, M.A., Baset, A.A., Bassiouny, M., Kasrawi, M.A. & Attia, M. (2009). Omega-3 fatty acids, vitamin C and Zn supplementation in asthmatic children: a randomized self-controlled study. *Acta Paediatrica,* Vol.98, No.4, (April 2009), pp. 737-742

Buss, I.H., Senthilmohan, R., Darlow, B.A., Mogridge, N., Kettle, A.J. & Winterbourn C.C. (2003). 3-Chlorotyrosine as a marker of protein damage by myeloperoxidase in tracheal aspirates from preterm infants: association with adverse respiratory outcome. *Pediatric Research,* Vol.53, No.3, (March 2003), pp. 455-462, Erratum in: *Pediatric Research,* Vol.53, No.5, (May 2003), pp. 868

Caballero Balanzá, S., Martorell Aragonés, A., Cerdá Mir, J.C., Ramírez, J.B., Navarro, Iváñez, R., Navarro Soriano, A., Félix Toledo, R. & Escribano Montaner A. (2010). Leukotriene B4 and 8-isorostane in exhaled breath condensate of children with episodic and persistent asthma. *Journal of Investigational Allergology and Clinical Immunology,* Vol.20, No.3, pp. 237-243

Casp, C.B., She, J.X. & McCormack, W.T. (2002). Genetic association of the catalase gene (CAT) with vitiligo susceptibility. *Pigment Cell Research,* Vol.15, No.1, (February 2002), pp. 62-66

Chan, P. H. (2001). Reactive oxygen radicals in signaling and damage in the ischemic brain. *Journal of Cerebral Blood Flow and Metab.olism,* Vol.21, No.1, (January 2001), pp. 2-14

Chatham, M.D., Eppler, J.H. Jr,, Saunder, L.R., Green, D. & Kulle, T.J. (1987). Evaluation of the effects of vitamin C on ozone induced bronchoconstriction in normal subjects. *Annals of the New York Academy of Sciences,* Vol.498, (1987), pp. 269–279

Checkley, W., West, K.P. Jr,, Wise. R,A., Wu, L., Leclerq, S.C., Khatry, S., Katz, J., Christian, P., Tielsch, J.M. & Sommer, A. (2011). Supplementation with vitamin A early in life and subsequent risk of asthma. *The European Respiratory Journal,* (June 2011), Epub ahead of print

Comhair, S.A., Bhathena, P.R., Dweik, R.A., Kavuru, M. & Erzurum, S.C. (2000). Rapid loss of superoxide dismutase activity during antigen-induced asthmatic responce, Lacent, Vol.355, No.9204, (February 2000), pp. 624

Comhair, S.A., Xu, W., Ghosh, S., Thunnissen, F.B., Almasan, A,, Calhoun, W.J., Janocha, A.J., Zheng, L., Hazen, S.L. &Erzurum, S.C. (2005). Superoxide dismutase inactivation in pathophysiology of asthmatic airway remodeling and reactivity. *The American Journal of Pathology,* Vol.166, No.3, (March 2005), pp. 663-674

Corradi, M., Folesani, G., Andreoli, R., Manini, P., Bodini, A., Piacentini, G., Carraro, S., Zanconato, S. & Baraldi E. (2003). Aldehydes and glutathione in exhaled breath condensate of children with asthma exacerbation. *American Journal of Respiratory and Critical Care Medicine,* Vol.167, No.3, (February 2003), pp. 395-399

Cotton, S.C., Sharp, L., Little, J. & Brockton, N. (2000). Glutathione S-transferase polymorphisms and colorectal cancer: a HuGE review. *American Journal of Epidemiology,* Vol.151, No.1, (January 2000), pp. 7-32

David, G.L., Romieu, I., Sienra-Monge, J.J., Collins, W.J., Ramirez-Aguilar, M., del Rio-Navarro, B.E., Reyes-Ruiz, N.I., Morris, R.W., Marzec, J.M. & London, S.J. (2003).

Nicotinamide adenine dinucleotide (phosphate) reduced:quinone oxidoreductase and glutathione S-transferase M1 polymorphisms and childhood asthma. *American Journal of Respiratory and Critical Care Medicine,* Vol.168, No.10, (November 2003), pp. 1199-1204

Davies, K. J. (1987). Protein damage and degeneration by oxygen radicals. *The Journal of Biological Chemistry,* Vol.262, No.20, (July 1987), pp. 9895-9901

De Keulenaer, G.W., Alexander, R.W., Ushio-Fukai, M., Ishizaka, N. & Griendling, K.K. (1998). Tumor necrosis factor alpha activities a p22phox based NADPH oxidase in vascular smooth muscle. *The Biochemical Journal,* Vol.329, No.Pt.3, (February 1998). pp. 653-657

Desikan, R., A-H-Mackerness, S., Hancock, J.T. & Neill, S.J. (2001). Regulation of the Arabidopsis trancriptome by oxidative stress. Plant Physiology, Vol.127, No.1, (September 2001), pp. 159-172

Dhalla, N. S., Temsah, R. M. & Netticadan, T. (2000). Role of oxidative stress in cardiovascular diseases. *Journal of Hypertension, Vol.*18, No.6, (June 2000), pp. 655-673

Dinauer ,M.C., Pierce, E.A., Bruns, G.A., Curnutte, J.T. & Orkin, S.H. (1990). Human neutrophil cytochrome b light chain (p22-Phox): gene structure, chromosomal location, and mutations in cytochrome-negative autosomal recesive chronic granulomatous disease. *The Journal of Clinical Investigation,* Vol.86, No.5, (November 1990), pp. 1729-1737

Dittrich, A.M., Meyer, H.A., Krokowski, M., Quarcoo, D., Ahrens, B., Kube, S.M., Witzenrath, M., Esworthy, R.S., Chu, F.F. & Hamelmann, E. (2009). Glutathione peroxidase-2 protects from allergen-induced airway inflammation in mice. *The European Respiratory Journal,* Vol.35, No.5, (May 2009), pp. 1148–1154

Dworski, R., Murray, J.J., Roberts, L.J. 2nd, Oates, J.A., Morrow, J.D., Fisher, L. & Sheller, J.R. (1999). Allergen-induced synthesis of F(2)-isoprostanes in atopic asthmatics. Evidence for oxidant stress. *American Journal of Respiratory and Critical Care Medicine,* Vol.160, Vol.6, (December 1999), pp. 1947-1951

Emelyanov, A., Fedoseev, G., Abulimity, A., Rudinski, K., Fedoulov, A., Karabanov, A. & Barnes P.J. (2001). Elevated concentrations of exhaled hydrogen peroxide in asthmatic patients. *Chest.* Vol.120, No.4, (October 2001), pp. 1136-1139

Fitzpatrick, A.M., Brown, L.A., Holguin, F. & Teague W.G. (2009). Levels of nitric oxide oxidation products are increased in the epithelial lining fluid of children with persistent asthma. *The Journal of Allergy and Clinical Immunology,* Vol.124, No.5, (November 2009), pp. 990-996

Flekac, M., Skrha, J., Hilgertova, J., Lacinova, Z. & Jarolimkova, M. (2008). Gene polymorphisms of superoxide dismutases and catalase in diabetes mellitus. *BMC Medical Genetics,* Vol.9,No.30 (April 2008)

Fogarty, A & Britton, J. (2000). The role of diet in the eatiology of asthma. Current Opinion in Pulmonary Medicine, Vol.30, No.5, (May 2000), pp. 615-627

Fogarty, A., Lewis, S.A., Scrivener, S.L., Antoniak, M., Pacey, S., Pringle, M. & Britton, J. (2003). Oral magnesium and vitamin C supplements in asthma: a parallel group randomized placebo-controlled trial. *Clinical and Experimental Allergy,* Vol33, No.10, (October 2003), pp. 1355–1359

Foreman, R.C., Mercer, P.F., Kroegel, C. & Warner J.A. (1999). Role of the eosinophil in protein oxidation in asthma: possible effects on proteinase/antiproteinase balance. *International Archives of Allergy and Immunology,* Vol.118, No.2-4, (February-April 1999), pp. 183-186

Forsberg, L., Lyrenäs, L., de Faire, U. & Morgenstern, R. (2001). A common functional C-T substitution polymorphism in the promoter region of the human catalase gene influences transcription factor binding, reporter gene transcription and its correlated to blood catalase levels. *Free Radical Biology and Medicine,* Vol.30, No.5, (March 2001), pp. 500-505

Fu, S., Davies, J. & Dean, R. T. (1998). Molecular aspects of free radical damage to proteins. In *Molecular biology of free radicals in human diseases,* O.I. Aruoma, B. Halliwell (eds.), pp. 29-56, OICA International: Saint Lucia, ISBN 976-8056-15-0, London UK

Fukagawa, N. K. (1999). Aging: is oxidative stress a marker or is it causal? *Proceedings of the Society for Experimental Biology and Medicine,* Vol.222, No.3, (December 1999), pp. 293-298

Gilliland, F.D., Berhane, K., Rappaport, E.B., Thomas, D.C., Avol, E., Gauderman, W.J., London, S.J., Margolis, H.G., McConnell, R., Islam, K.T. & Peters, J.M. (2001). The effects of ambient air pollution on school absenteeism due to respiratory illnesses. *Epidemiology,* Vol.12, No.1, (January 2001), pp. 43-54

Gilliland, F.D., Berhane, K.T., Li, Y.F., Gauderman, W.J., McConnell R. & Peters J. (2003). Children's lung function and antioxidant vitamin, fruit, juice, and vegetable intake. *American Journal of Epidemiology,* Vol.158, No.6, (September 2003), pp. 576-584

Gilliland, F.D., Gauderman, W.J., Vora, H., Rappaport, E. & Dubeau, L. (2002b). Effects of glutathione-S-transferase M1, T1, and P1 on childhood lung function growth. *American Journal of Respiratory ans Critical Care Medicine,* Vol.166, No.5, (September 2002), pp. 710-716

Gilliland, F.D., Li, Y.F., Dubeau, L., Berhane, K., Avol, E., McConnell, R., Gauderman, W.J. & Peters, J.M. (2002a). Effects of glutathione S-transferase M1, maternal smoking during pregnancy, and environmental tobacco smoke on asthma and wheezing in children. *American Journal of Respiratory ans Critical Care Medicine,* Vol.166, No.4, (August 2002), pp. 457-463

Gilliland, F.D., Rappaport, E.B., Berhane, K., Islam, T., Dubeau, L., Gauderman, W.J. & McConnell, R. (2002c). Effects of glutathione S-transferase P1, M1, and T1 on acute respiratory illness in school children. *American Journal of Respiratory ans Critical Care Medicine,* Vol.166, No.3, (August 2002), pp. 346-351

Goodrich, G.G., Goodman, P.H., Budhecha, S.K. & Pritsos, C.A. (2009). Functional polymorphism of detoxification gene NQO1 predicts intensity of empirical treatment of childhood asthma. *Mutation Research,* Vol.674, No.1-2, (March 2009), pp. 55-61

Góth L. (1998). Genetic heterogeneity of the 5' uncoding region of the catalase gene in Hungarian acatalasemic and hypocatalasemic subjects. *Clinica Chimica Acta,* Vol.271, No.1, (March 1998), pp. 73-78

Góth, L., Vitai, M., Rass, P., Sükei, E. & Páy A. (2005). Detection of a novel familial catalase mutation (Hungarian type D) and the possible risk of inherited catalase deficiency for diabetes mellitus. *Electrophoresis,* Vol.26, No.9, (May 2005), pp. 1646-1649

Halliwell, B. & Gutteridge, J.M.C. (1999). Free radicals in biology and medicine, University Press, ISBN 0-198-50044-0, Oxford, UK

Hanafy, K. A., Krumenacker, J. S. & Murad, F. (2001). NO, nitrotyrosine, and cyclic GMP in signal transduction. *Medical Science Monitor,* Vol.7, No.4, (July-August 2001), pp. 801-819

Hanazawa, T., Kharitonov, S.A. & Barnes P.J. (2000). Increased nitrotyrosine in exhaled breath condensate of patients with asthma. *American Journal of Respiratory and Critical Care Medicine,* Vol.162, No.4Pt1, (October 2000), pp. 1273-1276

Hanene, C., Jihene, L., Jamel, A., Kamel, H. & Agnès, H. (2007). Association of GST genes polymorphisms with asthma in Tunisian children. *Mediators of Inflammation,* Vol.2007, ID:19564

Hatch, G.E. (1995). Asthma, inhaled oxidants, and dietary anti-oxidants. *The American Journal of Clinical Nutrition,* Vol.61, No. 3 Suppl, (March 1995), pp. 625S–630S

Hayes, J.D. & Pulford, D.J. (1995). The glutathione S-transferase supergene family: regulation of GST and the contribution of the isoenzymes to cancer chemoprotection and drug resistance. *Critical Reviews in Biochemistry and Molecullar Biology,* Vol.30, No.6, pp. 445-600

Horvath, I., Donnelly, L.E., Kiss, A., Kharitonov, S.A., Lim, S., Chung, K.F. & Barnes P.J. (1998). Combined use of exhaled hydrogen peroxide and nitric oxide in monitoring asthma. *American Journal of Respiratory and Critical Care Medicine,* Vol.158, Vol.4, (October 1998), pp. 1042-1046

Imboden, M., Downs, S.H., Senn, O., Matyas, G., Brändli, O., Russi, E.W., Schindler, C., Ackermann-Liebrich, U., Berger, W., Probst-Hensch, N.M. & SAPALDIA Team. (2007). Glutathone S-transferase genotypes modify lung function decline in the general population: SAPALDIA cohor study. *Respiratory Research,* Vol.8:2, (January 2007)

Ivanov, V.P., Solodilova, M.A., Polonikov, A.V., Khoroshaia, I.V., Kozhukhov, M.A. & Panfilov, V.I. (2008). Association of *C242T* and *A640G* polymorphisms in the gene for p22phox subunit of NADPH oxidase with the risk of bronchial asthma: a pilot study. *Genetika,* Vol.44, No.5, (May 2008), pp. 693-701

Jaiswal, A.K. (2000). Regulation of genes encoding NAD(P)H: quinone oxidoreductases. *Free Radical Biology and Medicine,* Vol.29, No.3-4, (August 1994), pp. 254-262

Jarjour, N.N. & Calhoun, W.J. (1994). Enhanced production of oxygen radicals in asthma. *The Journal of Laboratory and Clinical Medicine,* Vol.123, No.1, (January 1994), pp. 131-136

Jia, B., Park, S.C., Lee, S., Pham, B.P., Yu, R., Le, T.L., Han, S.W., Yang, J.K., Choi, M.S., Baumeister, W. & Cheong, G.W. (2008). Hexameric ring structure of a thermophilic archaeon NADH oxidase that produces predominantly H2O. The FEBS Journal, Vol.275, NO.21, (November 2008), pp. 5355-5366

Kabesch, M., Hoefler, C., Carr, D., Leupold, W., Weiland, S.K. & von Mutius E. (2004). Glutathione S transferase deficiency and passive smoking increase childhood asthma. *Thorax,* Vol.59, No.7, (July 2004), pp. 569-573

Kabesch, M., Hoefler, C., Carr, D., Leupold, W., Weiland, S.K. & von Mutius, E. (2004). Glutathione S transferase deficiency and passive smoking increase childhood asthma. *Thorax,* Vol.59, No.7, (July 2004), pp. 569-573

Kalayci, O., Besler, T., Kilinç, K., Sekerel, B.E. & Saraçlar Y. (2000). Serum levels of antioxidant vitamins (alpha tocopherol, beta carotene, and ascorbic acid) in children with bronchial asthma. *The Turkish Journal of Pediatrics,* Vol.42, No.1, (January-March 2000), pp. 17-21

Kamada, F., Mashimo, Y., Inoue, H., Shao, C., Hirota, T., Doi, S., Kameda, M., Fujiwara, H., Fujita, K., Enomoto, T., Sasaki, S., Endo, H., Takayanagi, R., Nakazawa, C., Morikawa, T., Morikawa, M., Miyabayashi, S., Chiba, Y., Tamura, G., Shirakawa, T., Matsubara, Y., Hata, A., Tamari, M. & Suzuki, Y. (2007). The GSTP1 gene is a susceptibility gene for childhood asthma and the GSTM1 gene is a modifier of the GSTP1 gene. *International Archives of Allergy and Immunology,* Vol.144, No.4, (July 2007), pp. 275-286

Kaplan, P., Babusikova, E., Lehotsky, E. & Dobrota, D. (2003). Free radical-induced protein modification and inhibition of Ca2+-ATPase of cardiac sarcoplasmic reticulum. *Molecullar Cellular Biochemistry,* Vol.248, No.1-2, (June 2003), pp. 41-47

Katsoulis, K., Kontakiotis, T., Leonardopoulos, I., Kotsovili, A., Legakis, I.N. & Patakas D. (2003). Serum total antioxidant status in severe exacerbation of asthma: correlation with the severity of the disease. *Journal of Asthma,* Vol.40, No.8, (December 2003), pp. 847-854

Kinnula, V.L., Lehtonen, S., Koistinen, P., Kakko, S., Savolainen, M., Kere, J., Ollikainen, V. & Laitinen, T. (2004). Two functional variants of the superoxide dismutase genes in Finnish families with asthma. *Thorax,* Vol.59, No.2, (February 2004), pp. 116-119

Kinnula, V.L., Pietarinen, P., Aalto, K., Virtanen, I. & Raivio, K.O. (1995). Mitochondrial superoxide dismutase induction does not protect epithelial cells during oxidant exposure in vitro. *The American Journal of Physiology,* Vol.268, No.1Pt1, (January 1995), pp. L71-77

Kinnula, V.L., Whorton, A.R., Chang, L.Y. & Crapo, J.D. (1992). Regulation of hydrogen peroxide generation in cultured endothelial cells. *The American Journal of Respiratory cell and Molecullar biology,* Vol.6, No.2, (February 1992), pp. 175-182

Kishimoto, Y., Murakami, Y., Hayashi, K., Takahara, S., Sugimura, T. & Sekiya T. (1992). Detectionof a common mutation of the catalase gene in Japanese acatalasemic patients. *Human Genetic,* Vol.88, No.5, (March 1992), pp. 487-490

Kneepkens, C.M., Lepage, G. & Roy C.C. (1994). The potential of the hydrocarbon breath test as a measure of lipid peroxidation. *Free Radical Biology and Medicine,* Vol.17, No.2, (August 1994), pp. 127-160

Kroncke, K. D. (2001). Cysteine-Zn2+ complexes: unique molecular switches for inducible nitric oxide synthase-derived NO. *The FASEB Journal,* Vol.15, No.13, (November 2001), pp. 2503-2507

Lands, L.C., Grey, V., Smountas, A.A., Kramer, V.G. & McKenna D. (1999). Lymphocyte glutathione levels in children with cystic fibrosis. *Chest,* Vol.116, No.1, (July 1999), pp. 201-205

Larson, R.A., Wang, Y., Banerjee, M., Wiemels, J., Hartford, C., Le Beau, M.M. & Smith, M.T. (1999). Prevalence of the inactivating 609C-T polymorphism in the NAD(P)H:quinone oxidoreductase (NQO1) gene in the patiens with primary and therapy-related myeloid leukemia. Blood, Vol.94, No.2, (July 1999), pp. 803-807

Lee, M., Kim, S., Kwon, O.K., Oh, S.R., Lee, H.K. & Ahn, K. (2009). Anti-inflammatory and anti-asthmatic effects of resveratrol, a polyphenolic stilbene, in a mouse model of allergic asthma. *International Immunopharmacology*, Vol.9, No.4, (April 2009), pp. 418–424

Li, Y.F., Tseng, P.J., Lin, C.C., Hung, C.L., Lin, S.C., Su, W.C., Huang, Y.L., Sung, F.C. & Tai, C.K. (2009). NAD(P)H: quinone oxidoreductase 1, glutathione S-transferase M1, environmental tobacco smoke exposure, and children asthma. *Mutation Research*, Vol.678, No.1, (August 2009), pp. 53-58

Liao, M.F., Chen, C.C. & Hsu M.H. (2004). Evaluation of the serum antioxidant status in asthmatic children. *Acta Paediatrica Taiwan*, Vol.45, No.4, (July-August 2004), pp. 213-217

Mak, J.C., Leung, H.C., Ho, S.P., Ko, F.W., Cheung, A.H., Ip, M.S. & Chan-Yeung, M.M. (2006). Polymorphisms in manganese superoxide dismutase and catalase genes: functional study in Hong Kong Chinese asthma patients. *Clinical and Experimental Allergy*, Vol.36, No.4, (April 2006), pp. 440-447

Marçal, L.E., Rehder, J., Newburger, P.E. & Condino-Neto A. (2004). Superoxide release and cellular gluthatione peroxidase activity in leukocytes from chldren with persistent asthma. *Brazilian Journal of Medical and Biological Research*, Vol.37, No.11, (November 2004), pp. 1607-1613

Montuschi, P., Corradi, M., Ciabattoni, G., Nightingale, J., Kharitonov, S.A. & Barnes, P.J. (1999). Increased 8-isoprostane, a marker of oxidative stress, in exhaled condensate of asthma patients. *American Journal of Respiratory and Critical Care Medicine*, Vol.160, Vol.1, (july 1999), pp. 216-220

Moreno ,M.U., San José, G., Orbe, J., Páramo, J.A., Beloqui, O., Díez, J. & Zalba, G. (2003). Characterization of the promoter of the human p22phox gene: identification of a new polymorphism associated with hypertension. The FEBS Letters, Vol.542, No.1-3, (May 2003), pp. 27-31

Nadeem, A., Raj H.G. &Chhabra S.K. (2005). Increased oxidative stress in acute exacerbations of asthma. *Journal of Asthma*, Vol.42, No.1, (February 2005), pp. 45-50

Nath, K.A., Grande, J.P., Haggard, J.J., Croatt, A.J., Katusic, Z.S., Solovey, A. & Hebbel, R.P. (2001). Oxidative stress and induction of heme oxygenase-1 in the kidney in sickle cell disease. *The American Journal of Pathology*, Vol.158, No.3, (March 2001), pp. 892-903

Nickel, R., Haider, A., Sengler, C., Lau, S., Niggemann, B., Deichmann, K.A., Wahn, U. & Heinzmann A. (2005). Association study of Glutathione S-transferase P1 (GSTP1) with asthma and bronchial hyperresponsiveness in two German pediatric population. *Pediatric Allergy and Immunology*, Vol.16, No.6, (September 2005), pp. 539-541

Novak, Z., Nemeth, I., Gyurkovits, K., Varga, S.I. & Matkovics. B. (1991). Examination of the role of oxygen free radicals in bronchial asthma in childhood. *Clinica Chimica Acta*, Vol.201, No.3, pp. 247-251

Ochs-Balcom, H.M., Grant, B.J., Muti, P., Sempos, C.T., Freudenheim, J.L., Browne, R.W., McCann, S.E., Trevisan, M., Cassano, P.A., Iacoviello, L. & Schünemann H.J. (2006). Antioxidants, oxidative stress, and pulmonary function in individuals diagnosed with asthma or COPD. *European Journal of Clinical Nutrition*, Vol.60, No.8, (August 2006), pp. 991-999

Okamoto, N., Murata, T., Tamai, H., Tanaka, H. & Nagai, H. Effects of alpha tocopherol and probucol supplements on allergen-induced airway inflammation and hyperresponsiveness in a mouse model of allergic asthma. *International Archives of Allergy and Immunology*, Vol.141, No.2, (August 2006), pp. 172–180

Otterbein, L.E. & Choi, A.M. (2000). Heme oxygenase: colors of defence against cellular stress. *American Journal of Physiology. Lung Cellular and Molecular Physiology*, Vol.279., No.6, (December 2000), pp. L1029-L1037

Ozaras ,R., Tahan, V., Turkmen, S., Talay, F., Besirli, K., Aydin, S., Uzun, H. & Cetinkaya, A. (2000). Changes in malondialdehyde levels in bronchoalveolar fluid and serum by the treatment of asthma with inhaled steroid and beta2-agonist. *Respirology*, Vol.5, No.3, (September 2000), pp. 289-292

Paredi, P., Kharitonov, S.A. & Barnes P.J. (2000). Elevation of exhaled ethane concentration in asthma. *American Journal of Respiratory and Critical Care Medicine*, Vol.162, No.2Pt.1, (August 2000), pp. 1450-1454

Paredi, P., Leckie, M.J., Horvath, I., Allegra, L., Kharitonov, S.A. & Barnes, P.J. (1999). Changes in exhaled carbone monoxide and nitric oxide levels following allergen challenge in patients with asthma. *The European Respiratory Journal*, Vol.13, No.1, (January 1999), pp. 48-52

Pollack, M. & Leeuwenburgh, Ch. (1999). Molecular mechanisms of oxidative stress in aging: free radicals, aging, antioxidants and disease. In *Handbook of Oxidants and Antioxidants in exercise*. C.K. Sen, L. Packer, O. Hänninen (eds.), pp. 881-923, Elsevier Science, ISBN 978-044-4826-50-3, Amsterdam, Holland

Polonikov, A.V., Ivanov, V.P., Solodilova, M.A., Kozhuhov, M.A. & Panfilov, V.I. (2009). Tobacco smoking, fruit and vegetable intake modify association between -21A>T polymorphism of catalase gene and risk of bronchial asthma. *Journal of Asthma*, Vol.46, No.3, (April 2009), pp. 217-224

Powell, C.V., Nash, A.A., Powers, H.J. & Primhak, R.A. (1994). Antioxidant status in asthma. *Pediatric Pulmonology*, Vol.18, No.1, (July 1994), pp. 34-38

Praticò, D., Lawson, J.A., Rokach, J. &FitzGerald G.A. (2001). The isoprostanes in biology and medicine. *Trends in Endocrinology and Metabolism*, Vol.12, No.6, (August 2001), pp. 243-247

Rahman, I. & MacNee, W. (2002). Oxidative stress and adaptive response of glutathione in bronchial epithelial cells. *Clinical and Experimental Allergy*, Vol.32, No.4, (April 2002), pp. 486-488

Rebbeck, T.R. (1997). Molecular epidemiology of the human glutathione S-transferase genotypes GSTM1 and GSTT1 in cancer susceptibility. *Cancer Epidemiology, Biomarkers, and Preventions*, Vol.6, No.9, (September 1997), pp. 733-743

Romieu, I., Ramirez-Aguilar, M., Sienra-Monge, J.J., Moreno-Macías, H., del Rio-Navarro, B.E., David, G., Marzec, J., Hernández-Avila, M. & London, S. (2006). GSTM1 and GSTP1 and respiratory health in asthmatic children exposed to ozone. *The European Respiratory Journal*, Vol.28, No.5, (November 2006), pp. 953-959.

Romieu, I., Sienra-Monge, J.J., Ramírez-Aguilar, M., Téllez-Rojo, M.M., Moreno-Macías, H., Reyes-Ruiz, N.I., del Río-Navarro, B.E., Ruiz-Navarro, M.X., Hatch, G., Slade, R. & Hernández-Avila, M. (2002). Antioxidant supplementation and lung functions among children with asthma exposed to high levels of air pollutants. *American Journal of Respiratory and Critical Care Medicine*, Vol.166, No5, (September 2001), pp. 703-709

Ruscoe, J.E., Rosario, L.A., Wang, T., Gaté, L., Arifoglu, P., Wolf, C.R., Henderson, C.J., Ronai, Z. & Tew, K.D. (2001). Pharmacologic or genetic manipulation of glutathione S-transferase P1-1 (GSTpi) influences cell proliferation pathways. *The Journal of Pharmacology and Experimental Therapeutics,* Vol.298, No.1, (July 2001), pp. 339-345

Samet, J.M., Hatch, G.E., Horstman, D., Steck-Scott, S., Arab, L., Bromberg, P.A., Levine, M., McDonnell, W.F. & Devlin, R.B. (2001). Effects of antioxidant supplementation on ozone-induced lung injury in human subjects. *American Journal of Respiratory and Critical Care Medicine,* Vol.164, No5, (September 2001), pp. 819–825

Sardana, M.K., Drummond, G.S., Sassa, S. & Kappas, A. (1981). The potent heme oxygenase inducing action of arsenic and parasiticidal arsenicals. *Pharmacology,* Vol.23, No.5, pp. 247-253

Schock B.C., Young I.S., Brown V., Fitch P.S., Shields M.D., Ennis M. (2003). Antioxidants and oxidative stress in BAL fluid of atopic asthmatic children. *Pediatric Research,* Vol.53, No.3, (March 2003), pp. 375-381

Schock, B.C., Young, I.S., Brown V., Fitch, P.S., Shields, M.D. & Ennis M. (2003). Antioxidants and oxidative stress in BAL fluid of atopic asthmatic children. *Pediatric Research,* Vol.53, No.3, (March 2003), pp. 375-381

Sedgwick, J.B., Geiger, K.M. & Busse W.W. (1990). Superoxide generation by hypodense eosinophils from patients with asthma. *The American Review of Respiratory Disease,* Vol.142, No.1, (July 1990), pp. 120-125

Shanmugasundaram, K.R., Kumar, S.S. & Rajajee S. (2001). Excessive free radical generation in the blood of children suffering from asthma. *Clinica Chimica Acta,* Vol.305, No.1-2, (March 2001), pp. 107-114

Siegel, D., Bolton, E.M., Burr, J.A., Liebler, D.C. & Ross, D. (1997). The reduction of alpha-tocopherolquinone by human NAD(P)H: quinone oxidoreductase: the role of alpha-tocopherolhydroquinone as a cellular antioxidant. Molecular Pharmacology, Vol.52, No.2, (August 1997), pp. 300-305

Smit, H.A., Grievink, L. & Tabak, C. (1999). Dietary influences on chronic obstructive lung disease and asthma: a review of the epidemiological evidence. The Proceedings of the Nutrition Society, Vol.58, No.2, (May 1999), pp. 309-319

Soutar, A., Seaton, A. & Brown, K. (1997). Bronchial reactivity and dietary antioxidants. *Thorax,* Vol.52, No.2, (February 1997), pp.166–170

Sprenger, R., Schlagenhaufer, R., Kerb, R., Bruhn, C., Brockmöller, J., Roots, I. &Brinkmann, U. (2000). Characterization of the glutathione S-transferase GSTT1 deletion: discrimination of all genotypes by polymerase chain reaction indicate a trimodular genotype-phenotype correlation. *Pharmacogenetics,* Vol.10, No.6, (August 2000), pp. 557-565

Stadtman, E. R. & Berlett, B. S. (1997). Reactive oxygen-mediated protein oxidation in aging and disease. *Chemical Research in Toxicology,* Vol.10, No.5, (May 1997), pp. 485-494

Stadtman, E. R. (1993). Oxidation of free amino acids and amino acids residues in proteins by radiolysis and by metal-catalyzed reaction. *Annual Review of Biochemistry,* Vol.62, pp. 797-821

Szlagatys-Sidorkiewicz, A., Korzon, M., Małaczyńska, T., Renkel, J., Popadiuk, S. & Woźniak M. (2005). The antioxidative-prooxidative balance in children with asthma treated with inhaled corticosteroids and long acting beta2-agonists. *Pneumonologia i Alergologia Poska,.* Vol.73, No.2, pp. 178-181

Tamer, L., Calikoğlu, M., Ates, N.A., Yildirim, H., Ercan, B., Saritas, E., Unlü, A. & Atik, U. (2004). Glutathione-S-transferase gene polymorphisms (GSTT1, GSTM1, GSTP1) as increased risk factors for asthma. Respirology, Vol.9, No.4, (November 2004), pp. 493-498

Tappel A.L. (1984). Selenium-glutathione peroxidase: properties and synthesis. *Current Topics in Cellular Regulation,* Vol.24, pp. 87-97

Teramoto, S., Shu, C.Y., Ouchi, Y. & Fukuchi Y. (1996). Increased spontaneous production and generation of superoxide anion by blood neutrophils in patients with asthma. *The Journal of Asthma,* Vol.33, No.3, pp. 149-155

Traver, R.D., Horikoshi, T., Danenberg, K.D., Stadlbauer, T.H., Danenberg, P.V., Ross, D. & Gibson, N.W. (1997). NAD(P)H:quinone oxidoreductase gene expression in human colon carcinoma cells: characterization of a mutation wich modulates DT-diaphorase activity and mitomycin sensitivity. *Cancer Research,* Vol.52, No.4, (February 1992), pp. 797-802

Trenga, C.A., Koenig, J.Q. & Williams, P.V. (2001). Dietary antioxidants attenuate ozone-induced bronchial hyperresponsiveness (BHR) in asthmatic adults. *Archives of Environtal Health,* Vol.56, No.3, (May-June 2001), pp. 242–249

Troisi, R.J., Willet, W.C., Weiss, S.T., Trichopoulos, D., Rosner, B. & Spiezer, F.E. (1995). A prospective study of diet and adult-onset asthma. *American Journal of Respiratory and Critical Care Medicine,* Vol.151, No.5, (May 1995), pp. 1401–1408

Ukkola, O., Erkkilä, P.H., Savolainen, M.J. & Kesäniemi, Y.A. (2001). Lack of association between polymorphisms of catalase, copper-zinc superoxide dismutase (SOD), extracellular SOD and endothelial nitric oxide synthase genes and macroangiopathy in patients with type 2 diabetes mellitus. *Journal of Internal Medicine,* Vol.249, no.5, (May 2001), pp. 451-459

Vasiliou, D., Ross, D. & Nebert, D.W. (2006). Update of the NAD(P)H:quinone oxidoreductase (NQO) gene family. Human Genomics, Vol.2, No.5, (March 2006), pp. 329-325

Veal, E.A., Toone, W.M., Jones, N. &Morgan, B.A. (2002). Distinct roles for glutathione S-transferases in the oxidative stress response in Schizosaccharomyces pombe. *The Journal of Biological Chemistry,* Vol.277, No.38, (September 2002), pp. 35523-35531

Venge P. (1995). Role of eosinophils in childhood asthma inflammation. *Pediatric Pulmonology,* Suppl. 11, pp. 34-35

Venge P. (2010). The eosinophil and airway remodelling in asthma. *The Clinical Respiratory Journal,* Vol.4, Suppl 1, (May 2010), pp. 15-19

Wood, L.G., Fitzgerald, D.A., Gibson, P.G., Cooper, D.M. & Garg, M.L. (2000). Lipid peroxidation as determined by plasma isoprostanes is related to disease severity in mild asthma. *Lipids,* Vol.35, No.9, (September 2000), pp. 967-974

Xu, S., Wang, Y., Roe, B. & Pearson, W.R. (1998). Characterization of the human class Mu glutathione S-transferase gene cluster and the GSTM1 deletion. *The Journal of Biological Chemistry,* Vol.273, No.6, (February 1998), pp. 3517-3527

Zhou, X.F., Cui, J., DeStefano, A.L., Chazaro, I., Farrer, L.A., Manolis, A.J., Gavras, H. & Baldwin, C.T. (2005). Polymorphisms in the promoter region of catalase gene and essential hypertension. *Disease Markers,* Vol.21, No.1, pp. 3-7

Part 7

Viral Infections

8

An Overview of Management of URTI and a Novel Approach Towards RSV Infection

J.R. Krishnamoorthy[1], M.S. Ranjith[2], S. Gokulshankar[3], B.K. Mohanty[4], R. Sumithra[5], S. Ranganathan[1] and K. Babu[6]
[1]*Dr JRK Siddha Research and Pharmaceuticals Pvt Ltd, Chennai,*
[2]*Microbiology Unit, Faculty of Medicine, Quest International University Perak, Ipoh*
[3]*Microbiology Unit, Faculty of Medicine, AIMST University,*
[4]*Pharmacology Unit, Faculty of Medicine, UniKL-Royal College of Medicine Perak, Ipoh*
[5]*Department of Microbiology, MGR-Janaki College of Science, Chennai,*
[6]*R&D Center, Cholayil Private Limited, Chennai,*
[1,5,6]*India*
[2,3,4]*Malaysia*

1. Introduction

Upper respiratory tract infection (URTI) is an acute infection involving nose, paranasal sinuses, pharynx, larynx, trachea, and bronchi. It is one of the commonest infectious disease affecting people of all age groups particularly children. In most of the cases it is of viral origin. Viruses like myxovirus, paramyxovirus, adenovirus, picornavirus, and coronavirus groups are some of the common viruses that cause cold and similar upper respiratory tract illnesses in adults (Hamre and Connelly, 1966; Mims et al., 1998). URTI are frequent as there are large numbers of different causative viruses and also re-infections may occur with the same type of virus because of its ability for antigenic drift/shift.

There are many different antigenic types in these viruses and new strains/immunotypes are being discovered newly especially in coronavirus group. With the use of currently available methods of detection, the cause of approximately one third to one fourth of colds in adults remains unknown (Makela et al., 1998). Some illnesses may be undiagnosed because of the low sensitivity of diagnostic methods currently in use for detection of known viruses (Monto, 1997).

The respiratory viruses have a worldwide distribution. An URTI epidemic usually tends to occur during rainy season in the tropics and colder months in the temperate regions. Some viruses have their own seasonality viz. rhinovirus infection has its peak in the autumn and coronaviruses in the winter. Apart from climate variation, relative humidity plays a vital role in survival of the viruses. Enveloped viruses survive better than non-enveloped virus in a low relative humidity (Gwaltney 1984).

The main reservoir of respiratory viruses is the upper airway in young children. Spread of URTI is most common in an enclosed surrounding like home, schools and daycare centers

(Frenck RW, Glezen, 1990). The mechanisms for the spread of URTI viruses have not been well established but possibly occur by direct contact with infectious secretions on skin and environmental surfaces or contact with airborne droplet/droplet nuclei of respiratory secretions suspended in the environment or its combinations. For some viruses, such as rhinovirus and RSV, physical contact is necessary for efficient spread. Respiratory viruses are produced primarily in the nose and are shed in highest concentrations in nasal secretions. Effective spread is achieved when these viruses are present in hands of adults/children (Gwaltney, 1980).

Bacterial origin of URTI is less common involving etiological agents such as beta-hemolytic streptococci, *Corynebacterium diphtheriae, Streptococcus pneumoniae, Haemophilus influenzae* and *Moraxella catarrhalis* (Richard and Garibaldi, 1985).

2. Pathophysiology of RSV

Respiratory syncytial virus (RSV) is an enveloped single-stranded RNA virus belonging to family Paramyxoviridae (genus *Pneumovirus*) and is related to the parainfluenza, mumps and measles virus. RSV is a highly infectious, ubiquitous and is one of the most contagious human pathogens, comparable to measles virus. The RSV outbreak was first documented in 1964 in a neonatal intensive care unit (Berkovich, 1964). RSV is a significant cause of acute upper respiratory tract disease in individuals of all ages occurring both in normal and immunocompromised individuals (Hall et al., 2001).

Globally, the World Health Organization (WHO, 2009) estimates that RSV causes 64 million infections and 160,000 deaths annually. Approximately two-thirds of infants are infected with RSV during the first year of life, and 90% have been infected one or more times by 2 years of age (Karron et al., 1999). RSV infects patients earlier in life with greater consequences than other respiratory viruses. Rhinoviruses, influenza viruses, parainfluenza virus commonly infect children <6 months of age but RSV causes more frequent and severe infections because of their small size and narrow airways which is susceptible to obstruction. The ability to infect infants very early in life increases the impact of RSV.

The risk factors for severe RSV (Welliver, 2003)

- young age (<6 months)
- premature birth (<35 weeks of gestation)
- bronchopulmonary dysplasia
- congenital heart disease
- immunodeficiency or immunosuppression
- low birth weight
- low titer of RSV-specific serum antibodies
- old age increased exposure to infection in day care center, hospitalization, multiple siblings
- genetic predisposition (family history of asthma, genetic polymorphisms in genes encoding cytokines, chemokines)

The two major strains of RSV are A and B. The A strain is responsible for the majority of more severe forms of RSV bronchiolitis (Martinello et al, 2002; Walsh et al, 1997). Martinello et al. (2002) found that a subgroup of the A strain (GA3) was associated with more severe disease. It is also important to know that the different strains of RSV often circulate at the same time, and season-to-season variation is found in the predominant strain (American Academy of Pediatrics [AAP], 2003; Martinello et al., 2002).

The virus is shed in nasopharyngeal secretions; infected patients can shed the virus for up to 21 days. The portal of entry of the virus is through the mucosal surfaces of the mouth, nose, and conjunctivae. The virus replicates in the nasopharynx with an incubation period of 2 to 8 days with replication cycle (*in vitro*) of 30 to 48 hours. G protein on the viral envelope mediates attachment of the virus to the superficial cells of the respiratory epithelium including type 1 pneumocytes in the alveoli which are major targets of infection in the lower airway and non-ciliated epithelium and intraepithelial dendritic cells (Beeler and van Wyke Coelingh, 1989)

RSV invades the bronchiolar epithelial cells causing inflammation and edema. The membranes of the infected cells fuse with adjacent cells to form a large, multinucleated cell creating large masses of cells or "syncytia" (McIntosh, 2000; Wong et al., 2003) formation due to F (fusion) viral envelope glycoprotein which facilitates URTI to spread to lower respiratory tract. There may be occasional proliferation of the bronchiolar epithelium, infiltrates of monocytes and T cells centered on bronchiolar and pulmonary arterioles, and neutrophils between vascular structures and small airways. Infection and tissue damage are patchy rather than diffuse. There are abundant signs of airway obstruction due to sloughing of epithelial cells, mucus secretion, and accumulated immune cells (Levine et al., 1987).

RSV URTI symptoms include coryza, cough, wheezing, low-grade fever (< 101°F), and loss of appetite. Symptoms of LTRI are common even in infants with mild disease. Clinical symptoms of bronchiolitis include increased airway resistance, air trapping, and wheezing.

Coryza (the prominent symptom) is the inflammation of the mucous membranes lining the nasal cavity which causes nasal congestion and anosmia. The 3 stages of coryza are;

- Dry Prodromal Stage (initial phase): nasal drying and irritation, low-grade fever, chills, general malaise, anorexia
- Catarrhal Stage (second stage): watery clear rhinorrhea, congestion, lacrimation, worsening of constitutional symptoms
- Mucous Stage: thickened rhinorrhea (greenish and foul smelling if secondarily infected), improved constitutional symptoms

Reinfection with RSV occurs at all ages; however, with recurrent infection and increasing age, RSV infections are more limited to the URT. RSV URTI is more severe in nature than the URTI caused by other common cold viruses. RSV can re-infect throughout life without considerable antigenic change in sharp contrast with the ability of influenza A virus requiring antigenic drift or shift (Falsey et al., 2005).

An uncomplicated URTI can also progress to complicated lower respiratory tract infection (LRTI). The pathogenesis of RSV-induced airway inflammation and hyperreactivity remain largely unknown. There is mounting evidence suggesting that young children who contract RSV infection are more likely to suffer from long-term respiratory complications like reactive airway disease later in life (Shaheen, 1995). It is also observed that severe infantile RSV and influenza virus LRT are characterized by inadequate adaptive immune responses.

There is no effective therapeutic option currently available for the management of acute and chronic clinical manifestations of RSV.

3. Treatment of acute URTI

Common cold is a self limiting illness and can resolve spontaneously. It has been rightly told that "treated cold lasts for 1 week and the untreated lasts for seven days". The treatment of common cold is directed for alleviating the symptoms associated with it and the infection can be taken care by body's own immunity

Acute rhinosinusitis is most often associated with common cold and can be treated by a first generation antihistamine and a decongestant like pseudoephedrine. Similarly acute cough associated with common cold may be resolved by first generation antihistamine like diphenhydramine and chlorpheniramine along with decongestants (Chest 2006). Patients suffering from common cold are reluctant to take first generation antihistamines because of fear of drowsiness and absence from their work and can be treated by second generation antihistamine like cetirizine or loratadine for relief of symptoms of rhinosinusitis and acute cough. Cough usually occurs due to viral inflammation of the throat and can also be managed by simple home remedies like warm saline gargling and taking honey which can reduce symptoms and improve sleep particularly in children. Other drugs which can be prescribed for cough are dexomethorphan and codeine but these drugs can cause drowsiness and constipation respectively.

Over the counter preparations for cough and cold has limited efficacy in relieving cough due to URTI (Braman 2006). They may have undesirable side effects like allergic reactions, sleep disturbances, hallucinations particularly in children and therefore they should be avoided in children. Rest is an important factor for treating URTI but usual activities such as working and light exercise may be advised as much as tolerated (Siamak, 2011). Increased intake of oral fluids is also encouraged to sustain the fluid loss from running nose, fever and poor appetite associated with URTI. (Siamak, 2011)

Other medications which can be helpful in relieving the symptoms of common cold (acute URTI) are as follows

- Acetaminophen or Paracetamol - It is a safe drug to be used in both adults and children to reduce fever and body ache which are often associated with acute URTI
- NSAIDs - Non Steroidal Anti Inflammatory Drugs like ibuprofen can be used for fever and body ache
- Nasal secretions can be reduced by using nasal ipratropium (topical)
- Many cough medications like dextromethorphan, guaifenesin and codeine are also commercially available and can be used to relieve cough, if it is not reduced by saline gargling or antihistamines and decongestants. However, these medications can cause drowsiness and codeine can cause constipation.
- Oxymetazolin nasal drops can be used to reduce nasal stuffiness but for a short period. It can cause after congestion. Very young children and infants may be relieved from nasal stuffiness by saline drops instilled into both the nostrils.
- Other groups of drugs indicated are bronchodilators like short acting $\beta_2$agonists and ipratropium bromide administered by metered dose inhaler (MDIs) which help reduce

mucous in lungs and relax smooth muscles of large and medium bronchi, if URTI is associated with wheeze and bronchospasm.

Antibiotics are not advised if the patient is otherwise healthy because the immune system can clear the viral infection. No benefit has been demonstrated in terms of overall improvement from the use of antibiotics compared to placebo in patients with acute URTI. (Arroll et al., 2008).

Treatment with antibiotics neither shortens the duration of illness nor prevents bacterial rhinosinusitis and patients with purulent green or yellow secretions do not get benefit from antibiotic treatment (Gonzales et al., 2001)

The following complications may need a course of antibiotics

- Acute bacterial rhinosinusitis - Acute bacterial rhinosinusitis may develop in only 2% of cases (Hickner et al., 2001). Bacterial sinusitis may be present if symptoms persist for more than 7 days and pus is localized to the maxillary sinus (Hansen et al., 1995). Patients with mild symptoms need only symptomatic treatment with topical and oral decongestants. Patients with moderate or severe symptoms may be benefited by the use of narrow spectrum antibiotic like amoxicillin which can cover *Streptococcus pneumoniae* and *Hemophilus influenzae*. Alternatively Amoxicillin-clavalunic acid combination, third generation cephalosporins and for penicillin allergy, cotrimoxazole and extended spectrum macrolide or respiratory fluroquinolone may be considered if no improvement or worsening of symptoms after 72 hours.
- Pharyngitis may occur due to infection by group A beta hemolytic streptococci (GABHS) and routine respiratory viruses. Antibiotics are indicated if the symptoms persist for more than 7 days or there is increased severity particularly with GABHS infection manifested by sore throat, fever, head ache, tonsilopharyngeal erythema and exudates, palatal petecheae and anterior cervical lymphadenopathy and absence of cough (Cooper et al., 2001). The diagnosis of GABHS may be confirmed by throat culture and rapid antigen testing before using antibiotics.
  First line therapy includes penicillin V or benzathine penicillin G
  Alternative therapy may be instituted by amoxicillin, oral cephalosporins and erythromycin incase of patients allergic to penicillin.

Duration of treatment with suitable antibiotics is usually 10 days and the treatment guideline is same for adult as well as pediatric patients.

- Otitis media in children – another indication for the use of antibiotics complicating URTI. In case of non severe illness, high dose of amoxicillin is the first line therapy. If this treatment fails, the combination of amoxycillin and clavulanic acid in high doses may be tried. Alternative therapy includes oral third generation cephalosporins and in penicillin allergic patients macrolides. Bacterial agents complicating URTI with
- Acute bronchitis - Bacterial agents complicating are *Bordetella pertussis, Mycoplasma pneumoniae* and *Chlamydia pneumoniae*. Uncomplicated acute bacterial bronchitis does not need treatment with antibiotics even if the patient complains of purulent sputum. 95% of patients with purulent sputum do not have pneumonia (Diehr et al., 1984). The evaluation and treatment of the patient should be focused on excluding severe illness particularly pneumonia (Metlay et al., 1997). Treatment with antibiotics is reserved for

patients having acute bacterial exacerbation of chronic bronchitis and COPD most often in smokers. Antibiotics preferred in this group are amoxicillin, cotrimoxazole or doxycycline. In case of *B. pertussis, C. pneumoniae* and *M. pneumoniae* erythromycin or doxycycline can be given. (Smucny et al., 2004).

In children less than 8 years suffering from acute bronchitis and presenting with prolonged unimproving cough lasting for more than 14 days and after exclusion of pneumonia, macrolides may be preferred but for older children tetracyclines are preferable. Bronchiolitis or non specific URTI characterized by sore throat, sneezing, mild cough, fever less than 102°F for less than 3days, rhinorrhea, nasal congestion, self limited typically 5-14days needs only symptomatic treatment with adequate fluid intake, rest and humidifier.

URTI arising due to influenza and RSV needs special mention. The diagnosis of influenza may be done by abrupt onset of fever, myalgias, headache, rhinitis, severe malaise, non productive cough and sore throat. The mainstay of treatment is supportive care to relieve symptoms. But antiviral drugs like oseltamivir and zanamavir can decrease the duration of illness if administered within first 36hours of onset of illness (Montalto et al., 2000)

Recently a number of studies have established RSV as a potential pathogen in certain adult population, particularly very elderly with underlying cardiopulmonary disease and immunocompromised individuals. But the disease remains undiagnosed in many situations because diagnosis is difficult during acute illness. Antibiotics may be used in selected RSV infected persons having bacterial pathogens isolated from their sputum. At present aerosolized ribavarin is the only approved treatment for RSV infection (AHRQ 2003, Falsy and Walsh 2000). But the use of ribavarin is controversial in case of infants and is indicated only in high risk patients. Two immunoglobulin preparations i.e., polyclonal high titred RSV immunoglobulin and a humanized F-specific monoclonal antibody can be used along with ribavarin. The treatment must be instituted promptly at the onset of the illness to effectively inhibit the replication of the virus. (Malhotra and Krilov 2000). But regular and wide spread use of immunoglobulins is not encouraging due to their high cost of each monthly dose and only high risk infants can get benefits from prophylactic treatment (Cooper , 2011).

Development of RSV vaccine has been unsuccessful and previously developed vaccine using inactivated whole virus caused infection in infants. Recently it was understood that RSV can invade or even alter immune system. Therefore, better understanding of the immunological role of the virus and development of either immunomodulatory drugs or a vaccine remains the challenge for the future for the effective prevention or treatment of RSV infection (Sorrentino et al., 2000).

4. A new strategy of management: Immunomodulation

With the traditional knowledge available in the literature of the Siddha system of medicine (an ancient system of complementary medical practice in India) and the intense research on medicinal herbs done at Dr JRK Siddha Research and Pharmaceuticals Pvt Ltd, Chennai, India, a unique polyherbal formulation (trade named as SIVA syrup) was made with the following herbs.

Indigofera aspalathoides
Celastrus paniculates
Corallocarpus epigaeus
Solanum trilobatum
Wrightia tinctoria
Bacoba monnieri
Piper longum
Piper nigrum
Zingiber officinale
Tinospora cordifolia
Leucas aspera
Piper betle

5. Plant details

Indigofera aspalathoides Vahl ex DC. (Papilionaceae)

Vernacular names: *Tamil* - Shiva malli, shivanarvembu.

Habit - Undershrubs, leaves digitately compound, flowers red, pods straight, turgid.

Distribution - South India, Sri Lanka.

Uses - Leaves, flower and tender shoots demulscent; their decoction used in cancerous lesions and leprosy. Leaves also applied in abscesses.

Celastrus paniculatus Willd. (Celastraceae)

Vernacular names: *Sanskrit* - Jyothismathi; *Tamil* - Vaaluluvai.

Habit - Scandent shrubs with lenticellate branches. Leaves crenate-serrate. Flowers yellow or greenish-white, in terminal panicles. Capsules sub-globose, yellow with scarlet fleshy aril closing the seeds.

Distribution - South Asia to Australia.

Uses - Bark - Abortifacient. Seeds tonic and aphrodisiac. Seed oil used as nerve stimulant and brain tonic; also used in rheumatic pain.

Chemical constituents - Plant contain sesquiterpene ester malkanguniol, malkangunin, celapanine, etc. and alkaloids celastrine and paniculatine.

Corallocarpus epigaeus (Rottl. ex Willd.) Cl. (Cucurbitaceae)

Vernacular names: *Sanskrit* - Shukanaasa; *Tamil* - Agasagarudan.

Habit - Prostrate or climbing herb with tuberous roots. Leaves sub-orbicular. Flowers unisexual; female flowers usually solitary. Fruits ellipsoid, pulpy; seeds with a reddish margin.

Distribution - Tropics.

Uses - Roots used in chronic mucous enteritis and dysentery. It is also used as liniments for rheumatism.

Chemical constituents - Roots contains bitter principle bryonin.

Solanum trilobatum Linn. (Solanaceae)

Vernacular names: *Sanskrit* - ; *Tamil* - Thoothuvalai.

Habit - Much branched spiny scandent shrubs. Leaves deltoid or triangular, irregularly lobed. Flower purplish blue, in cymes. Berry globose, red or scarlet.

Distribution - Peninsular India and Malaysia.

Uses - Roots used for consumption in the form of electuary, decoction or powder. Berries and flowers used to relief cough.

Chemical constituents - Fruits and leaves contains alkaloid solasodine.

Wrightia tinctoria (Roxb.) R.Br. (Apocynaceae)

Vernacular names: *Sanskrit* - Svetakutaja; *Tamil* - Vetpalai.

Habit - Small deciduous tree with light grey, smooth, scaly bark. Leaves elliptic-lanceolate. Flowers fragrant white, in lax, dichotomously branched terminal cymes. Follicle cylindrical, acute, cohering when young.

Distribution - India, Sri Lanka.

Uses - Bark and seeds used in flatulence and bilious troubles. Seed aphrodisiac and anthelmintic.

Chemical constituents - Bark contains β–sitosterol, α- amyrin and its acetate and lupeol.

Bacopa monnieri (L.) Penn. (Scrophulariaceae)

Vernacular names: *Sanskrit* - Brahmi; *Tamil* - Neerbrahmi.

Habit - Decumbent or creeping herbs rooting at nodes. Flowers solitary, bluish or pinkish.

Distribution - Almost all districts in Tamilnadu, India and tropics.

Uses - used in epilepsy, insanity and other nervous diseases.

Chemical constituents - Plant contains nicotine, luteolin bacogenin A1, A2, A3, betulinic acid, bacoside A, A3, B & β–sitosterol.

Piper longum Linn. (Piperaceae)

Vernacular names: *Sanskrit* - Pippali; *Tamil* - Thippili.

Habit - Aromatic climbers with stout roots; stem jointed. Leaves ovate, cordate. Spikes cylindrical, peduncled. Fruits ovoid, yellowish-orange.

Distribution - India, cultivated in many places.

Uses - Roots and fruits used in respiratory tract diseases, as a counter irritant and analgesic for muscular pains and inflammations; as snuff in coma.

Chemical constituents - Roots contains alkaloids - piperlongumine, piperlonguminine, piperine, sesamine, piperolactum A & B. fruits yiels essential oil contains piperidine alkaloids, piperononaline, piperundecalidine etc.

Piper nigrum Linn. (Piperaceae)

Vernacular names: *Sanskrit* - Maricha; *Tamil* - Milagu.

Habit - Much branched climbing shrub rooting at nodes. Leaves entire, cordate. Flowers minute in spikes. Fruit ovoid or globose, bright red when ripe.

Distribution - south - west India, largely cultivated.

Uses - fruits used in fever, anaemia, cough, diarrhoea, as stimulant, in weakness due to fever, as a stomachic, and malaria. Externally applied as rubefacient for sore throat, piles.

Chemical constituents - Stem contains sesquisabinene , piperine, hentriacontane, β-sitosterol. Fruits contains piperine, oleoresin and volatile oil.

Zingiber officinale Rosc. (Zingiberaceae)

Vernacular names: *Sanskrit* - Sunthi; *Tamil* - Inji.

Habit - Slender aromatic rhizomatous herbs with leafy stem. Leaves linear-lanceolate, distichous, subsessile. Flowers greenish-yellow with dark purple or purplish black tip, in spikes.

Distribution - Extensively cultivated in many places all over the world.

Uses - Carminative and stimulant and also given in flatulence and colic.

Chemical constituents - Rhizomes contains diarylheptanoids, essential oil, zingiberene, zingiberenol, sesqui-thujene, cumene, myrcene, limonene, gingerol, shagoal, zingerone and paradol.

Tinospora cordifolia (Wild.)Hk.f. & Th. (Menispermaceae)

Vernacular names: *Sanskrit* - Guduchi; *Tamil* - Seenthilkodi.

Habit - Large climbing shrubs; bark greyish-brown or creamy-white, warty. Leaves membranous broadly ovate, cordate at base. Flowers greenish-yellow, appearing when the plant is leafless, in axillary and terminal racemes or panicles. Drupe ovoid, shining, succulent, light red when ripe.

Distribution - India, Srilanka.

Uses - Stem is an ingredient of several ayurvedic preparations used in general debility, dyspepsia, fever and urinary diseases. Leaf decoction given in gout.

Chemical constituents -Plant containe quaternary alkaloids - magnoflorine, tembestarine and isoquinoline alkaloid - jatrorrizine, furanoid diterpene, clerodane, tinosporidine, tinosporoside etc.

Leucas aspera (Wild.) Link (Lamiaceae)

Vernacular names: *Sanskrit* - Dronapushpi; *Tamil* - Thumbai.

Habit - Erect herbs with diffuse quadrangular branches. Leaves linear-lanceolate. Flowers white, in verticils. Nutlets oblong.

Distribution - India and Malaysia.

Uses - Juice of leaves applied externally in psoriasis, chronic skin eruptions and painful swellings. Flowers given with honey in coughs and cold.

Chemical constituents - plant contains sterol, alkaloids, galactose, oleanolic acid, ursolic acid etc.

Piper betle Linn. (Piperaceae)

Vernacular names: *Sanskrit* - Tambulavalli; *Tamil* - Vettrilai.

Habit - woody climber with adventitious roots. Leaves broadly ovate, slightly cordate and often obliqual at base. Male flowers in dense spike; female spikes pendulous. Fruits black in the fleshy spike.

Distribution - Native of Malaysia, cultivated in india.

Uses - decoction of leaves used for healing wounds. Roots with black pepper used to produce sterility in woman. Leaves yield essential oil which is used in repiratory catarrh and diphtheria, also as a carminative.

Chemical constituents - Leaves contains iodine, vitamin B, essential oil contains - chavibetol, chavibetol acetate, caryophyllene, allylpyrocatechol, camphene, eugenol etc.

These plants possess properties to modulate the immune system by induction, expression, amplification or inhibition of any part or phase of the immune response. Plants like *Solanum trilobatum, Wrightia tinctoria, Tinospora cordifolia* and *Leucas aspera* has been extensively used in Siddha preparations. Crude extracts of these plants possess wide range of properties like increase in total WBC count, boosting the phagocytic index of macrophages, polyclonal B cell activation, increase secretion of Interleukin-1 and tumor necrosis factor (TNF). Immunomodulation through plants provide inexpensive, safe, viable and natural means of seeking an effective alternate treatment.

6. Study methods

6.1 Virus preparation and assay

High-titer stocks of RSV were prepared on HEp2 cell monolayers. Virus titers were determined by plaque assay on STAT1_/_ mouse fibroblasts. Equivalent number of plaques was counted on STAT1_/_ fibroblast and HEp2 monolayers, but they appeared much more rapidly on the knockout murine cells: 36 h versus 5 days, respectively (Gitiban et al, 2005).

6.2 Study animals and infection

Juvenile chinchillas (*Chinchilla lanigera*) 3 months of age and weighing 300 to 350 g, were used. Male and female BALB/c mice were also used for the study. Mice were infected i.n.

following methodologies that were developed to deliver an inoculum specifically to the upper airway using a very small volume (Johnson et al., 1996, Visweswaraiah et al., 2002). Briefly, each mouse was mildly anesthetized, placed in a supine position, and given 10^3 PFU of RSV in a 20-µl volume. Two microliters per naris were delivered at 0, 2, 7, 9, and 11 min. Chinchillas were also inoculated i.n. with RSV, again delivered specifically to the upper airway. The dosages (in total PFU delivered), 10^3 were administered by passive inhalation of droplets of viral suspension delivered to the nares of chinchillas that were lightly anesthetized with xylazine (2mg/kg of body weight) and were lying in a prone position. (Gitiban et al, 2005).

6.3 Treatment with polyherbal formulation

The feed and water were provided to the animals *ad libitum*. The animals were grouped into two groups of 3 animals each as polyherbal formulation treated and non treated control. However, both groups were infected with RSV. The animals were infected only after 10 days of treatment with polyherbal formulation. After 5 days of infection, the animals from both groups were euthanized and the visceral regions were examined to assess the rate of infection.

6.4 Lavages and recovery of tissues for quantitative viral culture

RSV-infected mice under treatment and control groups were sacrificed at various time points by CO_2 inhalation. For virus titration, lungs and nasal mucosa were immediately frozen in liquid nitrogen. Prior to plaque assay, tissues were weighed and homogenized in 1 ml phosphate-buffered saline (PBS). Tissue homogenates were assayed as described above (Gitiban et al, 2005).

6.5 Serum neutralization assay

RSV (500 PFU/ml) was mixed with serial dilutions of chinchilla serum and incubated at room temperature for 30 min. These mixtures (100µl) were used to inoculate confluent monolayers of mouse STAT1_/_ fibroblast cells grown in 24-well plates. After 1-h incubation at 37°C, infected cells were washed and fed with growth medium plus 0.5% methylcellulose. After 2 days, plates were stained with crystal violet and plaques counted. The neutralizing titer was defined as the serum dilution that resulted in 50% reduction in plaque number compared to controls that had no serum (Gitiban et al, 2005).

7. Histology study

Sections through the NP of mice were obtained following formalin fixation and decalcification. For immunohistochemistry, sections were blocked with a Vector Avidin/Biotin blocking kit. Sections were visualized using a biotinylated mouse anti-goat secondary antibody, streptavidin-horseradish peroxidase, the chromogen AEC and a hematoxylin counterstaining.

8. Predisposition of Chinchilla to infection of the upper airway with RSV following i.n. challenge

A dose-effect was clearly detectable in chinchillas inoculated with increasing doses of RSV. At the lower dosages assayed, no signs of illness were noted at any time of post challenge. Conversely, animals that received higher dosages of the virus without polyherbal formulation treatment showed signs of acute respiratory tract infection. The symptoms of viral infection like ruffling of fur and lethargic behavior were observed by day 3-4 after challenge in all the animals that did not receive pre-treatment with polyherbal formulation.

In addition, nasal lavage fluids recovered from the RSV-infected chinchillas (control) had an abnormal yellowish-green tint and was notably turbid. There was no such change observed in polyherbal formulation treated group of animals. This latter observation is consistent with histopathological evaluations that showed hypersecretion of mucus into the ET lumen in tissues recovered from untreated chinchillas; such change was not seen in the case of polyherbal formulation treated group. Plaque assays conducted with homogenized NP mucosa and NP lavage fluids indicated that the chinchilla was permissive to RSV infection. Both NP mucosal tissue homogenates and NP lavage fluid specimens were positive on days 4 and 8 after challenge. Preliminary evidence in support of restriction of viral replication to the uppermost airway following i.n. challenge was supported by the absence of viral plaques when tracheal mucosa and lung tissue recovered 4 days after challenge in the treatment group even after receiving highest dose of RSV. This clearly indicates that the polyherbal formulation pretreatment prevent viral multiplication within 4 day of challenge.

9. RSV infection results in goblet cell hyperplasia, hypersecretion of mucus, and the clear presence of RSV within cells lining the ET

Examination of NP and ET mucosae from control animals showed the presence of mild inflammation. Periodic acid-Schiff–Alcian Blue staining showed sparse mononuclear submucosal infiltrate with eosinophils, marked goblet cell hyperplasia with mucus hypersecretion into the lumen of the ET. However no such abnormalities were observed in the polyherbal formulation treated animals. The relative abundance of mucus in the ET lumen, the number of heavily stained goblet cells, and the intensity of staining of submucosal glands in an RSV-infected chinchilla treated vs untreated with polyherbal formulation was observed. Clear distinction in the histological findings in the treated and control group was seen.

10. Conclusion

RSV is the chief cause of most of the upper respiratory infections in human being. The focus of the present study was to evaluate the immunomodulatory effect of polyherbal formulation (SIVA syrup) against RSV infection in animal model. Immunomodulatory potential of medicinal plants have been extensively studied by several researchers. (Benny et al., 2004; Kripa et al., 2011; Sunila & Kuttan, 2004). We have established the immunoprotective/immunomodulating effect can be achieved using polyherbal formulation earlier in our studies (Ranjith et al., 2010). Polyherbal formulation increases the phagocytosis index to several times over control when tested against murine phagocytes *in vitro* (Ranjith et al., 2008). Further, the effect of polyherbal formulation on the humoral antibody production in animal model by using SRBC as an antigen was also established (Ranjith, 2009). Candidal infections are quite common when the first line of host's defence mechanism get abrogated. Revalidation of the immune protection effect of polyherbal formulation in preventing experimental candidal infection in animal model was also confirmed (Ranjith, 2009). Findings of all the above studies clearly suggest that polyherbal formulation of medicinal plants is a very potent immunomodulator and has a significant role in the health and well being.

Several compliments have been received from various practitioners of alternative medicines in India for the role of SIVA in the management of upper respiratory tract infections especially in children, particularly of viral origin. The present study clearly established that polyherbal formulation has very specific effect of immune protection against upper respiratory tract infection caused by RSV in animal model. Comparative viral and hematological examinations of pretreated and control animals reveal that polyherbal formulation offers strong protection against RSV infection.

One of the plant compounds in the polyherbal formulation is *Indigofera asphalathoides* which is extremely bitter in taste. Most of the bitter principles viz., *Azadirachta indica, Phyllanthus niruri, Terminalia chebula* are known to have high antiviral activity. Further the therapeutic role of the bitter fraction in the bitter-gourd is also well known. The use of the bitter plant - *Indigofera aspalathoides* in the traditional drug preparations date back to Siddha era which is around 2000 BC. In the recent years, modern science has proved the role of bitter principles and bitter yielding plants have high therapeutic value including antiviral activity.

The exact mode of action of polyherbal formulation on RSV is not clearly understood. However, the protection of the polyherbal formulation treated group against the RSV infection could be attributed to its antiviral and immunomodulatory properties of the constituent medicinal plants in the formulation. A detailed clinical study is inevitable to substantiate the antiviral and immunomodulatory effect of the polyherbal formulation. Nevertheless immunomodulation would be the futuristic approach for the management of upper respiratory viral infections.

11. References

American Academy of Pediatrics (AAP). (2003). Respiratory syncytial virus. In: *2003 red book: Report of the Committee on Infectious Diseases* (26th ed., pp. 523-528). Elk Grove Village, IL: AAP

Arroll, B; Kenealy, T. & Falloon, K. (2008). Are antibiotics indicated as an initial treatment for patients with acute upper respiratory tract infections? A review. *The New Zealand Medical Journal,*121,1284

Beeler, JA. & van Wyke Coelingh K. (1989). Neutralization epitopes of the F glycoprotein of respiratory syncytial virus: effect of mutation upon fusion function. *Journal of Virology,*63:2941-2950.

Benny, KH.; Tan &Vanitha, J. (2004). Immunomodulatory and antimicrobial effects of some traditional Chinese medicinal herbs: *A Review Current Medicinal Chemistry,* 11, 1423-1430

Berkovich, S. (1964). Acute respiratory illness in the premature nursery associated with respiratory syncytial virus infections. *Pediatrics,*34:753-760.

Braman, SS. (2006). Chronic Cough Due to Acute Bronchitis. ACCP Evidence-Based Clinical Practice Guidelines. *Chest*,129;95S-103S

Cooper AC, Banasiak NC, Allen PJ (2011) Management and Prevention for Respiratory Syncytial Virus RSV)http://www.medscape.com/viewarticle/466839_11

Cooper, RJ.; Hoffman, JR.; Bartlett, JG.; Besser, RE.; Gonzales, R.; Hickner, JM. & Sande, MA. (2001). Principles of appropriate antibiotic use for acute pharyngitis in adults: background. *Annals of Internal Medicine*,134(6):509-17.

Diehr P, Wood RW, Bushyhead JB, Krueger L, Wolcott B, Tompkins RK. Prediction of pneumonia in outpatients with acute cough -- a statistical approach. J Chronic Dis 1984;37:215-225

Falsey, AR. & Walsh, EE. (2000). Respiratory Syncytial Virus Infection in Adults *Clinical Microbiology Reviews*,13(3),371-384

Falsey, AR.; Hennessey, PA.; Formica, MA.; Cox, C. & Walsh, EE. (2005). Respiratory syncytial virus infection in elderly and high-risk adults. *New England Journal of Medicine*, 352(17):1749-59

Frenck, RW. & Glezen, WP. (1990). Respiratory tract infections in children in day care. *Seminars* in *Pediatric Infectious Diseases*,1:234–244.

Garibaldi, RA. (1985). Epidemiology of community-acquired respiratory tract infections in adults: Incidence, etiology, and impact, *The American Journal of Medicine*, 78(6) Supplement 2,1985 32-37

Gitiban, N.; Jurcisek, JA.; Harris, RH.; Mertz, SE.; Durbin, RK,; Lauren, OB. & Durbin, JE. (2005) Chinchilla and murine models of upper respiratory tract infections with respiratory syncytial virus, *Journal of Virology*,79(10), 6035-6042.

Gonzales, R.; Bartlett, JG.; Besser, RE.; Hickner, JM.; Hoffman, JR. & Sande, MA. (2001). Principles of appropriate antibiotic use for treatment of nonspecific upper respiratory tract infections in adults: background. *Annals of Emergency Medicine*,37(6):698-702

Gwaltney Jr., JM. (1980). Epidemiology of the common cold. *Annals of the New York Academy of Sciences*,353:54.

Gwaltney Jr., JM. (1984). The Jeremiah Metzger lecture: Climatology and the common cold. *Transactions of the American Clinical and Climatological Association Journal*,96:159

Hall, CB.; Long, CE. & Schnabel, KC. (2001). Respiratory syncytial virus infections in previously healthy working adults. *Clinical Infectious Diseases*, 33:792-796.

Hamre, D.; Connelly Jr, AP. & Procknow, JJ. (1966). Virologic studies of acute respiratory disease in young adults: IV. Virus isolations during four years of surveillance. *American Journal of Epidemiology*,83:238

Hansen, JG; Schmidt, H; Rosborg, J; Lund, E: Predicting acute maxillary sinusitis in a general practice population. British Medical Journal 311: 233 (1995)

Hickner, JM.; Bartlett, JG.; Besser, RE.; Gonzales, R.; Hoffman, JR. & Sande, MA. (2001). Principles of appropriate antibiotic use for acute rhinosinusitis in adults: background. *Annals of Internal Medicine*,20;134(6):498-505.

Johnson, SA.; Ottolini MG.; Darnell, ME.; Porter, DD. & Prince GA. (1996). Unilateral nasal infection of cotton rats with respiratory syncytial virus allows assessment of local and systemic immunity. *Journal of General Virology*, 77:101–108.

Karron, RA.; Singleton, RJ.; Bulkow, L.; Parkinson, A.; D. Kruse, DeSmet, I.; Indorf, C.; Petersen, KM.; Leombruno, D.; Hurlburt, DM,; Santosham & Harrison, HL. (1999).

Severe respiratory syncytial virus disease in Alaska native children. *Journal of Infectious Diseases*, 180:41-49.

Kripa, KG.; Chamundeeswari, D.; Thanka, J. & Uma Maheswara Reddy C.(2011). Modulation of inflammatory markers by the ethanolic extract of *Leucas aspera* in adjuvant arthritis. *Journal of Ethnopharmacology*,134(3):1024-1027.

Levine, S.; Klaiber-Franco, R. & Paradiso, PR. (1987). Demonstration that glycoprotein G is the attachment protein of respiratory syncytial virus. *Journal of General Virology*, 68:2521-2524.

Makela, MJ.; Puhakka, T.; Ruuskanen, O.; Maija Leinonen, M.; Saikku, P.; Kimpimäki, M.; Blomqvist, S.; Hyypiä, T. & Arstila, P. (1998). Viruses and bacteria in the etiology of the common cold. Journal of Clinical Microbiology,36(2):539–542

Malhotra, A. & Krilov, LR. (2000). Influenza and respiratory syncytial virus. Update on infection, management, and prevention. *Pediatric Clinics of North America*,47(2):353-72

Martinello, R.A., Chen, M.D., Weibel, C., & Kahn, J.S. (2002). Correlation between respiratory syncytial virus genotype and severity of illness. *The Journal of Infectious Diseases, 186*, 839-849.

McIntosh, K. (2000). Respiratory syncytial virus. In R.E. Behrman, R.M. Kliegman, & H.B. Jenson (Eds.), *Nelson textbook of pediatrics* (16th ed., pp.991-993). Philadelphia: W.B. Saunders Company.

Metlay, JP.; Kapoor, NW. & Fine, MJ. (1997). Does This Patient Have Community-Acquired Pneumonia? Diagnosing Pneumonia by History and Physical Examination *Journal of the American Medical Association*,278(17):1440-1445.

Mims, C; Playfair, J; Roitt, I; Wakelin, D; & Williams, R. (1998). Upper respiratory tract infections, In: Medical Microbiology, (2nd edn) Mosby, London.

Montalto, NJ.; Gum KD. & Ashley, JV. (2000). Updated Treatment for Influenza A and B. *American Family Physician*,62:2467-76

Monto, AS. (1997). Coronaviruses. In: Evans AS, ed. Viral Infections of Humans: Epidemiology and Control. 4th ed. New York: Plenum, 211–227

Ranjith, MS.; Ranjitsingh, AJA.; Gokul Shankar, S.; Vijayalaksmi, GS.; Deepa,K.; Babu, K. & Harcharan Singh Sidhu. (2010). *Solanum trilobatum* in the management of atopy: Through inhibition of mast cell degranulation and moderation of release of interleukins. *Pharmacognosy Research*,2(1): 10–14.

Ranjith, MS.; Ranjitsingh, AJA.; Gokul Shankar, S.; Vijayalaksmi, GS.; Deepa, K. & Harcharan Singh Sidhu. (2008). Enhanced phagocytosis and antibody production by *Tinospora cordifolia* - A new dimension in immunomodulation. *African Journal of Biotechnology*,7(2),081-085

Ranjith, MS. (2009). A study on immunomodulatory properties of certain plant metabolites, PhD thesis, Manonmanium Sundaranar University, Trinelveli, India

Shaheen, SO. (1995). Changing patterns of childhood infection and the rise in allergic disease. Cl in Exp Allergy 1995;25:1034-7.

Siamak T. Nabili (2011). Upper respiratory infection ed. William C. Shiel http://www.medicinenet.com/upper_respiratory_infection/article.htm

Smucny, J.; Fahey, T.; Becker, L. & Glazier, R. (2004). Antibiotics for acute bronchitis. The most robust assessment of the evidence from clinical trials of antibiotic prescribing for acute bronchitis. *Cochrane Database Systematic Review* (4):CD000245.

Sorrentino, M., Powers, T., & The Palivizumab Outcomes Study Group. (2000). Effectiveness of palivizumab: Evaluation of outcomes from the 1998 to 1999 respiratory syncytial virus season. *Pediatric Infectious Disease Journal, 19*(11), 1068-1071.

Sunila, ES. & Kuttan, G. (2004). Immunomodulatory and antitumor activity of Piper longum Linn. and piperine. *Journal of Ethnopharmacology*,90(2-3):339-346.

Visweswaraiah, A., Novotny, LA.; Hjemdahl-Monsen, EJ.; Bakaletz, LO. and Thanavala, Y. (2002). Tracking the tissue distribution of marker dye following intranasal delivery in mice and chinchillas: a multifactorial analysis of parameters affecting nasal retention. *Vaccine* 20:3209–3220.

Walsh, E.E., McConnochie, K.M., Long, C.E., & Hall, C.B. (1997). Severity of respiratory syncytial virus infection is related to virus strain. *The Journal of Infectious Diseases, 175,* 814-820.

Welliver, RC. (2003). Review of epidemiology and clinical risk factors for severe respiratory syncytial virus (RSV) infection. *Journal of Pediatrics,* 143:S112-S117

World Health Organization, Acute Respiratory Infections (Update September 2009) http://www.who.int/vaccine_research/diseases/ari/en/index2.html

Wong, DL.; Hockenberry, MJ.; Wilson, D.; Winkelstein, M.L. & Kline, NE. (2003). Respiratory syncytial virus (RSV)/bronchiolitis. In *Nursing care of infants and children* (7th ed., pp. 1366-1368). St. Louis, MO: Mosby, Inc.

9

Variability of Respiratory Syncytial Virus Seasonality and Mortality

Michael J. Light
Ross University Medical School, Commonwealth of Dominica

1. Introduction

The importance of RSV is well recognized, especially in the first few months of life. It is the most prevalent cause of lower respiratory tract infection during infancy causing both bronchiolitis and pneumonia. The spectrum of RSV illness varies from a mild upper respiratory infection that is clinically similar to a cold, all the way to respiratory failure and death from a LRTI. RSV has been demonstrated to cause dual infection both with another virus as well as not uncommonly being associated with a bacterial infection.

Our appreciation of the variety of patterns of seasonality has improved in the last 10 to 15 years because it is more feasible to confirm the presence of RSV than it was 25 years ago. Despite this, there are still many issues because most studies, particularly outside the USA are with small numbers so that assumptions are made when the data is extrapolated to a larger area. As has been demonstrated with the seasonality in Southeast Florida (see below) this may result in misleading conclusions.

Seasonality in the majority of areas in the USA is predictable and follows a similar pattern that is repeated fairly consistently and also is similar in temperate areas around the world. The RSV season in these areas starts in the fall (autumn) and tends to last 4-5 months into the winter. This pattern is evident in both Northern and Southern hemispheres. Various factors impact the seasonality of RSV in other communities and geographic and climactic differences likely are the reason for some of these differences.

Early onset LRTI caused by RSV has also been implicated in the development of disorders of wheezing in children including allergic asthma.

Morbidity and mortality as a result of RSV is a complicated subject because of a multiplicity of issues. This is especially so in the developing countries as well as the impact on the population over 65 years of age.

2. Impact of RSV

At one year of age approximately 69% of infants will demonstrate serologic evidence of RSV infection and by 2 years almost all infants will have been infected [1], of whom 50% will have been infected twice [2]. Repeat infections are common throughout life as there are multiple serologic forms and immunity is short-lived. Subsequent infections tend to be milder [1].

During the first year of life approximately 22% of infants are diagnosed with a lower respiratory tract infection [1]. Bronchiolitis is the most common cause of hospitalization of infants, with more than 120,000 cases annually in the USA [3]. It is impossible to document how many of these are truly a result of RSV infection because the etiology is often not confirmed but more than 50% of the hospitalizations for LRTI are related to RSV [4] and during the RSV season in some communities up to 90-95% of the hospitalizations are caused by RSV.

The World Health Organization and the Bill and Melinda Gates Foundation funded a study to calculate the global incidence of and mortality from episodes of LRTI due to RSV in children younger than 5 years of age in 2005 [5]. This study was published in the Lancet in 2010. The group performed a systematic review of studies published between January 1995 and June 2009.

The major findings state that in 2005, an estimated 33.8 million new episodes of RSV-associated LRTI occurred worldwide in children younger than 5 years with a least 3.4 million severe enough to require hospitalization [5].

The estimations were calculated based on the 36 studies reviewed and the locations are shown in fig. 1. It can be seen from this map that there are many studies in Europe and the USA but there are large gaps worldwide.

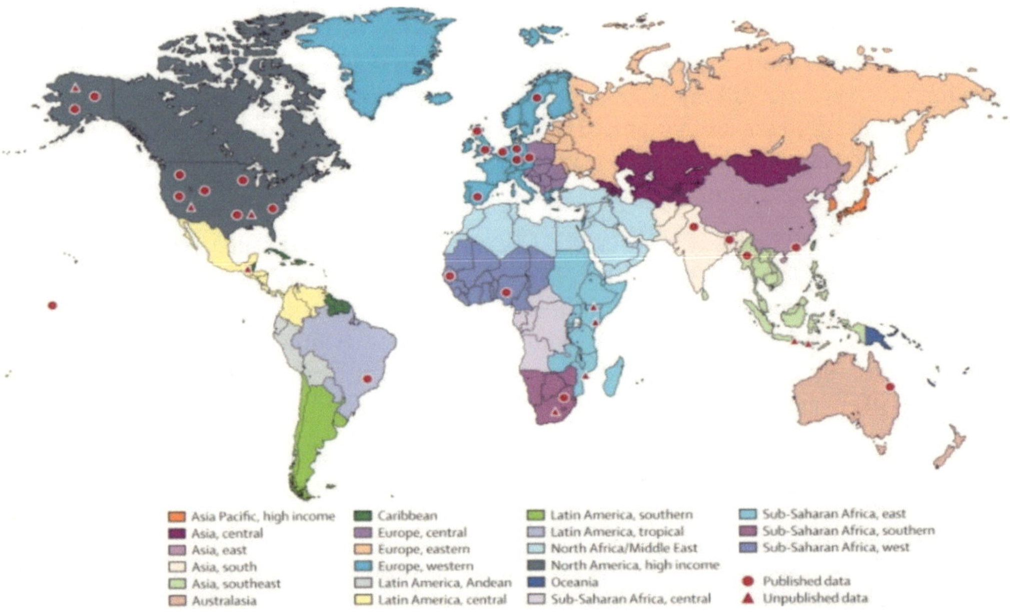

Fig. 1. Global map with circles (published) and triangles (unpublished) indicating the locations of the 36 studies.

2.1 Diagnosis of RSV

Respiratory syncytial virus is an enveloped, negative-sense, ssRNA virus that belongs to the Paramyxoviridae family. The virus has 10 genes that result in the production of 2 separate proteins. The RSV attachment (G) protein mediates attachment to the host cell via cell surface glycosaminoglycans [6]. The fusion (F) protein mediates virus entry by directing the fusion of the virion envelope with the plasma membrane of the host cell. The F protein has been demonstrated to activate Toll-like receptor (TLR)4 [7], and human studies have shown a correlation between the TLR4 receptor and susceptibility to severe RSV-induced respiratory disease [8].

There are several diagnostic assays that are used to confirm the diagnosis of RSV. The 4 primary methods include virus culture, serology, immunofluorescence antigen detection, and nucleic acid PCR-based tests. Major hospital laboratories use the IFA/DFA which is indirect/direct fluorescent antibody assay. This is a rapid test and so is clinically and practically useful. There are additional tests that can be used in the office or clinic setting using optical immunoassay, for example the BinaxNOW RSV or Clearview RSV. The most accurate test is the PCR or polymerase chain reaction. The PCR is being used more widely because of the accuracy, but it has to be remembered that identification of a particular virus does not necessarily imply that it is causing disease. Samples are usually collected by swab from the nasopharynx or by nasal wash.

Other viruses that cause respiratory infections in children include rhinovirus, coronavirus, adenovirus and parainfluenza and influenza. The identification of viruses causing lower respiratory infections is further complicated by the presence, uniquely or in combination, of a number of recently recognized viruses. Most important of these is human metapneumovirus (hMPV) that has a similar clinical profile to RSV. The two viruses may be present at the same time but the major differences between RSV and hMPV are that the latter produces milder disease and later in the season. Co-infection with RSV and hMPV has been shown to increase the intensive care unit rate of admission.

hMPV was first discovered in 2001 in the Netherlands [9]. Shortly thereafter it was described in the USA [10]. There is a range of clinical manifestations from mild upper respiratory symptoms similar to the common cold, to severe pneumonia and respiratory failure. Presentation is with cough, and fever may be present and wheeze and myalgia occur.

A more recently identified virus which causes respiratory illness in children is human bocavirus (HBoV). It was shown to have a prevalence of carriage of 3.1% among children with lower respiratory infection [11]. A study in San Diego, California [12], which consisted mainly of hospitalized patients, identified HBoV in 82 children, yielding a prevalence of 5.6% over a continuous 21-month period, with a peak prevalence as high as 14% in the spring and a virtual absence of activity during the summer months. San Diego has a temperate, dry climate. This study demonstrated a significant number of infants with paroxysmal cough which raised the clinical suspicion of pertussis. Additionally they reported a number of infants also had diarrhea.

2.2 Spread of infection

RSV is a virus that is easily spread from an infected individual, especially by touch and transfer from hand to mouth, nose or eyes. People who are infected with RSV may transmit the virus for 3 to 8 days and infants and those with weakened immune systems have the potential to be contagious for as long as 4 weeks. Schools, daycare centers and hospitals are important reservoirs for spreading the virus. In addition to direct contact with infected secretions the virus can be spread by sneezing or coughing and the virus particles that are inhaled or spread into the mouth, nose or eyes have the potential to infect. RSV may reside on hard surfaces for up to 24 hours or even longer.

RSV infection during the first 4 weeks of life is relatively infrequent in healthy term newborns. Transplacentally derived RSV-specific neutralizing antibody is present in the sera of newborns. The level of passive antibody in the term newborn is similar to the maternal level. Preterm infants have less antibody and the earlier the baby is delivered the lesser antibody is present.

Janssen [13] demonstrated that RSV susceptibility is complex, but that the strongest associations were with polymorphisms in the genes of the innate immune response. This included the transcriptional regulator Jun, alpha interferon (IFN-α), nitric oxide synthase, and the vitamin D receptor. The more recent study of preterm children by the same group [14] also indicated a critical association with innate immune system genes and bronchiolitis susceptibility.

The following table (1), shows some of the risk factors for the acquisition and spread of RSV infection.

Family size
Crowded living conditions
Older siblings in school or day-care
Attendance in day-care
Lack of breast feeding
Exposure to cigarette smoke
Birth in the months prior to the onset of the RSV season
Healthcare workers
Elderly patients in nursing homes
Genetic factors

Table 1. Risk factors for acquiring and spreading RSV.

2.3 Risk of increased severity

There are multiple factors that are associated with more severe disease including the following list shown in Table 2.

Although prematurity is at the top of this list, there are more full-term cases of RSV hospitalized because of the number delivered at each gestational age. Family history of asthma and genetic factors also correlate with more severe RSV disease.

In addition infants in developing countries are at increased risk because of malnutrition and possibly vitamin deficiency, especially vitamins A and D [15]. It also appears that repeated infections requiring hospitalization are more common in developing countries.

RSV, influenza virus, adenovirus, human metapneumovirus, parainfluenza virus and rhinovirus can all cause bronchiolitis, necessitating hospitalization. Second, of these viruses,

RSV has most commonly been reported to be the main cause of hospitalization due to bronchiolitis and increased disease severity, followed by rhinovirus and then by influenza virus. Third, viral coinfection is relatively common, occurring in about 20% of cases. However, there is no consensus on the effect of coinfection on disease severity. The effect may depend upon which viruses coinfect together.

Prematurity
Age less than 3 months
Male gender
Low socioeconomic status
Multiple births
Indoor smoke pollution
Malnutrition
Chronic lung disease of infancy (bronchopulmonary dysplasia)
Hemodynamically significant congenital heart disease
Immune deficiency problems especially severe combined immunodeficiency disorder (SCID) and HIV/AIDS
Severe neuromuscular disorders
Transplant patients
Hematopoietic transplants (bone marrow and stem cell)
Malignancy

Table 2. Factors associated with more severe disease.

3. Influenza

The influenza virus is spread rapidly from person to person. The result may be an influenza pandemic. A pandemic implies a worldwide epidemic that infects a large proportion of the total human population. Epidemic patterns of influenza occur most winters. The pandemic of influenza occurs irregularly. Although the pandemic of 1918 is probably the most well-known there have been about 3 pandemics in each of the last 3 centuries. The 1918 pandemic is also known as the Spanish Flu and resulted in an estimated worldwide mortality of perhaps 30 to 40 million people. Pandemics start when a new strain of the influenza virus is transmitted from an animal species hence the designation of swine flu and bird (avian) flu in recent times.

In February 2010 the CDC updated the recommendation for annual influenza shot to all persons greater than 6 months of age. For persons aged 65 and older the high-dose influenza vaccine (Fluzone), licensed in 2010, is mentioned as an option for this age group. Despite this recommendation the number of people who regularly get a flu shot is dismally low probably around 10%. In undeveloped countries the situation is much worse as there is no public health infrastructure in place to vaccinate large populations.

In 1997 a new subtype of influenza was found in humans, designated H5N1. This virus had only previously been described in birds and its effect on chickens led to the label of "Chicken Ebola". The population of Hong Kong found out in 1997 that it had the potential to be just as deadly in humans. The entire poultry population of ducks, geese and chickens in Hong Kong was destroyed.

The H1N1 strain of swine flu demonstrated the unpredictable nature of potential influenza pandemics in 2009. In the Spanish Flu of 1918 the population that was most threatened by the virus was not the usual population. Typically, the seasonal flu virus results in significant mortality to the very young and the very old. The Spanish Flu was more devastating to the younger adult population. The H1N1 strain also affected a different population with pregnant patients demonstrating the highest rate of mortality.

3.1 Influenza and RSV

Despite the numbers in the young (infants) and old (greater than 65 years) population we do not describe infection with RSV as pandemic. There is however, concern that there is potential for greater numbers of more severe disease with the combination of RSV and influenza virus. When H1N1 was circulating in 2009, it was noted that there was increased RSV transmission.

A comparison was made between the impact of seasonal RSV and influenza for young children locally and nationally [16]. In this study the impact of RSV for children less than 7 years of age was greater than influenza for emergency department visits and hospitalizations. The study evaluated health care resources and impact for 2 winter seasons between 2003 and 2005 in the USA. They estimated that 10.2 emergency department visits per 1000 children were attributable to influenza and 21.5 visits per 1000 to RSV. Children who were aged 0 to 23 months and infected with RSV had the highest rate of emergency department visits with 64.4 visits per 1000 children. Significantly more children required hospitalization as a result of an RSV infection compared with influenza, with calculated national hospitalization rates of 8.5 and 1.4 per 1000 children, respectively. The total number of workdays missed yearly by caregivers of children who required ED care was 246,965 days for influenza infections and 716,404 days for RSV infections.

4. RSV and bacterial infection

Much of the early literature relating RSV and bacterial infection considered the non-respiratory infections. Both otitis media and urinary tract infections were evaluated and the recommendation made that antibiotics were not routinely needed for RSV infections. In 1998 the etiology of childhood pneumonia was evaluated in children less than 5 years of age by Heiskanen-Kosma [17] stressing the relationship of RSV and *Streptococcus pneumoniae* with community acquired pneumonia. The pulmonary aspect of viral LRTI was addressed by Hament [18] who discussed the implication that viral infections facilitate bacterial colonization, adherence and translocation through the epithelial barrier, paving the way for bacterial disease.

The importance of secondary bacterial infection in children with severe RSV bronchiolitis was stressed by Thorburn [19]. The group in Liverpool followed 165 children with median age of 1.6 months admitted to the pediatric intensive care unit. 42.4% of these children, all of whom required mechanical ventilation, had lower airway secretions that were positive for bacteria. Laboratory evaluation, including white cell count, neutrophil count and C-reactive protein, did not distinguish between those who only had RSV and those who had bacterial infection.

5. Seasonality

The RSV season is defined in various ways. The season is most often described in the USA as the week in which 10% of the laboratory tests are positive for RSV. Tests that are referred for RSV testing from that community will define the season in that community. Some studies have included a positive rate of only 5% to define the season. An alternative approach is to define the season as the period in which there are increased hospitalizations for LRTI especially bronchiolitis. The season usually has a defined onset, from a few or no cases to multiple cases, and an offset which defines the end of the season.

Most communities with temperate climates have a well-defined season of 3 to 5 months usually starting in the Northern hemisphere in October or November and continuing until February or March. It is common for there to be a biennial change from one season to the next whereby the subsequent season is milder or more severe than the preceding. However, this is not predictable and the differences may be more related to climactic changes.

5.1 USA

The Center for Disease Control (CDC) in Atlanta Georgia has reported the seasonality of RSV based on the 10% threshold. The National Respiratory and Enteric Virus Surveillance System (NREVSS) is a voluntary laboratory-based system that tracks trends in RSV and other viruses. They reported 4 regions of the United States from July 2, 2004 to December 3, 2005 as shown in Fig. 2. This demonstrates a clear consistent seasonal pattern with onset between October and December and offset mid-February to April. Of note the South demonstrated at that time an onset of at least a month ahead of the other 3 regions.

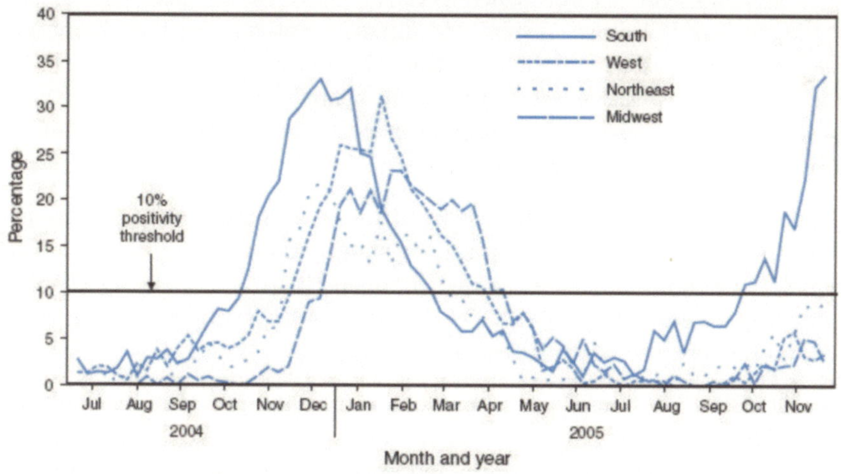

**Northeast:* Connecticut, Maine, Massachusetts, New Hampshire, New Jersey, New York, Pennsylvania, Rhode Island, and Vermont; *Midwest:* Illinois, Indiana, Iowa, Kansas, Michigan, Minnesota, Missouri, Nebraska, North Dakota, Ohio, South Dakota, and Wisconsin; *South:* Alabama, Arkansas, Delaware, District of Columbia, Florida, Georgia, Kentucky, Louisiana, Maryland, Mississippi, North Carolina, Oklahoma, South Carolina, Tennessee, Texas, Virginia, and West Virginia; *West:* Alaska, Arizona, California, Colorado, Hawaii, Idaho, Montana, Nevada, New Mexico, Oregon, Utah, Washington, and Wyoming.

Fig. 2. RSV season for 4 areas of USA defined by 10% positive for years 2004-2005. From CDC (NREVSS).

Clinicians in Florida recognized that the season for RSV was not in the same months as the data from CDC suggested. In order to define the seasonality in Florida a retrospective analysis of RSV surveillance data and hospitalizations was conducted for 5 regions of Florida from 2001 to 2004 [20]. The 5 regions within the State of Florida capture data from strategically placed laboratories in the southeast, southwest, central, northwest and north regions. As noted, data from these regions is reported on the Florida Department of Health website (http://www.doh.state.fl.us/disease_ctrl/epi/RSV/rsv.htm). The onset of the RSV season for the purpose of this study was when at least 10% of the RSV specimens submitted were positive during a surveillance week. The majority of the tests were by rapid tests although the specific number identified by rapid test, culture or PCR is not documented.

The evaluation procedures to define RSV season are based on the reporting from regional laboratories. Of necessity the validity of the data is dependent upon the number of samples submitted because if the number is too low then there may be a false positive conclusion. Also the use of hospitalization data is dependent on the accuracy of the patient discharge records which forms the basis of most calculations. In previous studies of hospitalization rates the International Classification of Diseases, 9th revision, clinical modification (ICD-9-CM) codes are used. These include 466.11 - RSV bronchiolitis, 480.1 - RSV pneumonia, and 079.6 - other RSV. Review of several studies report admission rates of 13 to 40.8 per 1000 children less than 1 year of age. The majority of studies reporting national data range from 22.8 to 27.4 per 1000 births.

Information pertinent to hospitalization in the State of Florida can be obtained from The Florida Agency for Health Care Administration (AHCA). Regional discharge sets from AHCA for the years 2001 through 2004 were reviewed for the primary and secondary discharge diagnosis of RSV lower respiratory illness for patients less than 12 months of age as well as 12 to less than 24 months of age. The discharge diagnosis of RSV is only documented if there is a positive test for RSV in the chart. The primary objective of the study was to compare the RSV seasonal data from the laboratories with the incidence of ICD-9-CM coded admissions for RSV lower respiratory illness.

The results of this study defined the RSV seasons for the 5 regions in Florida and the percent monthly positive RSV tests and hospitalizations statewide are shown in Fig. 3. There were an additional 27,140 hospitalizations caused by unspecified bronchiolitis (ICD-9-CM code 466.19) and unspecified pneumonia (ICD-9-CM code 486) during this same period. It is likely that a portion of these were also caused by RSV.

The season for RSV varied from year to year and during the period of the study there was circulation of RSV year round in some years and some regions. The longest season was in the southeast and the shortest in the north and northwest. The RSV season, on the basis of positive RSV tests and the hospitalizations for RSV illness are shown for the southeast region in Fig. 4. This shows the prolonged RSV season and the correlation between positive tests and hospitalization.

During this 4-year period there were more than 23,000 admissions of children less than 24 months of age of which 20,000 (86%) were less than 12 months of age. There were 23 hospitalizations yearly per 1000 live births. More than 90% of the hospital discharges occurred during the defined RSV season.

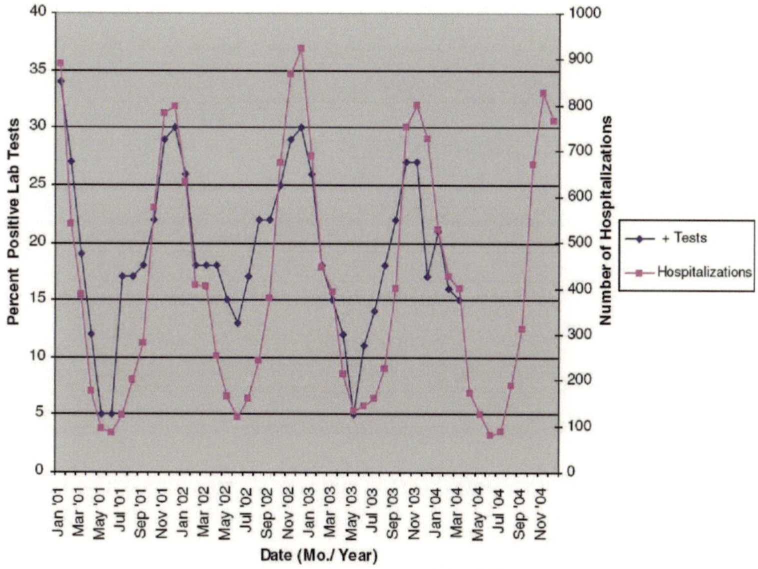

Fig. 3. Total RSV positive tests and hospitalizations for the State of Florida from January 2001 to November 2004.

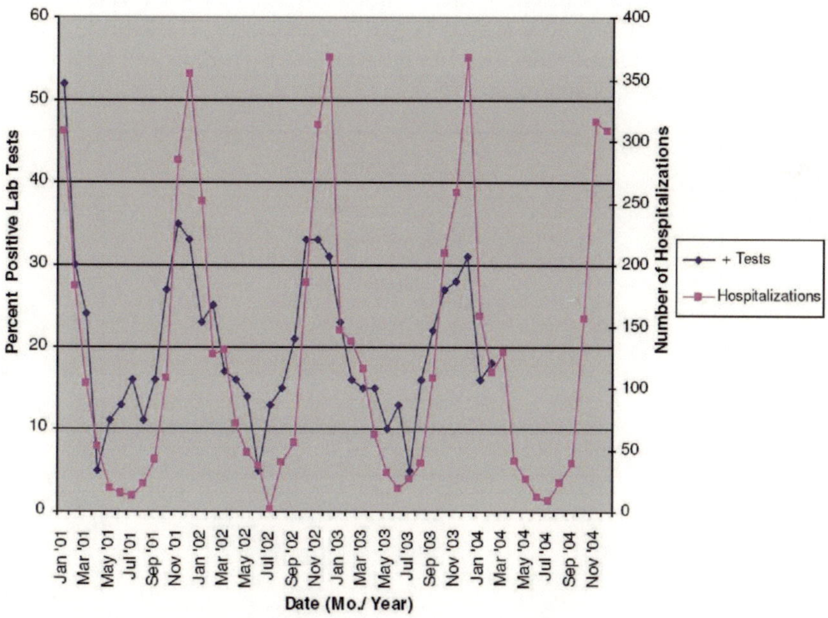

Fig. 4. RSV test data and hospitalization in southeast Florida.

The impact of Florida is demonstrated on the NREVSS of RSV for July 9 2005 to November 18, 2006 in Fig 5. Unlike the majority of the USA, the onset in Florida was in July, peaking in October and offset in April. Further evaluation of the Florida data reveals that the major contributor to the early onset is the tri-county area of Southeast Florida comprising Palm Beach, Broward and Miami-Dade counties [20].

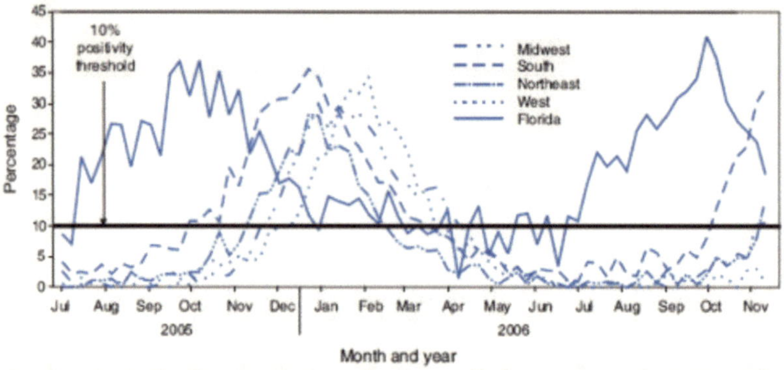

* *Northeast:* Connecticut, Massachusetts, New Hampshire, New Jersey, New York, and Rhode Island; *Midwest:* Illinois, Indiana, Minnesota, Missouri, Nebraska, North Dakota, Ohio, South Dakota, and Wisconsin; *South:* Alabama, Arkansas, Delaware, District of Columbia, Georgia, Kentucky, Louisiana, Maryland, Mississippi, North Carolina, Oklahoma, South Carolina, Tennessee, Texas, and Virginia; *West:* Alaska, Arizona, California, Colorado, Hawaii, Montana, Washington, and Wyoming; Florida. Data from Florida were presented separately because they differed substantially from RSV-detection data from the remainder of the South region.

Fig. 5. RSV data for 5 areas of USA with Florida separated, for years 2005-2006. From CDC (NREVSS).

The data for July 2008 to June 2009 with 10 regions and the addition of Florida and the National average are shown in Fig. 6. 238 laboratories from 45 states are included in this summary which included 404,798 tests of which 60,793 were positive. The national data showed onset in the first week of November, continuing for 20 weeks. When the data from Florida is excluded the national RSV season began 2 weeks later. These findings support the position that individual communities need to be aware of their data and how it impacts the onset and duration of the RSV season.

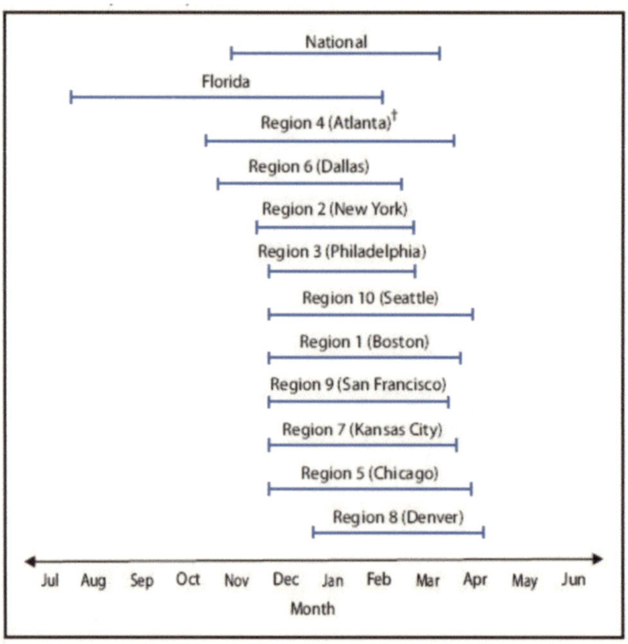

Fig. 6. RSV data for all of USA and 10 regions with Florida separated for the period July 2008 to June 2009. Each line represents the months of RSV season. From CDC (NREVSS).

Weekly updates which show RSV national, regional and state trends are available form the NREVSS website: http://www.cdc.gov/surveillance/NREVSS.

The most recent data from the USA and from Florida are shown in fig. 7a and 7b respectively.

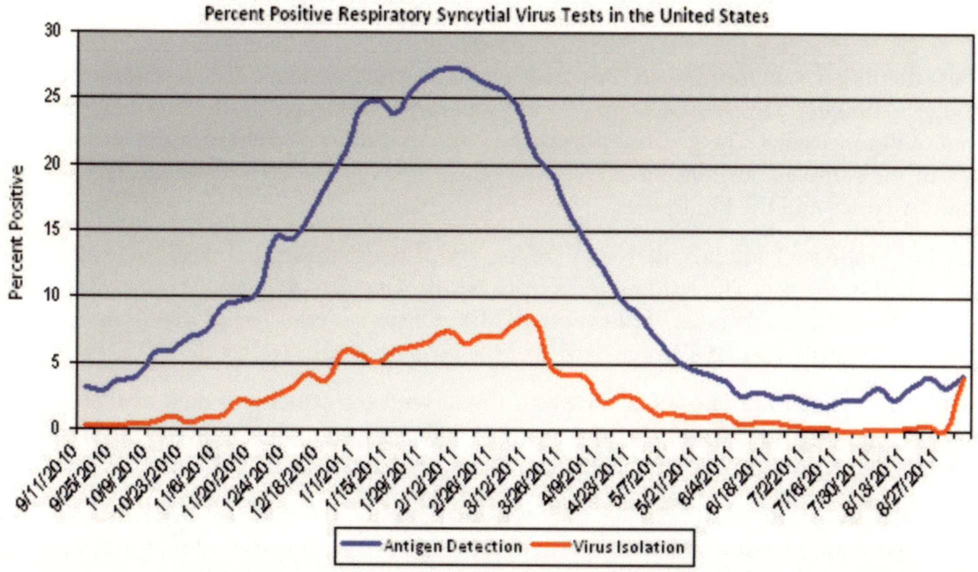

Fig. 7a. Percent positive RSV tests (antigen detection and virus isolation) in the United States. From CDC (NRVESS).

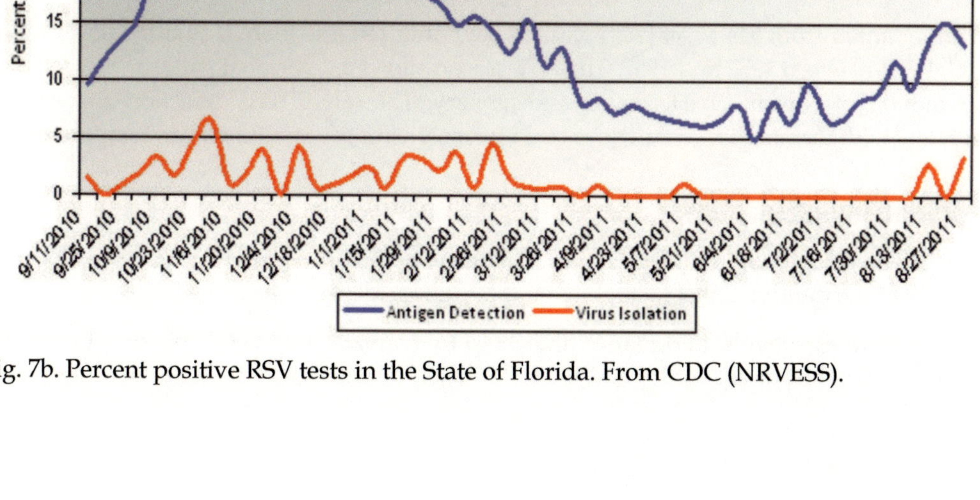

Fig. 7b. Percent positive RSV tests in the State of Florida. From CDC (NRVESS).

6. Developing countries

The impact of seasonality and mortality in tropical and developing countries was reviewed in 1998 [18] . This report was the first of many reviews that have scrutinized the literature to demonstrate the extent of RSV in a global sense. They found that RSV was the predominant viral cause of LRTI in childhood being responsible for 27-96% of hospitalized cases (mean 65%) in which a virus was found. Further that 39% of hospital patients with RSV were under 6 months of age.

They identified community studies and hospital-based studies. The community based studies, ranging from 1963 to 1989 reported RSV positivity by culture and immunofluorescence. The greatest number of patients studied was from India with less than 10% of the samples positive for RSV. The highest rates of positive RSV culture were from South America and the Phillipines.

The hospital-based studies that they reviewed also demonstrated RSV by culture and immunofluorescence. The studies were from South America, Asia and Africa from 1972 to 1990 with very variable rates of positivity to RSV. Of the samples tested that demonstrated a virus, RSV contributed an average of 65% of the positive results (range 27-96%).

Trying to demonstrate rates of LRTI was difficult with the paucity of data available at that time. The reported incidence varied from 10/1,000 children under one year hospitalized in Israel to 198/1000 child years from birth to 18 months in a study from Colombia.

In tropical and subtropical climates with seasonal rainfall, the outbreaks of RSV were more associated with the rainy season rather than the cold season. They found that the peak of the RSV season occurred one to two months after the onset of the rains [21].

In temperate climates, as well as Mediterranean and desert climates, the RSV season corresponds to the cold season.

In Singapore, the seasonal trends of viral respiratory infections were reviewed by Chew [22]. They reviewed the viral isolates from 1990 to 1994 and 3904 positive viral reports. RSV was the most dominant with 72% of the total. The RSV trends were associated with higher environmental temperature, lower relative humidity and higher maximal day-to-day temperature variation. There was a definite season noted related to these climate features. Although the influenza A outbreaks were not associated with meteorological factors, influenza B isolates were positively associated with rainfall.

A larger study from Malaysia [23] included 5691 children less than 24 months hospitalized with LRTI between 1982 and 1997. The RSV season showed a seasonal pattern with peaks in the months of November, December and January. The rate of RSV infection appeared to correlate with the number of rain days and inversely with the monthly mean temperature.

7. Variability of seasons

The differences in reported incidence of RSV infection are of necessity difficult to elucidate because of the multiplicity of factors that impact the incidence.

Various studies provide information that help to evaluate the overall picture. Brazil is a tropical and subtropical country and the RSV season peaks in the fall (autumn) and extends into the winter with a corresponding increase in hospital admissions for lower respiratory illnesses. This study [24] showed that in 1995-1996 RSV was the most prominent virus causing severe lower respiratory disease including bronchiolitis and pneumonia. It was found in 41.8% of the cohort. A further study in the same area [25] performed indirect immuofluorescent assay and demonstrated that RSV contributed 73% of the viruses that were identified in the population less than 5 years of age admitted for severe respiratory illness. Although the studies were different in terms of enrollment the point is made that there is variability in diagnosis of viral infection in the same location at differing time periods.

8. Climate

Year round prevalence of RSV in the USA has been reported in Florida, Hawaii, Texas and Alaska. Certainly warm equatorial areas demonstrate a long season of RSV especially if rainfall persists throughout the year.

To try and explain the climactic differences, this study [26] compared the data at several large cities which are geographically and climactically diverse. The cities were 1. near Bethel, Alaska, USA, 2. Mexico City, Mexico, 3. Delhi, India, 4. Miami, Florida, USA, 5. Houston, Texax, USA, 6. Tucson Arizona, USA, 7. Buffalo, New York, USA 8. Winnipeg, Canada and 9. Santiago, Chile. The sites were chosen because of their interest in defining seasonality and climate differences between the communities.

Data concerning mean temperatures, dew point, relative humidity and precipitation was obtained for the nine cities and is shown in Table 3.

City	Lat[1]	Temp[2]	Dew[3]	Hum[4]	Prec[5]
Mexico City	19.2 N	22.5	6.3	52.4	16.3
Miami Florida	25.8 N	24.2	19.1	56.7	18.0
Delhi India	28.4 N	23.9	13.9	52	13.5
Houston Texas	29.6 N	20.4	15	49.5	13.0
Tucson Arizona	32.1 N	20.2	1.9	19.3	2.5
Santiago Chile	33.2 S	14.4	7.8	66	0.3
Buffalo New York	42.6 N	8.9	3.2	54	9.7
Winnipeg Canada	49.5 N	14	-3.8	71.5	0.5
Bethel Alaska	60.5 N	-1.6	-3.8	n.a	0.4

[1]Latitude, [2]Mean temperature, centigrade, [3]Dew point [4]Humidity [5]Precipitation, mm per week

Table 3. Data concerning climate and humidity for the 9 cities.

The cities were warm and wet (Miami, Mexico City, Delhi and Houston), warm and dry (Tucson), cold and wet (Buffalo) and cold and dry (Winnipeg and Bethel). Santiago, Chile is in the Southern hemisphere with intermediate weather conditions. The relationship of mean temperature to RSV activity showed that the number of RSV cases increased when the mean temperature was 24-30^{0}C and again when the temperature was in the range 2-6^{0}C. In relation to humidity, RSV activity increased when the mean relative humidity was between 45 and 65% and ultraviolet B radiance was inversely related to the number of RSV cases. The dewpoint, which indicates relative humidity, correlated significantly with RSV activity.

Published reports from prior studies were discussed in this article [26] by Yusuf and tended to confirm their findings. In Singapore and Malaysia where temperatures are constant and rainfall is generally heavy, there is RSV activity throughout the year. In Gambia (West Africa) and Vellore, (India) it is hot and the rainfall is directly associated with RSV activity. In Riyadh, which is hot and dry, RSV activity occurs in the winter when there is some rainfall and lower temperature. In colder climates they further speculate that cold temperatures are more important than humidity.

Interesting speculation from this article [26] propose that high humidity and stable high temperatures enable RSV to be sustained well enough in large-particle aerosols to permit year round transmission of the virus. Onset of drier weather appears to reduce aerosol transmission of the virus.

9. Management of RSV bronchiolitis

The American Academy of Pediatrics convened a committee and partners to develop an evidence-based clinical practice guideline with recommendations for diagnosis and management of first onset RSV bronchiolitis [27].

It can be seen from Table 4 that the management is essentially supportive.

1a. Clinicians should diagnose bronchiolitis and assess disease severity on the basis of history and physical examination. Clinicians should not routinely order laboratory and radiologic studies for diagnosis (recommendation).
1b. Clinicians should assess risk factors for severe disease such as age less than 12 weeks, a history of prematurity, underlying cardiopulmonary disease, or immunodeficiency when making decisions about evaluation and management of children with bronchiolitis (recommendation).
2a. Bronchodilators should not be used routinely in the management of bronchiolitis (recommendation).
2b.A carefully monitored trial of α-adrenergic or ß-adrenergic medication is an option. Inhaled bronchodilators should be continued only if there is a documented positive clinical response to the trial using an objective means of evaluation (option).
3. Corticosteroid medications should not be used routinely in the management of bronchiolitis (recommendation).
4. Ribavirin should not be used routinely in children with bronchiolitis (recommendation).
5. Antibacterial medications should only be used in children with bronchiolitis who have specific indications of the coexistence of a bacterial infection. When present, bacterial

infection should be treated in the same manner as in the absence of bronchiolitis (recommendation). 6a. Clinicians should assess hydration and ability to take fluids orally (strong recommendation). 6b. Chest physiotherapy should not be used routinely in the management of bronchiolitis (recommendation). 7a. Supplemental oxygen is indicated if SpO_2 falls persistently below 90% in previously healthy infants. If the SpO_2 does persistently fall below 90%, adequate supplemental oxygen should be used to maintain an SpO_2 at or above 90%. Oxygen may be discontinued if SpO_2 is at or above 90% and the infant is feeding well and has minimal respiratory distress (option). 7b. As the child's clinical course improves, continuous measurement of SpO_2 is not routinely needed (option). 7c. Infants with a known history of hemodynamically significant heart or lung disease and premature infants require close monitoring as oxygen is being weaned (strong recommendation). 8a. Clinicians may administer palivizumab prophylaxis for selected infants and children with CLD or a history of prematurity (less than 35 weeks' gestation) or with congenital heart disease (recommendation). 8b. When given, prophylaxis with palivizumab should be given in 5 monthly doses, usually beginning in November or December, at a dose of 15 mg/kg per dose administered intramuscularly (recommendation). 9a. Hand decontamination is the most important step in preventing nosocomial spread of RSV. Hands should be decontaminated before and after direct contact with patients, after contact with inanimate objects in the direct vicinity of the patient, and after removing gloves (strong recommendation). 9b. Alcohol-based rubs are preferred for hand decontamination. An alternative is hand-washing with antimicrobial soap (recommendation). 9c. Clinicians should educate personnel and family members on hand sanitation (recommendation). 10a. Infants should not be exposed to passive smoking (strong recommendation). 10b.Breastfeeding is recommended to decrease a child's risk of having LRTD (recommendation). 11. Clinicians should inquire about use of CAM (option).

Table 4. Recommendations for diagnosis and management of bronchiolitis

Following the AAP Guideline there has been additional information. A promising new development is the use of hypertonic saline inhalation. A recent trial of this treatment, which has been successfully used for patients with cystic fibrosis, reported a reduction of 26% in the length of hospitalization for infants with acute viral bronchiolitis [28].

10. RSV Prevention

The history of development of a vaccine against RSV is complicated. Infants may respond inadequately because of immunologic immaturity or suppression because of maternal antibodies. In the 1960's a formalin inactivated RSV vaccine was studied in infants.

Unfortunately, not only did it not provide protection, but it also resulted in worse disease in vaccinated infants. 80% of the study infants were subsequently hospitalized and 2 died despite the fact that the RSV vaccine was an inactivated virus [29].

Palivizumab is the only FDA approved monoclonal antibody for RSV. It targets the F (fusion) glycoprotein, inhibiting viral entry into host cells. It was approved following a randomized, double-blind placebo-controlled trial that was conducted at 139 centers in the USA, the United Kingdom and Canada during the 1996-1997 RSV season. The patient population included prematurity (less than 35 weeks gestation) or bronchopulmonary dysplasia (BPD). They were randomized to receive 5 injections of either palivizumab, 15 mg/kg or a placebo. Children were followed for 150 days and the primary endpoint was hospitalization with confirmed RSV infection. Palivizumab prophylaxis resulted in a 55% reduction in hospitalization for RSV (10.6% of the placebo group and 4.8% of the treated group). Premature infants who did not have BPD had a reduction in hospitalization for RSV (8.1% placebo, 1.8% palivizumab).

As noted above, the majority of infants admitted with LRTI caused by RSV are full-term. More severe disease is associated with prematurity, chronic lung disease and congenital heart disease as major co-morbidities. There continues to be controversy concerning the optimal recommendations for the prescription of palivizumab. Several studies have been performed to evaluate the cost effectiveness of prophylaxis with palivizumab. The selection of infants who qualify for prophylaxis is defined in the Red Book from the Section of Infectious Diseases of the American Academy of Pediatrics [30]. The most recent iteration of the Red Book has this update which indicates which infants are eligible for 3 doses of palivizumab rather than the previously recommended 5 doses (Table 5). The other issue relates to the onset of the season that indicated the north central and southwest regions of Florida, onset of RSV occurs in late September to early October. Regions of southeast Florida have an onset of RSV in July. Children in these communities should receive palivizumab during the 3-5 months when they will be most likely to need coverage against peak RSV activity. Children with co-morbidities may require more than 3 or 5 doses because they are at higher risk for mortality.

Infants Eligible for a Maximum of 5 Doses
Infants younger than 24 months of age with chronic lung disease and requiring medical therapy
Infants younger than 24 months of age and requiring medical therapy for congenital heart disease
Preterm infants born at 31 weeks, 6 days of gestation or less
Certain infants with neuromuscular disease or congenital abnormalities of the airways
Infants Eligible for a Maximum of 3 Doses
Preterm infants with gestational age of 32 weeks, 0 days to 34 weeks, 6 days with at least 1 risk factor and born 3 months before or during RSV season.

*Data taken from Table 3.60. *Red Book 2009: p.560 [31]*

Table 5. Criteria for eligibility for 5 or 3 palivizumab doses.

The difficulty of only permitting 5 doses relates to those infants with chronic lung and cardiac disease that may be at risk for the first 2 years of life and perhaps even longer. In southeast Florida the season is longer than 5 months.

Also infants who are at risk for severe RSV who undergo cardiopulmonary bypass and are receiving palivizumab should receive palivizumab after surgery because the antibody will be "washed out" during bypass.

Prophylaxis in immunocompromised children has not been studied in randomized trials. The AAP policy states that these patients may also benefit from prophylaxis, however, more specific recommendations are not made at this time. Although the Cystic Fibrosis Foundation has recommended: "for infants with cystic fibrosis (CF) under 2 years of age that the use of palivizumab be considered for prophylaxis of respiratory syncytial virus", the Red Book suggests that "there is insufficient data to determine the effectiveness of palivizumab use in this patient population. Therefore, a recommendation for routine prophylaxis in patients with CF cannot be made."

11. Morbidity and mortality

The relationship between RSV infection in infancy and subsequent development of wheezing disorders has also been difficult to define. Again, there are probably a multiplicity of reasons that wheezing is impacted by RSV lower respiratory infection. Stein [32] reported in the Tucson respiratory study that RSV LRTI was an independent risk factor for wheezing up to 11 years of age, but not at 13 years. On the other hand Sigurs [33] showed that RSV infection requiring hospitalization in infancy was a risk factor for allergic asthma in early adolescence.

11.1 Mortality

Developed countries

In the developed countries the mortality from RSV induced respiratory infection in children is less than 1%. There are specific conditions that are associated with increased mortality and these are shown in Table 6 which is similar to Table 2 which showed the population at risk for severe disease. The first three are most important during infancy, the next group is important in childhood, and the population over 65 years of age is at risk for morbidity and mortality. Older children, and adults less than 65 years of age, who have no co-morbid conditions should not be at risk for severe RSV-associated illness.

Prematurity
Chronic lung disease (bronchopulmonary dysplasia)
Hemodynamically significant congenital cardiac disease
Immune deficiency
Complication of hematopoietic transplantation
Malignancy
Age over 65 years

Table 6. Factors associated with increased mortality.

There is significant mortality from RSV infection in both solid and hematologic transplants. Bone marrow and stem cell transplant patients are at especially significant risk for the development of difficult to treat RSV infection.

Intensive care units for newborns and children have lowered the mortality from RSV associated illness in developed countries to less than 1% of severe RSV LRTI. Children with significant lung and cardiac disease have reported mortality due to RSV LRTI of approximately 3% of intensive care admissions and this number continues to improve. Reported mortality rates of complications of hematopoietic transplant illness secondary to RSV have approximated 50%.

The paediatric intensive care unit at the Royal Liverpool Children's Hospital, U.K. admitted 406 RSV positive patients from 1999 to 2007 [34]. Of the deaths that were attributed to RSV, all of them had pre-existing medical conditions: chromosomal abnormalities 29%, cardiac lesions 27%, neuromuscular 15%, chronic lung disease 12%, large airway abnormality 9% and immunodeficiency 9%. Nosocomial and hospital-acquired disease comprised a significant proportion of morbidity and mortality related to RSV.

11.2 Globally

In 1992 the World Health Organization estimated that one third of the 12.2 million annual deaths in children under 5 years of age are the result of acute respiratory infections dominated by RSV, *Streptococcus pneumoniae* and *hemophilus influenzae* [35]. In developing countries calculations of mortality rates from lower respiratory tract infection are based on extrapolations of regional studies. It is difficult to calculate the impact of RSV because there are additional factors that are involved. Before the introduction of measles vaccination the measles virus was responsible for considerable morbidity and mortality related to pulmonary disease. The countries that have strong programs to provide protection against measles have demonstrated a shift in the etiologies and outcomes of lower respiratory infections.

Bacterial infection overshadows RSV in developing countries with *Streptococcus pneumoniae, Staphylococcus aureus* and *Hemophilus influenzae* playing major roles in morbidity and mortality of lower respiratory infections.

The Lancet study, discussed earlier [5], estimated that 66,000 to 199,000 children younger than 5 years of age died from RSV associated acute lower respiratory infection in 2005 with 99% of these occurring in developing countries.

11.3 Adults

RSV is definitely one of the most important respiratory viruses in children, especially during the first year of life. Children older than 2 years of age without confounding medical conditions continue to be reinfected with RSV. The infection usually results in an upper respiratory infection that is very similar to the common cold. Children who have hyperactive airways may have wheezing associated with this upper respiratory illness. This also applies to the healthy adult who may have cold symptoms and some may wheeze.

The importance of influenza virus in the elderly population is well known. Although RSV may coexist with influenza, the data supports the notion that RSV is a major contributor to mortality in the population greater than 65 years of age. The impact of RSV is difficult to evaluate because the rapid antigen detection tests are relatively insensitive in adults and few tests are ordered by medical practitioners in this age group. It has been suggested that deaths attributed to influenza in the past may more correctly be a result of RSV infection.

Falsey [36] reported that according to the National Center for Health Statistics of the CDC, in 1999 the numbers of discharges from USA hospitals for pneumonia was 1.3 million, chronic obstructive pulmonary disease, 0.76 million and asthma 0.35 million. It was then calculated that 177,525 admissions per year were accounted for by RSV and that the death rate from RSV would be 8% which comes to 14,000 annual deaths. An earlier study by Thompson [37] reported a similar finding of 11,321 deaths.

RSV pneumonia is a major complication of adults who are immunocompromised. Ebber [38] reported the results of bronchoalveolar lavage in 11 patients aged 21 to 77 years of age who were undergoing treatment for leukemia or lymphoma, or who were post-bone marrow transplant. The 11 patients had proven RSV and the mortality was 55% (6 patients). Of interest, 8 of the 11 had also bacterial or fungal infection.

It is important to be aware that although RSV infection in the immunocompromised patient is more likely during the RSV season of the community, it is well known that this population, as well as the solid organ transplant population may be infected with RSV outside the defined season.

IgA is considered to play an important role in the protection of initial infection with RSV. It is possible that reduced levels of IgA may impair the protective effect of subsequent RSV infections. Older individuals have reduced virus-specific antibodies and decreased T-cell numbers compared to younger individuals after inactivated influenza immunization. Elderly individuals do have similar neutralizing antibody titers which suggests that the reduction in neutralizing antibodies is not the cause of the more severe disease in the population over 65 years of age.

Increased susceptibility of the elderly to RSV infection may lie within the CD8 T-cell arm of the adaptive immune system. The numbers of RSV-specific CD8 T cells is decreased in old age which limits the ability to produce cytokines.

12. RSV vaccine

It has been challenging to find an appropriate vaccine against RSV. The extremes of age, the very young and the very old are the populations that stand to benefit most from a vaccine. The young infant has an immature immune system that is dominated by Th2-type response and in the presence of maternal antibody response to the vaccine is unpredictable. Older people have decreased numbers of T cells which would reduce the response to the vaccine.

13. Conclusion

Frequent handwashing is probably the greatest public health intervention that is available at the present time. Awareness of the season of RSV both in the hospital or clinic and in the community allows for interventions including cohorting and avoidance measures to reduce the spread of the virus.

Awareness of the seasonality of RSV permits appropriate timing of preventive programs that have the potential to reduce the impact of RSV. The RSV season that is repeated each year in temperate climates during the winter, may vary significantly in terms of onset, duration and severity from year to year. In tropical and sub-tropical climates it appears that the humidity is more of a dominant factor in terms of timing of the season, usually peaking 2-3 months after onset of the season, and varying with the temperature.

The number of health care dollars (and other currencies) that are spent as a result of the impact of RSV, is in the billions. It is clear that the development of a vaccine that reduces the morbidity and mortality of RSV-associated disease has the potential to save money and save lives.

14. Abbreviations

CDC: Centers for Disease Control and Prevention

RSV: respiratory syncytial virus

LRTI: lower respiratory tract infection

15. References

[1] W.P. Glezen. Risk of primary infection and reinfection with respiratory syncytial virus. *American Journal of Diseases of Children*. Vol. 140(6): pp. 543-6. June 1986.

[2] F.W. Henderson. The etiologic and epidemiologic spectrum of bronchiolitis in pediatric practice. *Journal of Pediatrics*. Vol. 95(2): pp. 183-90. Aug, 1979.

[3] D.K. Shay, Bronchiolitis-associated hospitalizations among U.S. children, 1980-1996. *Journal of the American Medical Association*, Vol. 282, pp.1440-6, 1999.

[4] S. Leader. Respiratory syncytial virus-coded pediatric hospitalizations, 1997 to 1999. *Pediatric Infectious Disease*. Vol. 21(7): pp. 629-32, Jul 2002.

[5] H. Nair Global burden of acute lower respiratory infections due to respiratory syncytial virus in young children: a systematic review and meta-analysis. *Lancet*. Vol.1;375(9725): pp. 1545-55.

[6] M.R. Olson. Pulmonary immunity and immunopathology: lessons from respiratory syncytial virus. *Expert Review of Vaccines*. Vol. 7(8): pp. 1239-1255, Oct 2008.

[7] L.M.Haynes. Involvement of Toll-like receptor 4 in innate immunity to respiratory syncytial virus. Journal of Virology. Vol. 75(22): pp.10730–10737, 2001.

[8] G. Tal Association between common Toll-like receptor 4 mutations and severe respiratory syncytial virus disease. *Journal of Infectious Disease*. Vol. 189(11): pp. 2057–2063, 2004.

[9] B.G.van den Hoogen. A newly discovered human pneumovirus isolated from children with respiratory tract disease. *Nature Medicine* Vol. 7: pp.719–24, 2001.

[10] T.C.Peret. Characterization of human metapneumoviruses isolated from patients in North America. *Journal of Infectious Diseases*. Vol. 185: pp. 1660–3, 2002.

[11] T. Allander T. Cloning of a human parvovirus by molecular screening of respiratory tract samples. *Proceedings of the National Academy of Sciences of the United States of America*. Vol. 102: pp. 12891-6, 2005.

[12] J.C. Arnold. Human bocavirus: prevalence and clinical spectrum at a children's hospital. *Clinical Infectious Diseases*. Vol. 1;43(3): pp. 283-8. Aug 2006.

[13] R. Janssen. Genetic susceptibility to respiratory syncytial virus bronchiolitis is predominantly associated with innate immune genes. *Journal of Infectious Diseases.* Vol. 196(6): pp. 826-34. Sep. 2007.

[14] C.L. Siezen. Genetic susceptibility to respiratory syncytial virus bronchiolitis in preterm children is associated with airway remodeling genes and innate immune genes. *Pediatric Infectious Disease Journal.*Vol 28(4): pp. 333-5. Apr. 2009.

[15] Holick MF. The vitamin D deficiency pandemic and consequences for nonskeletal health: mechanisms of action. *Molecular Aspects of Medicine.* Vol. 29(6): pp. 361-8. Dec 2008.

[16] F. T. Bourgeois, Relative Impact of Influenza and Respiratory Syncytial Virus in Young Children. *Pediatrics.* Vol. 124 No. 6 pp. e1072 -e1080, December 1, 2009.

[17] T. Heiskanen-Kosma, Etiology of childhood pneumonia: serologic results of a prospective, population based study. *Pediatric Infectious Diseases Journal.* Vol. 17, pp.986–991, 1998.

[18] J-M. Hament. Respiratory viral infection predisposing for bacterial disease: a concise review. *FEMS Immunology and Medical Microbiology.* 1999 Dec;26(3-4):189-95.

[19] K. Thorburn. High incidence of pulmonary bacterial co-infection in children with severe respiratory syncytial virus (RSV) bronchiolitis. *Thorax.* Vol. 61(7): pp. 611–615. July 2006.

[20] M. Light Correlation between respiratory syncytial virus (RSV) test data and hospitalization of children for RSV lower respiratory tract illness in Florida. *Pediatric Infectious Disease Journal.* Vol. 27: pp. 512-8, 2008.

[21] M.W.Weber Respiratory syncytial virus infection in tropical and developing countries. *Tropical Medicine and International Health.* Vol. 3:4, pp. 268-80, 1998.

[22] F.T. Chew. Seasonal trends of viral respiratory tract infections in the tropics. *Epidemiology and Infection.* Vol. 121(1): pp. 121-8. Aug 1998

[23] P.W. Chan. Seasonal variation in respiratory syncytial virus chest infection in the tropics. *Pediatric Pulmonology.* Vol. 34(1): pp. 47-51. Jul 2002.

[24] S.E. Vieira. Clinical patterns and seasonal trends in respiratory syncytial virus hospitalizations in São Paulo, Brazil. *Revista do Instituto do Medicina Tropical Sao Paulo.* Vol. 43(3): pp. 125-31, May-Jun 2001.

[25] R. Pecchini. Incidence and clinical characteristics of the infection by the respiratory syncytial virus in children admitted in Santa Casa de São Paulo Hospital. *Brazilian Journal of Infectious Diseases.* Vol. 12(6): pp.476-9, Dec 2008.

[26] S. Yusuf. The relationship of meteorological conditions to the epidemic activity of respiratory syncytial virus. *Epidemiology and Infection.* Vol.135(7): pp.1077-90. Oct 2007.

[27] American Academy of Pediatrics Subcommittee on Diagnosis and Management of Bronchiolitis. Diagnosis and management of bronchiolitis. *Pediatrics.* Vol. 118(4): pp1774-93; Oct 2006.

[28] A. Mandelberg. Nebulized 3% hypertonic saline solution treatment in hospitalized infants with viral bronchiolitis. *Chest.* Vol. 123(2): pp. 481-7. Feb 2003.

[29] H.W. Kim. Respiratory syncytial virus disease in infants despite prior administration of antigenic inactivated vaccine. American Journal of Epidemiology. Vol. 89(4): pp.422-34. Apr 1969.

[30] American Academy of Pediatrics. Respiratory syncytial virus. In: Pickering LK, Baker CJ, Kimberlin DW, Long SS, eds. Red book: 2009 Report of the Committee on Infectious Diseases. 28th ed. Elk Grove Village, IL: American Academy of Pediatrics; pp. 560—9, 2009.

[31] American Academy of Pediatrics Committee on Infectious Diseases. Modified recommendations for use of palivizumab for prevention of respiratory syncytial virus infections. *Pediatrics*. Vol. 124: pp.1694 –701, 2009.

[32] R.T. Stein. Respiratory syncytial virus in early life and risk of wheeze and allergy by age 13 years. *Lancet.*; Vol. 354(9178):pp. 541-5, 1999.

[33] N. Sigurs. Severe respiratory syncytial virus bronchiolitis in infancy and asthma and allergy at age 13. *American Journal of Respiratory and Critical Care Medicine.* 171(2):137-41, 2005.

[34] K. Thorburn. Pre-existing disease is associated with a significantly higher risk of death in severe respiratory syncytial virus infection. *Archives of Disease in Childhood.* Vol. 94(2): pp. 99-103. Feb 2009.

[35] M. Garenne The magnitude of mortality from acute respiratory infections in children under 5 years in developing countries. *World Health Statistics Quarterly.* Vol. 45(2-3): pp. 180-91. 1992.

[36] A. R. Falsey. Respiratory Syncytial Virus Infection in Elderly and High-Risk Adults. *New England Journal of Medicine*. Vol. 352: pp. 1749-1759, 2005.

[37] Thompson WW. Mortality associated with influenza and respiratory syncytial virus in the United States. *Journal of the American Medical Association.* Vol. 8;289(2): pp.179-86. Jan 2003.

[38] J.O. Ebbert. Respiratory Syncytial Virus Pneumonitis in Immunocompromised Adults: Clinical Features and Outcome. *Respiration.* Vol. 72; pp. 263-9, 2005.

10

Start of a Pandemic: Influenza A H1N1 Virus

Ma. Eugenia Manjarrez[1], Dora Rosete[1],
Anjarath Higuera[1], Rodolfo Ocádiz-Delgado[2],
José Rogelio Pérez-Padilla[1] and Carlos Cabello[1]
[1]*Instituto Nacional de Enfermedades Respiratorias Ismael Cosío Villegas,*
[2]*Departamento de Genética y Biología Molecular;*
Centro de Investigación y de Estudios Avanzados del Instituto Politécnico Nacional,
Mexico

1. Introduction

In Mexico, Influenza virus infections occur more frequently during the winter with small peaks throughout the year. In April 2009, an epidemic arose from the emergence of a new Influenza A virus, whose devastating effect reflected significantly in Mexico city. Numerous patients with Influenza-like severe symptoms were attended at the Instituto Nacional de Enfermedades Respiratorias Ismael Cosio Villegas, Mexico (INER) and in many cases required hospitalization. The INER, in collaboration with the Dirección General de Epidemiología (Mexico) and the Instituto Nacional de Referencia Epidemiológica, Mexico (INDRE) marked the first guidelines for the management, diagnosis and treatment of Influenza-illness in Mexico. The INER is considered one of the leading centers for the care of critically respiratory-ill patients, and was one of the first institutions to describe the clinical presentation and death in the initial period of outbreak (Acuña, 2010; Manjarrez et al., 2003). The pandemic that occurred in 2009 in Mexico, took a different tack in contrast to other countries with respect to the frequency, severity and number hospitalized patients with mortality and greater affection in healthy young people. Influenza is a respiratory illness caused by viruses of the same name. Each year, seasonal flu viruses originate occasional epidemics. The name "influenza" comes from the belief that disease was caused by a negative supernatural influence, that is, a malign influence, or that the stars have influence on the occurrence of the disease (Acuña, 2010; Manjarrez & Arenas 1999).

In Mexico, there exist accurate records of 13 severe epidemics occurred during: 1667, 1734, 1805, 1806, 1826, 1837, 1846, 1891, 1899, 1918, 1920, 1957 and 1969, being reported the highest rates of mortality in the year of 1919 (Acuña, 2010). Infections are most common during the winter and small outbreaks over the year (Manjarrez et al., 2003, 2010).

2. Characteristics of the influenza virus

2.1 Classification and nomenclature

Influenza viruses are grouped in the Orthomyxoviridae family including three types: A, B and C. The A gender is the most common, infecting birds and mammals, including humans;

it can causes epidemics and pandemics with high rates of morbidity and mortality. Influenza viruses B and C are less frequent, mainly infecting humans and causing moderate epidemics or outbreaks (Manjarrez & Arenas 1999; Manjarrez et al., 2010; Souza, 2011; Zambon, 1999). According to the antigenic characteristics of hemagglutinin (HA) and neuraminidase (NA) proteins, influenza viruses are subdivided into subtypes. To date, it has been characterized sixteen HA subtypes and nine NA antigenic subtypes, all of which are found in aquatic wild birds. The international nomenclature used to describe the different influenza virus is to appoint the following characteristics: a) gender of the virus A, B or C; b) host type is ignored when it comes from human c) place of isolation; d) case number in the laboratory; e) year of isolation; f) HA and NA subtype of the virus which is written in parentheses. An example of a human virus isolated in Mexico in 2009 was described as "A / Mexico / INDRE / 4487 / 2009 (H1N1)" (Dawood et al., 2009; López-Cervantes et al., 2009; WHO, 2009a).

2.2 Structure

Viruses range in size from 80 to 120 nm in diameter having a pleomorphic or spherical form. They have a segmented genome (7 and 8 fragments) of single stranded RNA of negative polarity, encoding 11 proteins being two glycoproteins. Fragments 1, 2 and 3 encode proteins PB1, PB2 and PA those are part of the polymerase complex and are involved in the synthesis of RNA. Segment 4 encodes the HA protein which is the receptor that binds to the cell. It is synthesized as a monomer which undergoes posttranslational modifications and is activated by a host protease that cuts it into two fragments, HA1 and HA2, exposing the peptide fusion in the aminoterminal region of the HA2 fragment, allowing fusion of the viral envelope with the endosome in order to release the genome into the cytoplasm. The mature protein is a trimer formed by a stem that is inserted into the membrane and three globular regions. The globular region has an amino terminal region, where are localized the antigenic sites that are surrounding the receptor binding site (Manjarrez & Arenas, 1999; Zambon, 1999). The fragment 5 encodes the nucleoprotein (NP), forms a complex with RNA, protects the genome and is involved in replication. Segment 6 encodes for the neuraminidase (NA), the mature protein consists of a stalk and a globular head constituted of 4 subunits each with a catalytic site. Its role is to remove sialic acid residues of the membrane of the infected cell, allowing the newly synthesized virions were not clumping together and released properly. Segment 7 corresponds to the M1 and M2 proteins that are synthesized by a overlaid reading frame. M1 protein surrounds the nucleocapsid and M2 is located in the membrane and functions as an ion channel allowing the transport of protons to the endosome and is the target for antiviral drugs (e.g. amantadine). Segment 8 encodes for two nonstructural proteins: NS1 and NS2, that is, not belonging to the virion; these proteins are synthesized when the cell is infected. The NS1 protein inhibits the production of interferon; however, the function of NS2 protein is still unknown. Recently, it has been described the PB-1-F2 protein with a pro-apoptotic function (Manjarrez et al., 2010; Zambon 2001; WHO, 2002). Influenza viruses have a high rate of molecular variation, changes that can cause epidemics and pandemics. These changes are given by different factors: the nature of the virus (RNA replication needs of a RNA polymerase, which is inefficient to correct errors, so that mutations are common, in addition, the genome is segmented allowing increased recombination. Influenza A viruses infect humans as well as a variety of animals, this allows high levels of recombination between viruses from two or more hosts. Among the known mechanisms of variation there is the "antigenic drift", which are small changes that lead to mutations, mainly in the two viral glycoproteins (HA and NA). This variation allows an ineffective function of the host neutralizing antibodies, contributing to the need of renew vaccines annually. Other variation mechanism that is less frequent is the "antigenic shift". This mechanism allows the generation of new subtypes that can arise by recombination and rearrangement of entire segments of genes (Figure 1).

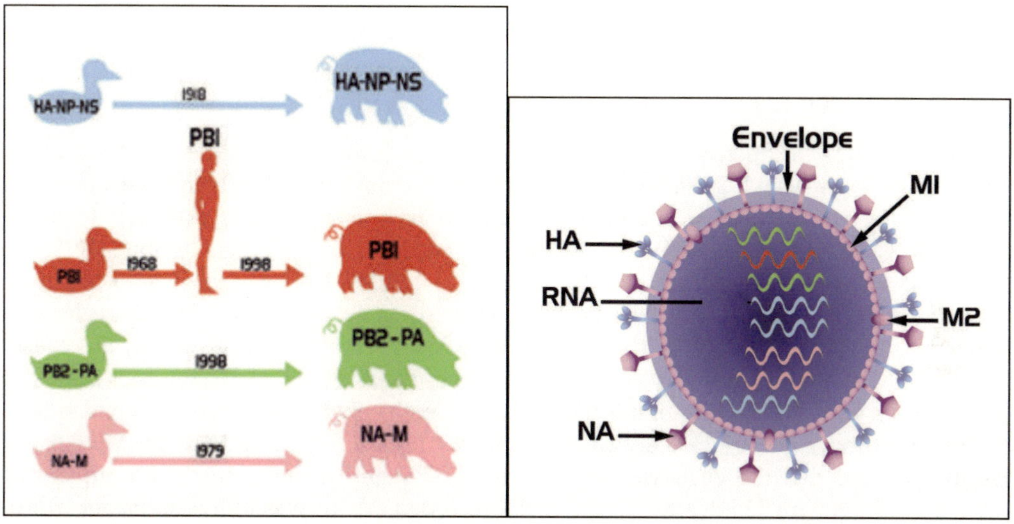

Fig. 1. Pandemic Influenza Virus. The new virus has a reassortant, the changes are shown in different colors: PB2, Classical North American Swine H1N1/Triple reassortant swine H3N2/A avian-like; PB1, Classical North American Swine H1N1/Triple reassortant swine H3N2/A avian-like; PA, Triple reassortant swine H3N2/A avian like; HA, Classical North American Swine H1N1; NP, Classical North American Swine H1N1/Triple reassortant swine H3N2; NA, Eurasian Swine N1; M Eurasian Swine; NS, Classical North American Swine H1N1/Triple reassortant swine H3N2.

2.3 Viral transmission and pathogenesis

The virus enters through the nasopharyngeal region for aerosols and droplets expelled to talking, coughing and sneezing, with hands and objects contaminated with aerosols and can last for hours or days on contaminated surfaces. The virus infects mucus-secreting epithelial cells and ciliates cells.

The HA binds to cell receptor, after incubation for one to three days, the virus replicates rapidly and infects neighboring cells. The virus causes cell damage, which alters the cilia activity, with increased secretion of mucus. To get out and infect other cells the NA reduces the viscosity of the mucus.

Desquamation on the epithelium causes respiratory symptoms and signs, involving the respiratory tract's natural response and promotes bacterial incorporation. Other damage is on the submucosal edema, which in turn may lead to hyaline membrane disease, emphysema and alveolar necrosis. The inflammatory process may break bronchi, bronchioles and alveolar regions. All these events originate characteristic initial symptoms of infection such as: fever, chills, and widespread pain, particularly muscle aches, headache, anorexia and prostration. The local monocytes and lymphocytes are the primary response and interferon is effective against the virus. The virus induces an effective humoral response, it is important in recovery, but should be considered that the antibody response is specific for each variant of the virus, while the T lymphocytes and macrophages is general and depending on the damage and the condition of host, epithelial repair can take up to a month. Start the virus infects upper respiratory tract but, it can reach low way causing bronchitis, bronchiolitis and pneumonia.

3. A new pandemic caused by a new influenza A virus in 2009

Usually in Mexico, Influenza infections occur in winter (Cabello et al., 2006; Vandale et al., 1997); however, in March 2009, began to be evident the first signs of influenza infections, an unusual time for the viral infection. The spread was fast and it was extended to many countries. On April 30th, the World Health Organization called officially an "H1N1/09 Pandemic Virus" (Dawood et al., 2009; Garten et al., 2009; López-Cervantes et al., 2009; Updated 2009; Vaillant et al., 2009; WHO, 2009). So, on June 11th, the WHO declared a pandemic. Mexico City showed the most serious cases with numerous deaths, the causal agent was found to be a new type of influenza virus. To June 15th, in 76 countries the virus was detected with 35,928 cases of infection and 163 deaths. By July 17th the virus had spread to 135 countries, with 101,250 confirmed cases. In Mexico, July 17th, Mexican Ministry of Health reported that the virus was present in all 32 states of the country; the number of cases was 13,646 with 125 deaths. Of the 70.4% recorded deaths was found in the age group of 20 to 54 years, the deaths accounted for 0.9% of total deaths, of which 52% were women, most of whom were housewives (Secretaria de Salud de Mexico, 2010b)

When the pandemic virus appears, there may be several periods of outbreaks with a range of 3 to 9 months between them. The pandemic in Mexico occurred in three outbreaks. The first began with the epidemiological alert on April 17th, and lasted for about a month. The second was in the months of June-July in the Southeast, although the magnitude was much smaller than the first outbreak. The third began in September 2009, mainly in northern and central Mexico.

On November 27th, the WHO informed that more than 207 countries had reported the presence of the new virus (Vaillant et al., 2009; WHO 2009). Here is a brief narrative of the activities, measures and experiences that took place in the INER at the onset of the influenza pandemia.

4. Approach of influenza medical cases at the respiratory emergency unit

It was received a disproportionate demand of patients showing severe acute respiratory infection (SARI) in addition to other possible influenza patients with other pathologies. Therefore, the mechanisms of classification, prioritization and selection of hospital management were reinforced. For the epidemic emerged in Mexico were implemented three phases of Triage:

1. **Initial Triage.** Patients with potentially SARI were separated from those with other diseases. Patients were required to fill an application form assessed by a physician.

2. **Second Triage**. Patients with respiratory symptoms related to influenza A H1N1 infection or potential epidemic/pandemic infection were removed from patients with infection by other viruses or bacteria.
3. **Third Triage**. It was defined the location of patient: home, hospital ward or intensive care.

Triage is useful for infection control and epidemiological monitoring, as well as the rationalization and organization of the Respiratory Emergency Unit overcoming potential responsiveness.

Classification systems include schemes to determine the severity of community-acquired pneumonia and influenza; this classification is not necessary when the risk groups are different so they could be misclassified probably conducing to an increased mortality in young patients during the pandemic. The proposed schemes should only be considered as a guide and do not replace the clinical criteria (Corrales, 2010; WHO, 2007). Among the schemes implemented are: Criteria for classification of patients; calculation Score: Pneumonia Severity Index for Adult (PSI/PORT), which consider the characteristics of patient demographic factors, comorbidity disease, findings on physical examination, laboratory and/or radiographic findings (ranked by points) (Corrales 2010, Osterholm 2006); Risk Rating PORT severity index of pneumonia, and Scoring System CURB-65 (See next box).

SCORING SYSTEM CYRB-65

FEATURES	POINTS
Confusion	+1
Urea> 7mmol/L (20 mg/dL)	+1
Respiratory rate > 30 breaths per min.	+1
Blood pressure (systolic > 90 or diastolic < 60 mm Hg)	+1
Age > 65	+1

Patient Score	Site Recommended care
0-1	outpatient
2	Ward
3-5	Hospital room or intensive care unit

Table 1. Criteria for classification of patients

Unfortunately, all efforts to use these scales in viral pneumonia, especially those caused by human influenza virus A H1N1 during the 2009 pandemic have been unsuccessful and unreliable.

5. Considerations for selection of patients on critical care medicine

It was considered two components of Triage: 1) prioritize patients and 2) management and resource optimization. This system is not error-free (overtriage or undertriage).

Experts in disaster situations have established a classification system or Triage at the Emergency Department or Intensive Care Unit. This system consists in to establish a color system for assessment and patient selection: green (patient will survive or not receiving support), yellow (patient will survive in case of delayed medical care); red (patient needs immediate intervention to survive), blue or black (patient will die despite the best efforts of Physicians).

However, the situation that we live during the first outbreak of pandemic influenza experienced at the INER during March to May was truly different and represented a challenge for the treatment of many patients with severe respiratory failure requiring mechanical ventilation or in shock.

Unable to attend all patients because the Department of Critical Medicine has only 9 intensive care beds (2 of them for pediatric patients) and 5 intermediate care beds, it was decided to transform the cubicles of pediatric patients into care beds for adults. This action allowed us to had 15 beds.

Moreover, the conversion took place in hospital besides enabling a pavilion, also allowing the use of this area for the care of patients with influenza A H1N1 pneumonia with or without need for mechanical ventilation in this situation; we had to suspend the no outpatient urgent and elective surgery activities in order to concentrate human resources in these areas. According to these conditions, patients most likely to survive (e.g. under 65 years old without comorbidity in end-stage cancer, without multiple organ failure and/or without terminal renal failure with requirement of replacement therapy because there was no equipment for (renal replacement T-Hemofiltration and hemodyalisis). They were accepted preferably in the Department of Critical Medicine, that was our initial triage system. We organized a committee Influenza Hospital (Bautista, 2010; Funk et al., 2010). Patients who were not chosen for their attention to a critical care area, represented a difficult situation because although they should be given immediate attention, establish a prognosis according to their severity and set neatly in the family may even be conflicting even among physicians in different areas within the hospital, but in a pandemic is only a problem in addition to a long list that puts the resource limit with which it has in every way, physical area, technology, inputs and humans. To decide which patients should be hospitalized and then locate them in the level of care they should receive may be more complex (outpatient observation in the emergency room, hospitalization, need for critical care or in spite of the latter by requiring extremely serious and not being able to triage proportions) creates a serious problem.

Regarding to resources, it was necessary to make a list indicating the available material and which must have, number of mechanical ventilators, beds, protective equipment for personnel, drugs and so on. It should be performed together involving CEOs, medical and administrative personnel, nursing, Medical Committee etc., for monitoring and troubleshooting. Several aspects of the strategy included area marking, media provide reports to the press and interested staff, health staff compare with that account and assign roles and responsibilities, flexibility of spaces, since in an emergency usually mechanical ventilators, beds in the different units and services which are not enough to make adaptations (Sandoval, 2010).

This indicates that the triage is necessary for the success of a medical contingency. Triage has medical basis for their development. It is necessary that each hospital unit set their standards according to their structure and needs (Sandoval, 2010; Rubinson et al., 2008).

6. Characteristics of the clinical cases

Clinical cases of influenza-like illness showed respiratory insufficiency and later was confirmed the infection with influenza A (H1N1) virus. Patients were mostly young individuals, in less than one year had the highest rates, with a gradual decrease in inverse proportion to the age (Figure 2). However, it was found that complications occurred in 10% of adults who were hospitalized. With increase age after 35 years, it was shown the highest percentage (20%); people over 65 years-old required hospitalization. Same behavior was observed with regard to lethality, with an increase on 20 to 35 years-old group as well as in the age group over 65 years-old. Because of the severity of respiratory damage, a large number of patients required intubation (mean age: 37 years-old). Fifty percent of all cases were female with no significant differences in mortality and hospitalization. Co-morbidities were frequent and varied in patients: the most common were diabetes mellitus, hypertension, chronic obstructive pulmonary disease, obesity, smoking and pregnancy (Bojorquez et al., 2010; Behazin et al., 2009; Cabello et al, 2012 in press). Patients who presented with a severe respiratory illness were immediately isolated.

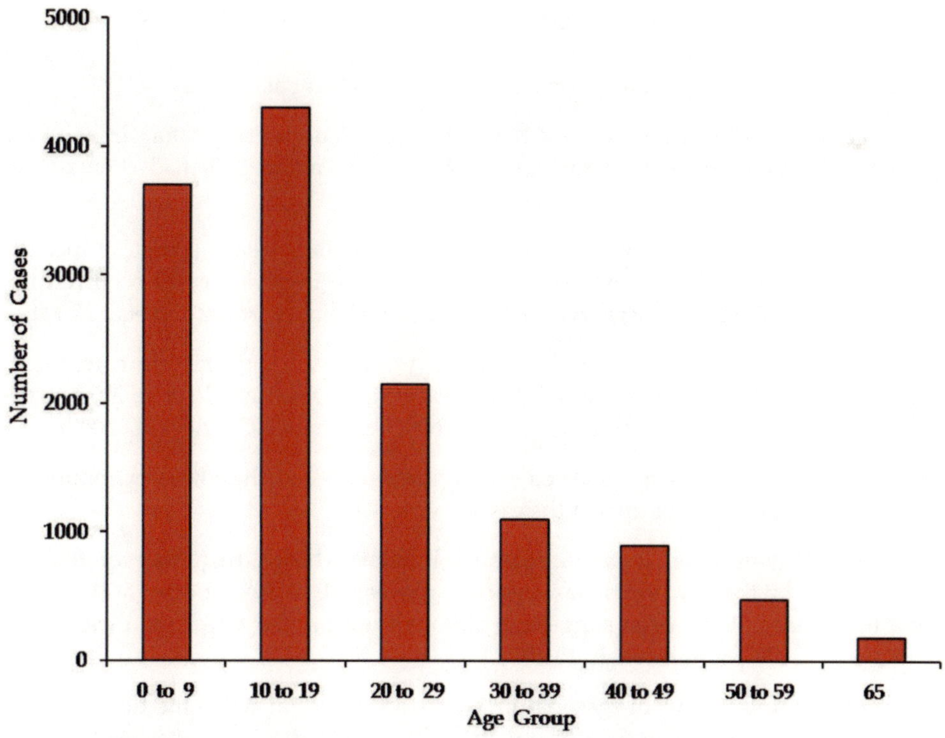

Fig. 2. Influenza cases in Mexico by age group from 11th March to 27th May, 2009. Data obtained from: Fajardo, et al. 2009.

7. Clinical manifestations

In general, the clinical manifestations observed during the infection tend to be similar with any subtype of influenza virus. The characteristics of the disease included signs and symptoms ranging from mild to severe manifestations. In Mexico, at the beginning of the pandemic of 2009, it was introduced a delay in diagnosis because the patients first consulted a general practitioner who were given treatment with antibiotics. Once identified the circulation of a new influenza virus, most patients (over 50%) had self-limiting illness without medical care. Complicated cases arrived at a hospital were treated with antiviral treatment, considering that if 72 hours after was not an improvement; illness were managed in accordance with the recommendations for progressive disease treatment. In mild cases, damage was mainly in upper respiratory tract, and the main symptom was dry cough. When the infection spreads to the lower airways, bronchus and lung parenchyma, it causes pneumonia with cyanosis and sometimes bloody sputum. Signs and symptoms were as follows:

Cough. Cough occurred between 90 and 100% of cases. Initially, illness was unproductive and then, in 33% of patients showed bloody sputum.

Dyspnea. It was presented in 65-73% of patients with complicated disease, so it was considered as the main symptom indicating the severity of the disease evolution. This symptom was presented in 86% of patients with pneumonia and in 90% of patients requiring management in the Intensive Care Unit (Cabello et al, 2012 in press; Pérez-Padilla et al., 2009; Echeverría-Zuno et al., 2009; Domínguez-Cherit et al., 2009). Sore throat and runny nose was observed in patients with upper respiratory tract infection (75% of patients) and in patients requiring hospitalization (35%) (Pérez-Padilla et al., 2009).

Sore throat and rhinorrhea. It was noted that patients with upper respiratory tract infection occurred in 75 and in patients requiring hospitalization, about 35% had (Pérez-Padilla, 2009).

Fever. Temperatures over 38°C were considered as the main systemic symptom increasing with the severity; in mild cases occurred in 40-50% while in severe cases occurred up to 100% (Cabello et al, 2012 in press; Pérez-Padilla et al., 2009; Echeverría-Zuno et al., 2009).

Headache. It was more common at the onset of the disease and was more frequent in outpatients than inpatients. We recorded 22 to 88% of the cases (Cabello et al, 2012 in press; Pérez-Padilla et al., 2009; Echeverría-Zuno et al., 2009; Domínguez-Cherit et al., 2009).

Myalgia and arthralgia. It was reported mainly in muscles of the lower extremities and occurred between 40 to 70% of total of the cases.

Gastrointestinal symptoms. Usually, seasonal influenza has a frequency of 5% while influenza caused by the new virus was reported between 10 to 30% of cases and was more common in children. It has been suggested, although not proven a fecal-oral transmission (Petrosillo et al., 2009; Ramírez et al., 2010).

Diarrhea, nausea and vomit. In seasonal influenza are rare, but when the disease is more severe it has been reported in 3 to 5% of the patients. At the INER the new virus was reported in 10% of severe cases in comparison with other medical centers in which it was reported a positive infection in 20 to 38% of cases.

At the beginning of the outbreak, there was a transmissibility rate of 1.2% and a mortality rate of 0.4%. Subsequently it was reported new ranges of mortality, from 0.20 to 1.23%, of which the lower ranks were in Europe and the highest in Mexico. It has been reported in Mexico during the pandemic that in Mexico city was the highest number of deaths in comparison with other countries, and the increased risk of death from pneumonia included people over 60 years of age. At the INER from April 17th to December 4th, 2009, it was reported a total of 763 cases of pneumonia with 138 deaths accrued. There have been some possible explanations for this situation: being the first country in which began the outbreak, the virus had an increased pathogenic activity and spread, therefore, patients to be unaware that this was a new virus, failed to get adequate medical care. In addition, medical staff was not aware of the existence of new viruses conducing to mismanagement of patients. In children, the clinical picture of the new virus influenza A (H1N1) infection was launched as seasonal flu-like infection, fever greater than 37.5°C, cough, chills, headache, nausea, hyperoxia, lethargy, muscle pain and fatigue, but added gastrointestinal symptoms such as diarrhea and vomiting. The clinical spectrum of symptoms was mild to progressive respiratory distress syndrome, requiring mechanical ventilation, associated with organ failure and death. Finally, the main causes of death were respiratory failure, sepsis, dehydration and electrolyte imbalance (Cabello et al, 2012 in press; Cano et al., 2010; Fajardo et al., 2009; Garrido et al., 2010).

8. Histopathological features of the disease detected in patients admitted to the INER

8.1 Tracheobronchial abnormalities

The seasonal influenza virus A and B have an affinity for epithelial cells and produce ciliated epithelial erosion and ulceration and inflammatory infiltrate in the subepithelial layer, initially neutrophils and later by lymphocytes. Macroscopic autopsy confirmed patients infected with influenza A (H1N1) virus showing extensive hemorrhagic tracheobronchitis, ciliated columnar epithelium with extensive necrosis, intraluminal desquamation of epithelial cells with partially eroded basement membrane, few epithelial cells with cytoplasmic vacuolization and deposition of hyaline membranes focally. In patients who died within hours after hospital admission showed no inflammatory cells. Patients with longer history had few neutrophils in the *lamina propia* of the mucosa while in patients with longer time of hospitalization, it was observed numerous lymphocytes infiltrating the tracheobronchial wall. Other findings observed were: vascular congestion and interstitial edema. In past pandemics caused by influenza virus infection, these observations have been described by other authors (Taubenberger & Moreno, 2008; Jeannette et al., 2006).

8.2 Pulmonary histopathological findings

While the new virus caused several deaths, macroscopic lung findings were not very different from those described in seasonal influenza. The *post mortem* biopsy specimens and autopsy cases showed massive pleural effusion predominantly on the right, lung weight and larger size, shiny outer surface, heterogeneous areas of congestion and hemorrhage of bright pink and red violet color; these lungs were poorly demarcated, confluent, giving a

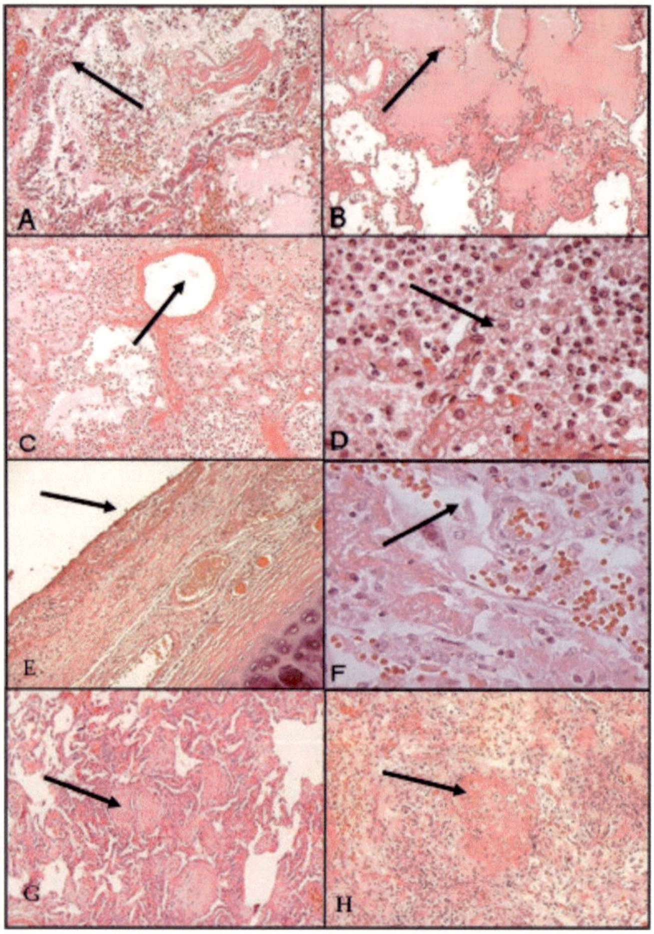

Fig. 3. **Micrographs of damage in the lung parenchyma and tracheal:** A) Respiratory bronchiole epithelial ulceration, fibrin plugs and scaling of columnar cells and macrophages; B) Alveolar edema and hemorrhage; C) Necrosis of the alveoli with deposits of hyaline membranes and alveolar edema with heavy infiltration by neutrophils and congestion of the capillaries; D) Interstitial edema with infiltration by neutrophils, capillary dilation and intraalveolar edema; E) Wall of the trachea is observed denudation of the respiratory mucosa; F) Hyperplasia of type II pneumocytes and cytomegaly; G) Areas of bronchiolitis obliterans due to proliferation of fibroblasts; H) necrotizing vasculitis surrounded by acute inflammatory infiltrate. Hematoxilyn and eosin stain (HE).

marbling pink to red-violet color, soft consistency and some consolidated areas; some cases showed lobar consolidation (Vázquez et al., 2010). Microscopically, most cases showed diffuse alveolar damage in exudative phase, with marked alveolar epithelial necrosis and hyaline membrane formation up to 5 microns thick, with focal dilatation of alveolar spaces, intra-alveolar hemorrhage, edema, hyperplasia and scaling of Type II pneumocytes and macrophages in the alveolar pinocytosis. In some macrophages and pneumocytes cytopathic damage was observed characterized by nucleomegaly, thrombosis with appearance of frosted glass capillary and necrosis of alveolar septa. It was identified areas of congestion and capillary alveolar wall thickening. According to the evolution time and complications, leukocyte infiltration between predominantly neutrophilic and lymphocytic lineage was little more intense in areas with few megakaryocytic intracapillary necrosis. Thrombosis of the capillary rise of the alveolar wall necrosis in large areas, confluent with fibrin exudate and loss of alveolar epithelium adjacent to the intra-alveolar hemorrhage and diffuse alveolar damage of acute lung inflammation was observed as well as occasionally peribronchial and bronchiolitis with necrosis and ulceration of the epithelium, which corresponds to the typical histological pattern of viral-induced lung damage. There were signs of tissue repair, regeneration of the bronchiolar and alveolar epithelial hyperplasia, and squamous metaplasia of pneumocytes (Vázquez et al., 2010). In the interstitium and bronchioles (bronchiolitis obliterans) was observed proliferation and reorganization of fibroblasts (Masson bodies) as well as large areas of fibrosis. Other authors (Guarner et al., 2000) detected influenza virus infection in bronchial epithelium and submucosal glands of the trachea, bronchi and bronchioles. Figure three shows some of the histopathological findings.

8.3 Findings using electron microscopy

By examining several sections of the lung, the ultrastructural changes that were detected were: alveolar capillaries with numerous erythrocytes and some leukocytes, airspaces with Type II pneumocytes, with projections in discrete cytoplasmic membrane and occasionally adjacent debris. In the cytoplasm of some macrophages phagocytosed erythrocytes and autophagosomes (electron concentric deposits) were observed. Type II pneumocytes have abundant cytoplasm with mitochondria-like swollen smooth endoplasmic reticulum which tend to lose their crests; in addition, round nuclei with little heterochromatin attached to the inner nuclear envelope and a prominent nucleolus were found. Low viral particle number, ranging from 93 to 150 nm in diameter, was visualized in the cytoplasm of some alveolar epithelial cells. At different stages of the viral cycle, it was observed vacuoles and endosomes emerging from the cytoplasmic membrane of the pneumocyte. Alveolar epithelial cells showed moderately dilated smooth endoplasmic reticulum, presence of electron-slightly larger vacuoles (compatible with pulmonary surfactant), round to oval nuclei with little heterochromatin in the nucleoplasm and prominent/eccentric nucleoli (Vázquez et al., 2010).

9. Imaging studies

The first choice study was simple plate-ray or chest X-ray; the techniques used were the portable X-ray and teleradiographs. The most frequent pattern was mixed alveolar and interstitial, predominantly axial and bilateral basal respecting the periphery. Cases with rapid progression were observed following the consolidation respecting upper lobes without associated lymphadenopathy or pleural effusion. In severe cases, the progression was rapid and affection pattern reverted to 18 to 30 days. Some patients underwent high-resolution computed tomography. Reconstructions were completed after 1 second, reconstruction algorithm and the high end of a forced inspiration, also took a series on forced expiration from lung apex to the diaphragmatic dome. The pattern found was mixed (interstitial and alveolar), predominantly interstitial type, characterized by areas of unpolished glass with a trend of consolidation, predominantly basal bilateral, axial compliance lung apices sometimes patchy pattern. Associated effusion or lymphadenopathy were not found. Expiratory phase showed areas of air trapping (Abella, 2009; Alva & Perdigón 2010; Chowell et al., 2009).

Figure four shows some of the findings in radiographic images.

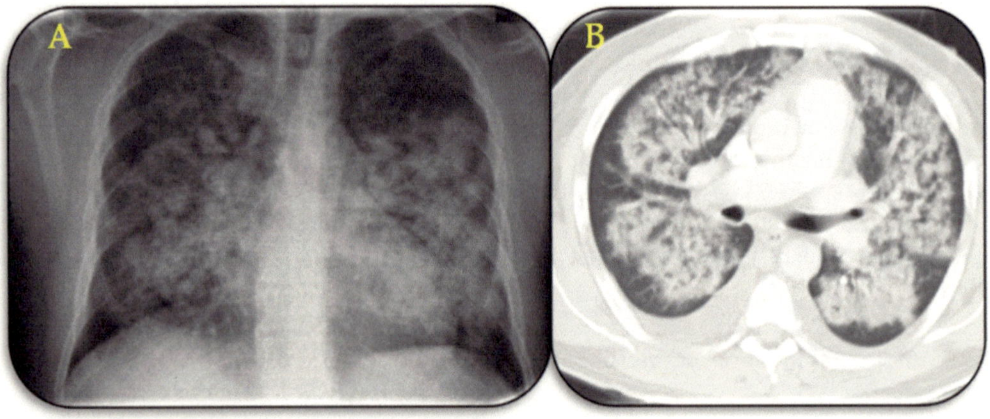

Fig. 4. Male patient 47 years of age diagnosed with H1N1 and 15 days earlier. A) The radiograph shows bilateral alveolar opacities; B) TAC Atypical pneumonia, and diffuse alveolar damage.

10. Respiratory therapy strategies for the management of patients with influenza A H1N1 virus

One of the important points in the respiratory therapy strategy involves knowing all the devices used in patients with some degree of respiratory failure and that includes everything from ways to deliver oxygen, nasal cannula, masks in all its varieties combining with moisture systems and the need to administer bronchodilators and/or inflammatory airway. In patients infected with the influenza A H1N1 virus, the use of bronchodilators and inhaled anti-inflammatory drugs is required. It is recommended the use of thermal units with systems of automatic filling and thermal self-regulation, reducing the handling of samples and the risk of dispersion of viral particles into the environment. Is important to avoid the use of thermal units that promote water condensation in the ventilator circuit. This situation requires the frequent disconnection of the circuit promoting environmental contamination with viral particles. Filters/nose or HME filter (Humidity Moisture Exchange) generate passive moisture and prevent the passage of bacteria into the patient allowing the safely change of filters every 7 days (Garcia & Garcia, 2010; Thorpe & Darcy 2009). We recommend active humidity systems for mechanically ventilated patients with high PEEP and are candidates for the use of bronchodilators. If the patient does not require the use of bronchodilators or other medications in nebulizer, nose/filter is a good choice. In the case of circuits of mechanical ventilation, the new generation ventilators compensate for leaks in the circuit. These systems can be cleaned safely each 7 days, even 15 days, in both cases, as long as the circuit does not show contaminating secretions. The interaction between the circuit and thermal units, and misting systems or aerosol delivery are important and we recommend a combination in the setting to the minimum necessary to disconnect or unplug it. Disconnection is suggested for each clamp on the tracheal cannula after the inspiratory phase, decreasing the risk of viral contamination into the environment. The processes of oxygenation in patients with influenza include devices such as nasal prongs, masks (opened and closed; high and low flow). All these systems have shown that in the process of exhaling, sneezing and coughing are generated particles including viral particles. The oxygen delivery systems in patients with influenza and respiratory failure depend on the severity of respiratory symptoms, the greater hypoxemia, and more oxygen is required. The administration by nasal cannula provides an inspired oxygen fraction up to 40% in order to maintain or improve oxygen saturation (oxygen partial pressure above 60 mmHg) (Garcia & Garcia, 2010; Tellier, 2009; Jefferson et al., 2009).

It still necessary studies to optimize the management of patients with influenza and to generate techniques to minimize risks to medical staff, nurses, technicians and anyone who interacts with the patient.

11. Extrapulmonary complications in pneumonia due to influenza A H1N1

Pneumonia caused by Influenza Virus A (H1N1) corresponds to Acute Respiratory Distress Syndrome (ARDS) with increased intra-alveolar hemorrhage. In ARDS, the increased mortality due to no respiratory complications is common in the critically ill patient; 16% of patients may develop a complication that includes: sepsis and septic shock, myocarditis and pericarditis, acute encephalitis, rabdomielitis, acute renal failure, liver failure and/or disseminated intravascular coagulation. In patients with chronic obstructive pulmonary disease or asthma, viral infections are frequent causes of complications.

12. Respiratory failure and multi-organ in Influenza-induced illness

In the first cases of influenza in Mexico, that included 18 patients, people required hospitalization, oxygen therapy and required mechanical ventilation due to ARDS. Among the reported data it can be included: elevated body mass index elevated LDH or CPK as well as history of smoking. Epidemiological data of patients with respiratory failure, who required intensive care, have been described in two series of patients in Mexico City and Canada (Echeverría-Zumo, 2010; Kumar et al., 2009). In both series the age groups are similar (40-50 years), showing, respect to seniors, a peak in early childhood and a significant variation in mortality for hospitalized patients (48 and 14% respectively) and oxygenation index [ratio of arterial oxygen pressure to fraction of inspired oxygen (PaO 2 / FoO2)], founding significant differences in the need for early mechanical ventilation (less than 10 hours), renal failure, hypotension at admission or shock refractory to intravenous fluids or need for vasoactive drugs and elevated values of lactic dehydrogenase, although the latter difference was not significant. Other interesting facts included decreased arterial oxygen saturation in patients who required mechanical ventilation (average 71%) and severe degree of hypoxemia in the group of nonsurvivors (41.5 mmHg) (Bautista et al., 2010; Dominguez-Cherit et al., 2009; Chavarría et al., 2010). For the proper management of patients with any acute or chronic lung disease exacerbated is important to integrate all data and knowledge.

13. Diagnosis

The speed with which the diagnosis is made is directly related to virological techniques employed. Techniques can be used to detect viral antigens using immunofluorescence or ELISA (Enzyme-linked immunosorbent assay) assays, which allows having a fast and reliable diagnosis. Novel detection technique such as Influenza A (H1N1)-real-time PCR (AH1N1-RTqPCR) was recommended recently by the WHO (CDC, 2009a, 2009b; Poon et al, 2009; Public Health 2009). This assay allows discriminating between different strains of seasonal and pandemic influenza. This technique uses specific primers to amplify specifically fragments of genes that codify the influenza virus Hemagglutinin or M2 proteins. The RTqPCR can detect up to 5,000 copies of a gene in each sample, and it can be used combined set of primers for determining different viral strains in a single biological sample. During the A (H1N1) pandemic, this technique was implemented as a main part of a diagnostic platform allowing the detection of new viral mutations of the recent A (H1N1) pandemic strain (Public Health, 2009; Pabbaraju et al., 2009; Balish et al., 2009). For the determination of neutralizing antibodies, the WHO suggested hemagglutination inhibition test (CDC, 2009).

The techniques used for early diagnosis of influenza directly dependent on the type, quality and quantity of biological sample and for the detection of viruses. On the recommendation of the WHO, we used different types of samples such as bronchoalveolar lavage samples, aspirates, nasal and nasopharyngeal swabs or aspirates (Balish et al., 2009; Ison, 2009; Thorpe & Darcy 2009). For patients who are intubated, it was considered the recollection of endotracheal aspirates (Balish et al., 2009; Thorpe & Darcy 2009).

In order to minimize the possible spread of disease, during the sampling was used appropriate work equipment. For the transport of biological samples was important to consider the use of specific culture media for viruses as well as the use of equipment or refrigerants to maintain a temperature of 4°C, which help to reduce the loss of virus collected.

14. Therapeutic management

Usually, the majority of flu cases showed mild and minor symptoms or manifestations, are self-limited not requiring antiviral treatment instead only symptomatic measures such as analgesics, antipyretics like acetaminophen or ibuprofen. During the influenza pandemic were considered for treatment the following clinical features: persistent fever, progressive symptoms, risk factors such as pregnancy, obesity, infants with alarm data. When not requiring antiviral therapy were given directions to go back to see if they have alarm data such as dyspnea, fever difficult to control, bloody sputum or changes in consciousness. In case of children, they were monitored to the presence of changes such as cyanosis, tachypnea and apnea. Before treatment and for the proper management of patients were considered some aspects: Treatment should be initiated as soon as influenza is suspected since when management delayed for more than 48 hours is not very effective, in severe cases should be initiated as soon as possible, even if have been more than 48 hours. In cases of pneumonia, it has been described that treatment was effective in patients who have symptoms for more than 6 days, helping to decrease mortality. Treatment will probably not prevent the development of ARDS, or cytokine storm, but prevents serious illness and death. Another important aspect is that treatment can reduce the need for hospitalization and length of hospital stay; in addition, there exists the need to know if comorbidity or data that might indicate a progressive evolution (Cabello et al, 2012 in press; CDC, 2009; Higuera et al., 2011; Sada, 2010; WHO, 2009b).

14.1 Antiviral drugs

The dose of oseltamivir administered to adult patients was 75 mg, every 12 hours for 5 days. In cases of pneumonia, it should use double dose, i.e. 150 mg every twelve hours, being able to prolong treatment for ten days. The adult dose of zanamivir was two doses of 10 mg by inhalation every twelve hours for 5 days having the disadvantage of producing irritation of the airway that could lead to bronchospasm, so caution should be exercised with patients with prior respiratory problems, such as asthma and chronic obstructive pulmonary disease. In some cases is recommended the prophylactic administration of bronchodilators prior to the application of zanamivir. In the case of intravenous neuraminidase inhibitor, peramivir, the recommended dose is 600 mg every 24 hours. Pediatric doses of oseltamivir should be calculated by age and weight, according to the following recommendations: 30 mg twice daily if ≤15 kg; 45 mg twice daily if weight is 15 to 23 kg; 60 mg twice a day for weight from 23 to 40 kg; 75 mg twice daily if weight > 40 kg. In children under 5 years is not recommended the use of zanamivir while in children over 5 years old, doses are similar to those of adults: two inhalations of 10 mg every twelve hours (CDC, 2010; Hanshaoworakui et al., 2009;Kidd et al., 2009; Sada, 2010; Updated, 2009; WHO 2009b).

During pregnancy, it has been shown that antiviral drugs are effective; however, it should be administered early to prevent the development of pneumonia; fortunately these drugs have not been associated with congenital malformations.

14.2 Antimicrobial treatment

In severe disease there may be some bacterial respiratory complications in these cases it can use the treatment guidelines for community-acquired pneumonia. In the schemes recommended by Mexican experts, it has decided that all patients with pneumonia should also receive antiviral drugs such as ceftriaxone at a dose of 2 g intravenous or intramuscular every 24 hours for 7 to 10 days. Patients who require mechanical ventilation are not exempt from acquiring a nosocomial infection, so antibiotics were used according results of bacteriological analyses (Sada, 2010; Updated, 2009a, 2009b). In specific cases of patients with influenza, in addition to specific antiviral treatment is recommended other symptomatic treatments such as antipyretics and anti-inflammatory drugs (paracetamol or ibuprofen) at useful doses. It was considered contraindicated the use of aspirin, especially in children and young people and their use in influenza is associated with development of Reye's syndrome.

15. Pre-pandemic phase

In Mexico, in 2003 it was created a multidisciplinary group to develop a National Plan for preparedness and response to pandemic avian influenza, which was completed in 2006 (Manjarrez, 2007; Secretaría de Salud de Mexico, 2010 a). For the situation that arose in 2009, this Plan was resumed (Figure 5) in accordance with the recommendations of the WHO, the

Ministry of Health participated through the National Epidemiological Surveillance and Disease Control (CENAVECE), the Department of Epidemiology (DGEPI), the Coordinating Committee of the National Institutes of Health and High Specialty Hospitals (CCIN Salud HAE) in collaboration with entities of the health sector and government sector. In this document is showed local actions for a possible pandemic of avian influenza, in order to reduce cases of human infection and mortality. Main action lines of action for strategic activities were: 1) Dissemination and information, 2) Epidemiological surveillance, 3) Confirmation of the diagnosis, 4) Care for the population, 5) Strategic reserve and 6) Research and development.

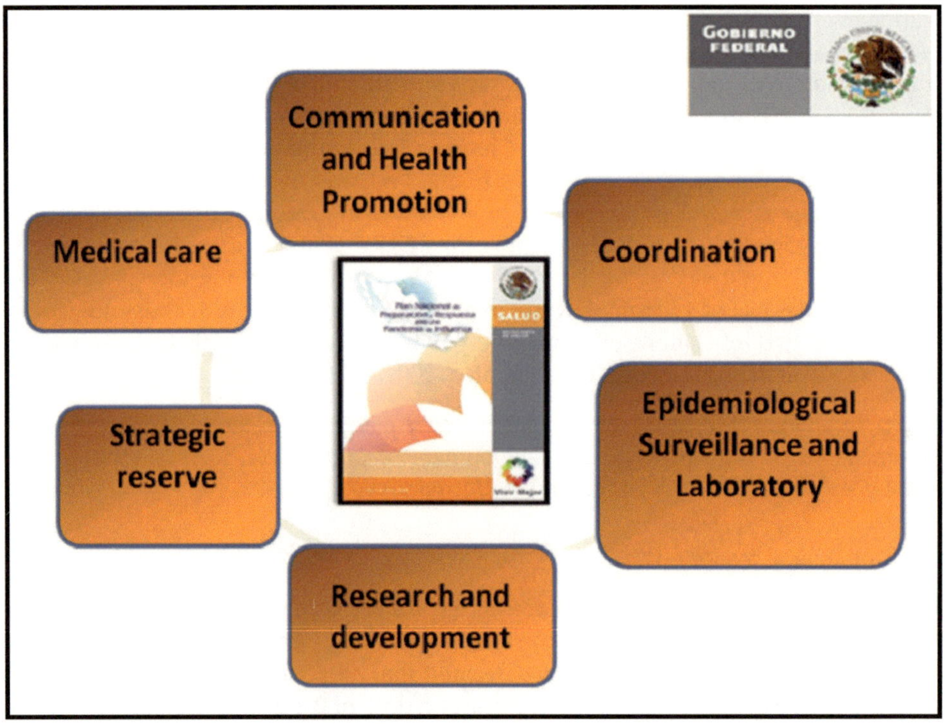

Fig. 5. National Plan for preparedness and response to pandemic influenza in Mexico.

15.1 Pandemic phase

The National Plan for preparedness and response to pandemic influenza in Mexico was not fully consolidated, requiring dissemination of guidelines and operational training as well as antiviral supplies in all health institutions in the country, including non-governmental health institutions. When detonated the alert in Mexico, it began negotiations for the preparation, packaging and distribution of oseltamivir to all healthcare facilities across the country, which reported suspected or confirmed cases of A (H1N1), which caused a delay in the timely administration of the first patients affected by the pandemic (Manjarrez, 2010; Secretaría de Salud de Mexico, 2010).

Among the most outstanding activities was the diagnosis as a crucial part of epidemiological surveillance to monitor the A (H1N1) virus circulation correlating with the occurrence of severe pneumonia cases. It could be proposed that this action was transformed to a vulnerable point of the health system and a point of discussion in the committees, because main resources and efforts were limited only to patients with pneumonia.

Hospital authorities adopted, as strategy, reference mechanisms since the facilities were inadequate, especially intermediate and intensive care units where many cases required mechanical ventilation; in addition, care activities from specialist staff was insufficient for local needs. Influenza committee sessions were performed daily in order to solve the main problems: the shortage of human and material resources. Other problems were: limited coverage of seasonal influenza vaccination, access to health services, availability of information on health, socioeconomic level, demographic characteristics, cultural background, educational level, government policies on health, etc. (Secretaría de Salud de Mexico, 2010). Mexico was the first country that gave international epidemiological alert in March and April 2009. According to official reports of surveillance were involved several states including San Luis Potosi, Hidalgo, Queretaro and Mexico City (Central Mexico). The Secretary of Health of Mexico reported the viral infection on April 24th (Secretaría de Salud de Mexico, 2010), therefore, social distancing measures were intensified to contain the pandemic, which included the closure of certain public places like restaurants, schools, kindergartens, cinemas, theaters, foot-ball stadiums, among others, these actions were extended until May 11th to Mexico City and May 18th for the rest of the states. In contrast to the global alert issued by WHO, Mexican pandemic rose to five on a scale of 6 on April 29th (fig.6).

15.2 Post pandemic phase

After the pandemic, there were disseminated, through various information media, criticism of the decisions taken by the authorities of the Ministry of Health in Mexico, because these radical actions to contain the dissemination of viral infection, National economy were crashed. However, this strategy played an important role in advancing on the field of epidemiology and public health that included:

- Improved hand hygiene in the population.
- Control of antimicrobials through medical prescription.
- Activation of epidemiological surveillance systems.
- Research resources.
- Investment in health infrastructure, including medical equipment such as mechanical ventilators.

It was developed several guidelines and rules to follow, including:

15.3 Precautions to prevent transmission in hospitals and health care

- Preventive isolation of patients, including a combination of standard and transmission precautions
  - Direct contact
  - Drop spread
  - Air spread
- According to the demands, ideally patients should stay in a room with negative pressure, or to use a single room whose door will remain closed most the time. When

institutions do not have these resources by the magnitude of the pandemic, patients should stay in multiple rooms or rooms specially designated for patients infected with influenza. The litters must be a minimum distance of 1 m.

- Health professionals, directly involved in patient care must use high efficiency masks as N-95 or its equivalent, long sleeved gowns with adjustable cuffs, face shield or goggles and gloves. This equipment is not recommended for administrative professionals that do not require direct contact with these patients as is recommended face masks only.
- It is necessary to limit the number of health professionals in direct contact with the patients and to limit the access to the patient environment.
- Health professionals who attend patients with pandemic influenza should not take care of patients diagnosed with other disease or young children.
- Restrict visits to a minimum.
- Give visitors the regulation of hospital safety and personal protective equipment with instructions for use.
- Encourage frequent hand washing, particularly in areas of risk by the presence of influenza patients.

15.4 Security measures at an unprotected exposure of health professionals or family members

1. Professionals who care for infected patients should monitor their temperature twice daily and report any febrile episode. If exist any sign or symptoms, the professional should not to participate in non-specific or direct care of patients.
2. Health professionals who have a fever (temperature > 38°C) and have been in contact with patients should undergo appropriate diagnostic tests. If no other cause is identified, it should be assumed an influenza infection and immediately start treatment with oseltamivir.
3. Healthcare professionals involved in high-risk procedures (e.g. procedures which generate aerosols) that begin with any signs or symptoms should consider the need for prophylaxis.

15.5 Precautions for the general population during an influenza contingency

1. Household contacts should take appropriate steps in terms of hygiene; not sharing utensils, avoid face to face contact with patients with confirmed or presumptive diagnosis and the use of high-efficiency masks and googles (e.g. N-95 type).
2. Contacts who have shared a particular environment: home, homes of other family members, hospitals, schools, workplace, recreation centers, mass transport, etc., with a patient with confirmed or suspected influenza A (H1N1) should monitor their temperature twice daily as well as the appearance of symptoms within 7 days after the last exposure.
3. Confirmed asymptomatic contacts should not receive oseltamivir.
4. Symptomatic household contacts with temperature > 38°C, cough, dyspnea, diarrhea or other systemic symptoms, should receive empirical antiviral therapy (e.g. a dose of 75 mg once daily for 5 days in adults and children) and undergo to diagnostic testing as soon as possible.

15.6 Preventive measures for travelers going to areas with Influenza alert

1. People who are traveling to areas with avian influenza activity should be immunized with trivalent human vaccine available (seasonal), two weeks before the trip.
2. Travelers should avoid direct contact with poultry, including chickens, ducks, or geese that appear healthy, in addition, these people should avoid farms or live animal markets, poultry, or touching surfaces contaminated with feces of poultry secretions.
3. Travelers should take preventive measures to reduce risks of exposure through proper hygiene and frequent hand washing with alcohol-gel. Also, avoid eating eggs or foods derived from poultry that haven poorly cooked or raw.
4. Hand washing is important when handling raw poultry for cooking, either at home or in business.
5. It is necessary to recommend to travelers to consult a physician if the traveler has fever and respiratory symptoms during the 10 days after of returning from an affected area.

15.7 End of the pandemic

Health Secretary lifts the state of epidemic alert on June 30th, 2010. The latest official data, published by the Ministry of Health on June 19th, 2010, indicated that Mexico recorded 72,548 confirmed cases and 1,316 confirmed deaths, representing a mortality of 1.8%. Seventy percent of deaths corresponded to the age group between 20 and 54 years old, and 39.8% of them did not find any pathological history relevant to death (Secretaría de Salud de México, 2010a, 2010b).

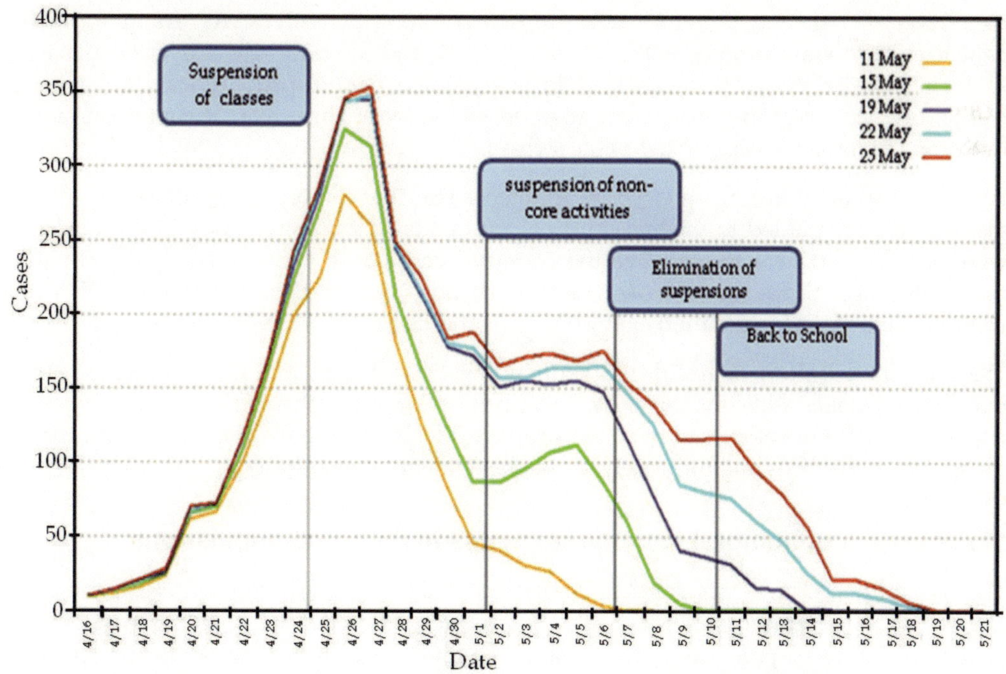

Fig. 6. Confirmed cases according to the date of symptoms on the population

16. Social response to the epidemic

The first manifestations of the epidemic in Mexico caused significant morbidity and mortality in the population, with implications for high psychological, social and economic impact (Cruz & Corrales 2010). With the emergence of a new influenza virus, the growth of reports of confirmed cases of illness and deaths caused the mass media fix their attention on it, the news spread very fast because it had little knowledge of the virus, generated a great concern throughout the population, disrupting social stability that had already been altered for several reasons.

The social response to an epidemic is given in circumstances that occur in time, space, era and culture, and serve to properly interpret phenomena according to social reality. An important aspect to understand this response is the psychosocial vulnerability, an internal condition of a subject or a group of subjects exposed to threatening or traumatic event, which corresponds to the perception of risk in which the person has to be damaged. Perception can be objective (real threat) or subjective (built by the subject, it may be consistent with reality or the risk can be distorted and exaggerated or minimized). Since the many kinds of risk perception, the situation led to a series of emotions and behaviors appropriate or inappropriate to the society. Adequate collective behaviors refer to protection measures that will allow reducing the spread of the virus and thereby reduce the number of cases, eliminating to fall into chaos. Inappropriate behaviors such as spreading rumors that encourage mass hysteria or that the situation is unreal will generate maladaptive behaviors that gradually lead to social disorganization (Cruz & Corrales 2010).

One of the feelings experienced by people was the collective fear, which is characterized by sharing an intense fear in a social group. This fear can be adaptive, allowing people to grade their level of risk and therefore take steps to protect themselves. As example, masks, antibacterial, vitamin supplements such as vitamin C and subsequently antiviral drugs were sold out. The collective fear can lead to exaggerated and disproportionate behavior of reality; one example: the population stopped eating pork since fear of contagion, as the initiation of pandemic was related to the swine flu.

Fear can turn into panic, manifested by an intense fear that can produce primitive reactions, messy and can take led to violence and discrimination (Cruz & Corrales 2010). Mexicans, who were abroad or want to leave the country, were badly treated and their individual rights breached. Some countries set restrictions on commercial and business flights that were suspended. Discrimination against Mexico and its people was very severe.

The coordinated effort of health workers, authorities, officials and civilians were able to maintain adequate adjustment mechanisms, promoting the restructuring of social welfare and allowing the development of active strategies for protecting the population and reduce the spread of the virus and ultimately, drive the epidemic successfully.

17. Detection of humoral immune response in different populations

The new influenza virus circulated and remained stable in the environment, easily entering the body. The immune system is activated to produce antibodies, which in any way prevent or reduce the development of the disease. For information from the presence of specific antibodies against the new influenza virus, we performed a multicenter study, which were obtained several results mentioned here only a brief summary of some of them.

1. Anti-virus influenza A (H1N1) pandemic in people at different levels of exposure to the virus, whose aim was to: Identify and compare the presence of specific serum Ab against the new virus influenza A (H1N1) and GEA INER staff at different levels of exposure. This study concluded that greater exposure, higher titers of antibodies and the application of the specific vaccine enhanced the response.
2. Prevalence of influenza virus A (H1N1) in blood donors. In this study analyzed 241 samples of sera from donors, by the method of hemagglutination inhibition (HI) for antibodies against influenza virus seasonal and pandemic virus. Samples were taken from November 2008 to May 2009. We found that in 65 (27%) were detected antibodies to the novel influenza virus and seasonal influenza virus 87 (36%). Found that only 26 (10%) samples were positive for both viruses. The titles ranged from 1:10 to 1:80. By comparing the results of the pre-pandemic period the epidemic found a statistically significant difference [OR 6.1,95% (2.34-14.1) p <0.0001]. Concluded that there are few studies showing the prevalence of the pandemic virus in a healthy population without recent illness. Although the results are few, indicate that the population was in contact with the new virus probably since 2008 the end of 2008 antibodies were detected and the prevalence in this population ranged from 9% pre-epidemic period and 36% epidemic period.
3. Another objective was to compare the presence of antibodies against the new influenza virus and seasonal influenza viruses INER staff and a Technology University of Tecamac (UT). This study concluded that the greatest number of people with antibodies to both viruses was INER, being significant in the case of the new virus, indicating that their exposure was greater when dealing with infected patients. It is interesting to note that INER staff is annually vaccinated against the virus, but number of people with seasonal virus antibodies was low.

The presence of antibodies may provide guidance on some aspects such as proximity or degree of exposure to the virus the ability to respond immunologically to viral stimulation, virus circulation:the possibility of partial or weak protection of a vaccine.

18. Acknowledgments

The authors acknowledge the financial support from CONACYT (SALUD-2009-C02-126832). The authors thank Dr. Ma. Eugenia Vázquez for the histological photographs. The authors also thank Dr. Edgar Bautista and Dr. Ignacio Paramo for technical assistance, comments and suggestions.

19. References

Abella HA. X-ray and CT offer predictive power for swine flu diagnosis. Diagnostic Imaging 2009. Available: http://www.diagnosticimaging.com/digital-x-ray/content/article/113619/1425699.

Acuña Rodolfo. 2010. Perspectiva histórica de las epidemias de influenza en México. In: *Influenza por el nuevo virus A H1N1, un panorama integral.* José R Pérez Padilla, Andrés Palomar Lever, Jorge Salas Hernández, Juan C Vázquez García. Pp 16-25. Graphimedic, 978-607-00-2720-8, Mexico.

Alva, L & Perdigón, G. 2010. Estudios de imagen en neumonía por influenza. In: *Influenza por el nuevo virus A H1N1, un panorama integral.* José R Pérez Padilla, Andrés Palomar Lever, Jorge Salas Hernández, Juan C Vázquez García. Pp 155-161. Graphimedic, ISBN, 978-607-00-2720-8, México.

Balish A, Warnes CM, Wu K, et al. 2009. Evaluation of rapid influenza diagnostic test for detection of novel influenza A (H1N1) virus-United States 2009. *MMWR. Morbid Mortal Wkly Report.* 58:826-829.

Bautista E, Arcos M, Monares E, Sandoval J, Rocha F. 2010. Influenza A H1N1: Neumonía severa y lesión pulmonar aguda; una guía del manejo de la ventilación mecánica. In: *Influenza por el nuevo virus A H1N1, un panorama integral.* José R Pérez Padilla, Andrés Palomar Lever, Jorge Salas Hernández, Juan C Vázquez García. Pp 301-316. Graphimedic, ISBN, 978-607-00-2720-8, México.

Behazin N, Jones SB, Cohen RT, et al. 2009. Respiratory restriction and elevated pleural and esophageal pressures in morbid obesity. *J Appl Physiol.* 108: 212-218

Bojorquez I, García C, Fernández M, Palacios E, López-Gatell H. 2010. Comportamiento de la pandemaia 2009 en México. In: *Influenza por el nuevo virus A H1N1, un panorama integral.* José R Pérez Padilla, Andrés Palomar Lever, Jorge Salas Hernández, Juan C Vázquez García. Pp 42-56. Graphimedic, ISBN, 978-607-00-2720-8, México.

Cabello C, Manjarrez ME, Rosete DP, Villalba J, Valle L, Paramo I. 2006. Frequency of viruses associated with acute respiratory infections in children younger than five years of age at a locality of Mexico City. *Mem Inst Oswaldo Cruz.* 101 (1): 21-24.

Cabello C, Rosete DP, Manjarrez ME. In press. Situación de la Influenza en México. In: *Avances en la Investigación de la Influenza en Mexico.* Elizabeth Loza-Rubio & Edith Rojas Anaya. Instituto Nacional de Investigaciones Forestales, Agrícolas y Pecuarias, and Instituto de Ciencia y Tecnología del D.F. México.

Cano M, Garrido C, Alejandre A. 2010. Manifestaciones Clínicas de influenza A H1N1 2009 en niños. In: *Influenza por el nuevo virus A H1N1, un panorama integral.* José R Pérez Padilla, Andrés Palomar Lever, Jorge Salas Hernández, Juan C Vázquez García. Pp 95-107. Graphimedic, ISBN, 978-607-00-2720-8, México.

Centers for Disease Control and Prevention. Protocol of realtime RT-PCR for influenza A (H1N1). Geneva: World Health Organization, April 2009. Accessed July 20, 2009. Available:http//www.who.int/csr/resources/publications/swineflu/CDCRealtimeRTPCR_swineH1assay-2009_20090430.pdf.

Centers for Disease Control and Prevention (2010) Updated Interim Recommendations for theUse of Antiviral Medications in the treatment and Prevention of Influenza for the 2009-2010 Season. Available:
http:// WWW.cdc.gov/h1n1 flu/recommendations.htm. Accessed 29 July 2010.

Chavarría U, Treviño M, Puente R, Acosta G, Mercado R. 2010. Falla Respiratoria y multiorgánica en influenza. In: *Influenza por el nuevo virus A H1N1, un panorama integral.* José R Pérez Padilla, Andrés Palomar Lever, Jorge Salas Hernández, Juan C Vázquez García. Pp 283-299. Graphimedic, ISBN, 978-607-00-2720-8, México.

Chowell G, Bertozzi SM, Colchero A, López GH, Alpuche AC, Hernández M, Miller MA. 2009. Severe Respiratory Disease Concurrent with the Circulation of H1N1 Influenza. *N Engl J Med.* 361:674- 79.

Corrales A. Criterios de valoración y selección de pacientes en un servicio de urgencias durante la epidemia. In: *Influenza por el nuevo virus A H1N1, un panorama integral.*

José R Pérez Padilla, Andrés Palomar Lever, Jorge Salas Hernández, Juan C Vázquez García. Pp 108-133. Graphimedic, ISBN, 978-607-00-2720-8, México.

Cruz, B & Austria, F. 2010. Impacto psicosocial de una epidemia. In: *Influenza por el nuevo virus A H1N1, un panorama integral.* José R Pérez Padilla, Andrés Palomar Lever, Jorge Salas Hernández, Juan C Vázquez García. Pp 443-449. Graphimedic, ISBN, 978-607-00-2720-8, México.

Dawood MD, Jain S, Finelli L, Shaw M, Lindstrom S, Garteb R. et al. 2009. Emergence of a novel swine-origin influenza A (H1N1) virus in humans.*New Engl J Med.* 360(25):2605-2615.

Domínguez-Cherit G, Lapinsky SE, Macia Ae, Pinto R, Espinosa-Pérez L, de la Torre A, Poblano-Morales M, Baltazar-Torres JA, Bautista E, Martinez A, Martinez MA, Rivero E, Valdez R, Ruiz- Palacios G, Hernandez M, Stewart TE, Fowler RA. 2009. Critically ill patients with 2009 influenza A (H1N1) in México. *JAMA.* 302 (17): 1880- 1887.

Echeverría-Zuno S, Mejía-Aranguré JM, Mar-Obeso AJ, Grajales-Muñiz C, Robles-Pérez E, Gonzáles León M, Ortega-Alvarez MC, González-Bonilla C, Rascón-Pacheco RA, Borja-Aburto VH. 2009. Infection and death from influenza A (H1N1) virus in México: A retrospective analysis. *Lancet.* doi: 10.1016/SO140-6736 (08)61345-8.

Fajardo GE, Hernández F, Santacruz J, Rodrígue J, Lamy P, Arboleya H, Gutiérrez R, Manuell G, Cordova JA. 2009. Perfil epidemiológico de la mortalidad por influenza humana A (H1N1) en México. *Sal Pub Mex.* 51 (5):361.371.

Funk DJ, Siddiqui F, Wiebe K, Miller RR, Bautista E, et al. 2010. Practical lessons from the first outbreaks: Clinical presentation, obstacles, and management strategies for severe pandemic (pH1N1) 2009 influenza pneumonitis. Crit Care Med. 38 (4) suppl.): e30-e35.

García, R & García, J. Estrategias de terapia respiratorias en influenza. In: *Influenza por el nuevo virus A H1N1, un panorama integral.* José R Pérez Padilla, Andrés Palomar Lever, Jorge Salas Hernández, Juan C Vázquez García. Pp 226-238. Graphimedic, ISBN, 978-607-00-2720-8, México.

Garrido C, Cano C, Salcedo M, Del Razo R, Alejandre A. 2010. Influenza A H1N1 influenza A en niños estudiados en el INER. *Acta Pediátrica.* 31 (4): 162-7.

Garten R, Davis CT, Russell CA, et al. Antigenic and Genetic Characteristics of swine-origin 2009 A (H1N1) influenza viruses circulating in humans. Sciencexpress/ www.sciencexpress.org/22may2009/Page 1/10.1126/science.1176225.

Guarner J, Wen-Ja S, Dawson J. 2000. Immunohistochemical and in situ hybridization studies of influenza A infection in human lungs. *Am J Clin Pathol.* 114:227-33.

Hanshaoworakui W, Simmerman JM, Narueponjirakul U, et al. 2009. Severe human influenza infections in Thailand: Oseltamivir treatmen and risk factors for fatal outcome. *Plos One.* 4(6): e6051.

Higuera A, Kudo K, Manabe T, Corcho A, Corrales A, Alfaro L, Guevara R, Manjarrez ME, Takasaki J, Izumi S, Shimbo T, Bautista E, Pérez R. 2011. Reducing Occurrence and Severity of pneumonia due to Pandemic H1N1 2009 by early Oseltamivir administration: A retrospective study in Mexico. *Plos One.* 6(7): e21838. doi:10.1371/journal.pone.0021838.

Ison MG. 2009. Influenza in Hospitalized Adults: Gaining Insigth into a Significant Problem. *J Infect Dis.* 200: 485-488.

Jeannette G, Christopher D, Wun-Ju S, Michelle M, Mitesh P, Sherif R. 2006. Histopathological and immunohistochemical features of fatal influenza virus infection in children during the 2004-2004 Season.*CID*. 43(15):132-40.

Jefferson T, Del Mar C, Dooley L et al. 2009. Physical interventions to interrupt or reduce the Spreads of respiratory virases: systematic review. *BMJ*. 339: b3675.

Kumar A, Zarychanski R, Pinto R, et al. 2009. Critically ill patients with 2009 influenza A H1N1 infection in Canada. *Jama*. 302(17)1872-79.

Kidd IM, Down J, Nastouli E, et al. 2009. H1N1 pneumonitis Treated with intravenous zanamivir. *Lancet*. 374: 1036.

López-Cervantes M, Venado A, Moreno A, Pacheco R, Ortega-Pierres G. 2009. On the Spread of the Novel Influenza A (H1N1) Virus in Mexico. *J Infect Dev Ctries*. 3:327-330.

Manjarrez, ME & Arena, G. 1999. Virus influenza: enigma del pasado y del presente. *Rev Inst Nal Enf Resp Mex*. 12:290-299.

Manjarrez ME, Rosete DP, Rincón VM, Villalba J, Cravioto A, Cabrera R. 2003. Cabrera. Comparative viral frequency in Mexican children under 5 years of Age with and without upper respiratory symptoms. *Journal of Medical Microbiology*. 52: 579-583.

Manjarrez ME. 2007. Antecedentes y Origen de la pandemia de influenza aviar H5 N1. *Neumología y Cirugía del tórax*. 66 (S1): S4- S11.

Manjarrez ME, Cabello C, Rosete DP. 2010. Biología del virus: familia Orthomyxoviridae. In: *Influenza por el nuevo virus A H1N1, un panorama integral*. José R Pérez Padilla, Andrés Palomar Lever, Jorge Salas Hernández, Juan C Vázquez García. Pp 26-41. Graphimedic, ISBN, 978-607-00-2720-8, México.

Manjarrez ME. 2010. Familia Orthomixoviridae. I*n Microbiología: Bacteriologia y Virología*. Molina José, Manjarrez ME., Tay J. Méndez Editores. Pp 483-501. ISBN-978-607-7659-11-2. México.

Osterholm MT. 2006. En prevención de la próxima pandemia. *Sal Pub Méx*. 48: 279-285.

Pabbaraju K, Wong S, Wong AA, Appleyard GD, Chui L, Pang XL, Yanow SK, Fonseca K, Lee BE, Fox JD, Preiksaitis JK. 2009. Desing and valdation of real-time reverse transcription- PCR assays for detection of pandemic (H1N1) 2009 virus. *J Clin Microbiol*. 47 (11): 3454-3460.

Pérez-Padilla R, de la Rosa-Zamboni D, Ponce de Leon S, Hernández M, Quiñones-Falconi F, et al. 2009. Pneumonia and respiratory failure from swine-origin influenza A (H1N1) in Mexico. *N Engl J Med*. 361 (7): 680-689.

Petrosillo N, Di Bella S, Drapeau CM, Grilli E. 2009. The novel influenza A (H1N1) virus pandemic: An update. *Ann Thorac Med*. 4 (4): 163-172.

Poon LL, Chan KL, Smith GJ, Leung CS,Guan Y, Yuen KY, Peirs JS. 2009. Molecular detection of a novel human influenza (H1N1) of pandemic potential by conventional and real-time quantitative RT-PCR assay. *Clin Chem*. 55 (8):1555-1558.

Public Health Agency of Canada: RT-PCR protocol for swine H1N1 influenza, April 2009. Ottawa Ontario: National Microbiology Laboratory, PHAC; 2009. Pp 1-7.

Ramírez A, Pérez O, Hernández D, Hernánde R, Flores F, Amaya L, Espinosa C, Sansores R. 2010. Cuadro clínico. In: *Influenza por el nuevo virus A H1N1, un panorama integral*. José R Pérez Padilla, Andrés Palomar Lever, Jorge Salas Hernández, Juan C Vázquez García. Pp 80-94. Graphimedic, ISBN, 978-607-00-2720-8, México.

Rubinson L, Hick JL, Hanfling DG, Devereaux AV, Dichter JR, Christian MD, Talmor D, Medina J, Curtis JR, Geiling JA. 2008. Task Force for Mass Critical Care. Definitive care for the critically ill during a disaster: a framework for optimizing critical care surge capacity: from a Task Force for Mass Critical Care summit meeting, January 26-27, 2007, Chicago, IL. Chest. 2008 May;133(5 Suppl):18S-31S.

Sada E. 2010. Manejo terapéutico. In: *Influenza por el nuevo virus A H1N1, un panorama integral.* José R Pérez Padilla, Andrés Palomar Lever, Jorge Salas Hernández, Juan C Vázquez García. Pp 215-225. Graphimedic, ISBN, 978-607-00-2720-8, México.

Sandoval, JL & Bautista, E. 2010. Consideraciones para selección de pacientes (triage) en medicina crítica en la contingencia por influenza. In: *Influenza por el nuevo virus A H1N1, un panorama integral.* José R Pérez Padilla, Andrés Palomar Lever, Jorge Salas Hernández, Juan C Vázquez García. Pp 137-143. Graphimedic, ISBN, 978-607-00-2720-8, Mexico.

Secretaría de Salud de México. Plan Nacional de Preparación y Respuesta ante una Pandemia de Influenza. Consultado 2010 (a), febrero 12]. Available: http://www.dgepi.salud.gob.mx/pandemia/FLU-aviar-PNPRAPI.htm

Secretaría de Salud de México. Situación actual de la epidemia. Consultado 2010 (b), noviembre 22]. Available: http://portal.salud.gob.mx/sites/salud/descargas/pdf/influenza/situacion_actual_epidemia_100210.pdf.

Taubenberger J & Moreno D. 2008. The pathology of Influenza Virus Infections. *AnnRev Pathol.* 3:499-522.

Tellier R. 2009. Aerosol transmission of influenza A virus: a review of Studies. *J R Soc Interface.* 6 (Suppl 6):S783-90.

Thorpe, C & Darcy, S. 2009. A/H1N1 flu pandemic. Consider bronchoalveolar lavage. *BMJ.* 339: b5094.

Update: swine influenza A (H1N1) infections_ California and Texas, April 2009 (a).MMWR Morb Mortal Wkly Rep 2009; 58:435-7.

Updated: situation of Pandemic (H1N1) 2009 (b).- Epidemiologic information for medical providers. April 23, 2010.Tokyo: Ministry of Health, Labour and Welfare - Japan, 2010 on lineat http://www.mhlw.go.jp/bunya/kenkou/kekkaku-kansenshou04/pdf/100423-01.pdf (Japanese).

Updated: Interim Recommendations for the Use of Antiviral Medications in the Treatment and Prevention of Influenza for the 2009-2010 Season, December 07, 2009.Atlanta: Centers for Disease Control and Prevention, 2010 (Accessed July 29, 2010)online at: http://www.cdc.gov/h1n1flu/recommendations.htm

Vaillant L, La Ruche G, Tarantola A, et al. 2009. Epidemic intelligence Team at InVS. Epidemiology of fatal cases associated with pandemic H1N1 influenza 2009. *Euro Surveill.* 14 (33): 19309.

Vandale S, Rascón-Pacheco R, Kageyama M. 1997. Time-trends and causes of infant, neonatal and postnatal mortality in Mexico, 1980-1990. *Sal Pub Méx.* 39 (1): 48-52.

Vázquez ME, Rivera RM, Peña E, Moshe H, Méndez A. 2010. Cambios histopatológicos en las vías aéreas y pulmón por El vírus de La influenza A H1N1. In: *Influenza por el nuevo virus A H1N1, un panorama integral.* José R Pérez Padilla, Andrés Palomar

Lever, Jorge Salas Hernández, Juan C Vázquez García. Pp 195-205. Graphimedic, ISBN, 978-607-00-2720-8, México.

WHO. 2002. Draft WHO guidelines on the use of vaccines and antivirals dirung influenza pandemics. *Wkly Epidemiol Rec.* 77:394-404.

WHO. 2007. Infection preventionand control of epidemic and pandemic prone acute respiratory diseases in Elath care. *Interim Guidelines.* June 2007.

WHO. 2009. (a) global alert and Response. Available: http://www.who.int/csr/disease/swineflu/updates/en/index.html (Access 27 de november 2009).

WHO. 2009. (b). Guidelines for pharmacologial management of pandemic (H1N1) 2009 influenza and others influenza viruses. Geneva world Health Organization. Available: http://www.who.int/csr/resources/publications/swineflu/h1n1_use_antivirals_20090820/en/index.htm/.

Zambon MC. 1999. Epidemiology and pathogenesis of influenza. *J Antimicrob Chemother.* 44(S-B):3-9.

Zambon MC. 2001. The pathogenesis of influenza in humans. *Rev Med Virol.* 11:227-41.